T0230617

Neuroanatomy

and

Physiology

of

Abdominal Vagal Afferents

Neuroanatomy
and
Physiology
of
Abdominal Vagal Afferents

Edited by

Sue Ritter
Robert C. Ritter
Charles D. Barnes
Department of Veterinary and Comparative Anatomy,
Pharmacology and Physiology
College of Veterinary Medicine
Washington State University
Pullman, Washington

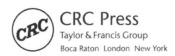

CRC Press
Taylor & Francis Group
Boca Raton London New York

CRC Press is an imprint of the
Taylor & Francis Group, an **informa** business

Library of Congress Cataloging-in-Publication Data

Catalog record is available from the Library of Congress.

Developed by Telford Press

Direct all inquiries to CRC Press, Inc., 2000 Corporate Blvd., N.W., Boca Raton, Florida, 33431.

1992 by CRC Press, Inc.

International Standard Book Number 0-8493-8881-3

CONTENTS

CHAPTER 1

COMPARATIVE ANATOMY OF MEDULLARY VAGAL NERVE
NUCLEI

CHAPTER 2

VISCEROTOPIC REPRESENTATION OF THE ALIMENTARY
TRACT IN THE DORSAL AND VENTRAL VAGAL COMPLEXES
IN THE RAT

CHAPTER 3

THE DORSAL VAGAL COMPLEX FORMS A SENSORY-MOTOR
LATTICE: THE CIRCUITRY OF GASTROINTESTINAL REFLEXES

CHAPTER 4

CENTRAL CONNECTIONS OF THE NUCLEI OF THE VAGUS NERVE

CHAPTER 5

CENTRAL REGULATION OF BRAINSTEM GASTRIC VAGO-VAGAL
CONTROL CIRCUITS

CHAPTER 6

VAGAL AFFERENT INNERVATION OF THE ENTERIC NERVOUS
SYSTEM

ABOUT THE EDITORS

Dr. Sue Ritter, Ph.D., is Professor of Physiology and Pharmacology in the Department of Veterinary and Comparative Anatomy, Pharmacology and Physiology (VCAPP) in the College of Veterinary Medicine at Washington State University.

Dr. Ritter graduated from Valparaiso University in 1968 with a BA in psychology. In 1970 she earned an M.S. and in 1972 received the Ph.D. from Bryn Mawr College in the area of psychopharmacology.

From 1972 to 1974 Dr. Ritter was a senior psychologist at Wyeth Laboratories in the Department of Psychopharmacology. She was appointed Assistant Professor of Physiology in the College of Veterinary Medicine in 1974. She advanced to Associate Professor of Physiology and Pharmacology in 1979 and was made a full professor in 1986. She is director of veterinary neuroscience teaching for the Department of VCAPP. In 1986 and 1987 she was a Fogarty International Fellow and Visiting Professor of Gastroenterology at the London Hospital Medical College of the University of London, England.

Dr. Ritter is a member of the Society for Neuroscience, the International Brain Research Organization, the North American Society for the Study of Obesity and the Society for the Study of Ingestive Behavior. She serves on the editorial advisory board of *Physiology and Behavior* and has served as a consultant and study section member for the National Institutes of Health. She has been the recipient of research grants from the National Institutes of Health, the American Heart Association and private foundations.

Dr. Ritter has authored more than 50 scientific papers and book chapters. Her two most active areas of research are metabolic controls of food intake and the use of specific toxins to study neuroanatomy.

Dr. Robert C. Ritter, VMD, Ph.D., is Professor of Physiology and Pharmacology in the Department of Veterinary and Comparative Anatomy, Pharmacology and Physiology, in the College of Veterinary Medicine at Washington State University.

Dr. Ritter graduated from Valparaiso University in 1967 with a B.S. in biology. He received a doctorate in veterinary medicine from the University of Pennsylvania in 1971. From 1971 to 1974 he was a postdoctoral fellow at the Institute of Neurological Sciences at the University of Pennsylvania, from which he received the Ph.D. in biology in 1974.

In 1974 Dr. Ritter became Assistant Professor of Veterinary Medicine in the WOI Regional Program in Veterinary Medicine at the University of Idaho. He was advanced to Associate Professor in 1979 and to Professor in 1984. In 1988 he was appointed Professor of Physiology and Pharmacology at the College of Veterinary Medicine at Washington State University. Dr. Ritter is Chairman of the Research Track in the veterinary curriculum. He was a Fogarty International Fellow and Visiting Professor of Gastroenterology at the London Hospital Medical College of the University of London, England, in 1986 and 1987. He was recently named a Jacob Javits Neuroscience Investigator by the National Institutes of Health.

Dr. Ritter is a member of the Society for Neuroscience, the International Brain Research Organization, the North American Society for the Study of Obesity, the Society for the Study of Ingestive Behavior and the Phi Kappa Phi academic honor society. He serves on the editorial board of the *American Journal of Physiology* and has served as consultant for the National Institutes of Health. Dr. Ritter has received research grants from the National Institutes of Health, National Institute of Alcohol, Drug Abuse and Mental Health, the USDA and private foundations.

Dr. Ritter has authored more than 40 scientific papers and chapters. His research focuses on neural and gastrointestinal interactions in the control of food intake.

Dr. Charles D. Barnes, Ph.D., is Professor and Chairman of the Department of Veterinary and Comparative Anatomy, Pharmacology and Physiology in the College of Veterinary Medicine at Washington State University.

Dr. Barnes received his B.S. degree from Montana State University in 1958 with double majors in biology and physics. In 1961 he received an M.S. degree in physiology and biophysics from the University of Washington, and in 1962 he earned his Ph.D. in physiology from the University of Iowa.

After two years as a postdoctoral fellow in the Department of Pharmacology at the University of California at San Francisco, he became Assistant Professor of Anatomy and Physiology at Indiana University in 1964. He advanced to Associate Professor in 1968, and in 1971 became Professor of Life Sciences at Indiana State University. In 1975 he was named Chairman of the Department of Physiology at Texas Tech University College of Medicine, where he remained until taking his present position in 1983.

Dr. Barnes is a member of the American Association for the Advancement of Science, American Association of Anatomists, American Institute of Biological Sciences, American Physiological Society, American Association of Veterinary Anatomists, American Society of Pharmacology and Experimental Therapeutics, American Society of Veterinary Physiologists and Pharmacologists, Association of Veterinary Anatomy Chairpersons, Association of Chairmen of Departments of Physiology, International Brain Research Organization, Society for Experimental Biology and Medicine, Society for Neuroscience, Society of General Physiologists, and the Western Pharmacological Society. He has been the recipient of many research grants from the National Institutes of Health and the National Science Foundation.

Dr. Barnes is the author of more than 150 papers and has been the author or editor of 16 books. His current research interests relate to the modulation of nervous system output by centers in the brainstem.

CONTRIBUTORS
(IN ORDER OF CHAPTER PRESENTATION)

THOMAS E. FINGER, Ph.D.
Professor
Department of Cellular and Structural Biology
University of Colorado Medical School
Denver, CO

STEVEN M. ALTSCHULER, M.D.
Acting Chief
Division of Gastroenterology Nutrition and Lipid-Heart Research
The Children's Hospital of Philadelphia
Assistant Professor of Pediatrics
University of Pennsylvania School of Medicine
Philadelphia, PA

LINDA RINAMAN, Ph.D.
Research Associate
Department of Behavioral Neuroscience
University of Pittsburgh
Pittsburgh, PA

RICHARD R. MISELIS, M.D., Ph.D.
Professor of Animal Biology
University of Pennsylvania
Philadelphia, PA

TERRY L. POWLEY, Ph.D.
Professor
Department of Psychological Sciences
Purdue University
West Lafayette, IN

HANS-RUDOLF BERTHOUD, Ph.D.
Associate Professor
Anatomy Institute
University of Zürich
Zürich, Switzerland

EDWARD A. FOX, Ph.D.
Postdoctoral Fellow
Department of Neuropharmacology
The Scripps Research Institute
LaJolla, CA

WATSON LAUGHTON, Ph.D.
Scientific Writer
Immunobiology Research Institute
Annandale, NJ

RONALD A. LESLIE, Ph.D., D.Phil.
Assistant Director and Research Manager
Oxford University Smith Kline Beecham Centre
    for Applied Neruopsychobiology
Department of Clinical Pharmacology
    and
Research Fellow
Green College
Oxford University, UK

D. JOHN M. REYNOLDS, M.A., B.M., B.Ch., MRCP
Clinical Lecturer
Department of Clinical Pharmacology
Oxford University
Oxford, UK

I.N.C. LAWES, MBBS
Lecturer
Biomedical Science
University of Sheffield
Sheffield, UK

R.C. ROGERS, Ph.D.
Professor
Department of Physiology
Ohio State University
Columbus, OH

GERLINDA E. HERMANN, Ph.D.
Postdoctoral Fellow
Department of Physiology
Ohio State University
Columbus, OH

CATIA STERNINI, M.D.
Associate Professor
Medicine and Brain Research Institute
Center for Health Sciences/Digestive Disease Center
University of California (UCLA)
Los Angeles, CA

TIMOTHY H. MORAN, Ph.D.
Associate Professor
Department of Psychiatry and Behavioral Science
Johns Hopkins University School of Medicine
Baltimore, MD

PAUL R. McHUGH, M.D.
Professor and Chairman
Department of Psychiatry and Behavioral Science
Johns Hopkins University School of Medicine
Baltimore, MD

DAVID GRUNDY, Ph.D.
Department of Biomedical Science
University of Sheffield
Sheffield, UK

HELEN E. RAYBOULD, Ph.D.
Adjunct Assistant Professor of Medicine
CURE/VA Wadsworth Medical Center
University of California (UCLA)
Los Angeles, CA

ROBERT C. RITTER, VMD, Ph.D.
Professor
Department of Veterinary and Comparative Anatomy, Pharmacology
    and Physiology (VCAPP)
College of Veterinary Medicine
Washington State University
Pullman, WA

LYNNE BRENNER, M.A.
Research Associate
Department of Veterinary and Comparative Anatomy, Pharmacology
    and Physiology (VCAPP)
College of Veterinary Medicine
Washington State University
Pullman, WA

DANIEL P. YOX, Ph.D.
Postdoctoral Fellow
SUNY Buffalo
Neurobiology Laboratory
Department of Physiology
School of Medicine
Buffalo, NY

SUE RITTER, Ph.D
Professor
Department of Veterinary and Comparative Anatomy, Pharmacology
    and Physiology (VCAPP)
College of Veterinary Medicine
Washington State University
Pullman, WA

NOEL Y. CALINGASAN, DVM, Ph.D
    Research Associate
    Department of Veterinary and Comparative Anatomy, Pharmacology
        and Physiology (VCAPP)
    College of Veterinary Medicine
    Washington State University
    Pullman, WA

BRUCE HUTTON, DVM
    Research Associate
    Department of Veterinary and Comparative Anatomy, Pharmacology
        and Physiology (VCAPP)
    College of Veterinary Medicine
    Washington State University
    Pullman, WA

THU T. DINH
    Research Associate
    Department of Veterinary and Comparative Anatomy, Pharmacology
        and Physiology (VCAPP)
    College of Veterinary Medicine
    Washington State University
    Pullman, WA

P.L.R. ANDREWS, Ph.D
    Reader in Physiology
    Department of Physiology
    St. George's Hospital Medical School
    Cranmer Terrace
    Tooting, London

PREFACE

The vagus nerve innervates nearly all of the thoracic and abdominal viscera. A majority of cervical vagal fibers, however, are destined for subdiaphragmatic target organs. In non-ruminant animals between 75–90% of these abdominal vagal fibers appear to be sensory rather than motor. Thus, the vagus nerve constitutes a veritable express route by which information from the gastrointestinal tract travels directly to the brain. This book surveys what sorts of information are carried by vagal sensory neurons, how the vagal sensory and motor components interact anatomically and physiologically in the brain, and the nature of vagal sensory participation in selected aspects of physiology and behavior.

Although the vagus of the rat is emphasized by most contributors to this book, the volume begins on a comparative note with Tom Finger's anatomical abstraction of an organizational plan of the vagus. The subsequent three chapters continue the focus on central vagal neuroanatomy. Dr. Altschuler and his coauthors provide a detailed portrayal of the viscerotopic organization of the vagal sensory and motor nuclei, while Dr. Powley and colleagues emphasize the neuroanatomical geometry that may facilitate integrative function in the dorsal vagal complex. Dr. Leslie *et al.* then summarize the interconnection of the vagal sensory and motor nuclei with other brain areas. Drs. Rogers and Hermann have placed the neuroanatomical information provided in the first four chapters in a functional context via a discussion of their work on central neural circuits involved in vago-vagal control of the stomach.

The next three chapters emphasize anatomical and functional aspects of the peripheral vagus. Dr. Sternini begins this grouping with her discussion of vagal sensory innervation of the enteric plexes. Her chapter is followed by a review of vagal expression of receptors for gastroenteric transmitters and hormones by Drs. Moran and McHugh. Dr. Grundy then discusses the nature of vagal reception of mechanical and chemical signals from the gastrointestinal tract.

The final four offerings in the volume are broadly functional in focus. Dr. Raybould's chapter examines the participation of the peripheral vagal sensory innervation in control of gastric function. R. Ritter *et al.* then review recent experimental evidence for control of food intake by vagal sensory signals from the stomach and intestine. S. Ritter and coauthors then review intriguing results that indicate that feeding behavior may be aroused by interaction of vagally sensed metabolic signals from below the diaphragm with metabolic cues sensed in the brain itself. The volume ends as it began, with an abstraction. In their concluding chapter, Drs. Andrews and Lawes provide a wide-ranging examination of familiar and novel vagal functions, culminating in the proposition that the function of the vagus is primarily one of protection of the organism from damage or deficit.

We hope that the flow of observations and opinions in this book will be as stimulating to other readers as it is to us. Certainly, the most difficult questions concerning the sensory functions of the abdominal vagi remain to be answered and, like most investigators, we anticipate the most exciting results concerning vagal afferent form and function are just over the next experimental ridge. Hopefully, this compilation will assist all of us who already are on the trail of vagal sensory functions in our respective areas of biology and medicine. In addition, perhaps it may serve as a chart to assist newer investigators in their efforts to uncover the workings of the great wanderer, the vagus.

Sue Ritter
Editor

Robert C. Ritter
Editor

Charles D. Barnes
Editor

ACKNOWLEDGMENTS

Like most books, this one would not have been completed without the hard work of people whose names do not appear on the cover or in the list of contributors. Chief among the unemblazoned but certainly not unappreciated people is our departmental editor, Jeanne Jensen, who formatted the entire book and took care of nearly all of the chores of correspondence with authors. We are much obliged for her high standards and dedication. During the early stages of work on this book, we also received valuable assistance from former members of our departmental word processing unit, Paula Perron-Bates and Catherine Smith. In addition we wish to thank the authors themselves, not only for their outstanding chapters, but for the patience that many of them exhibited during a publishing project that took longer than expected.

Chapter 1

COMPARATIVE ANATOMY OF MEDULLARY VAGAL NERVE NUCLEI

T.E. Finger

TABLE OF CONTENTS

LIST OF FIGURE ABBREVIATIONS

alar p = alar plate
basal p = basal plate
dVM = dorsal motor nucleus of the vagus
MLF = medial longitudinal fasciculus
Nsm = somatic motor nerve root
nST = nucleus of the solitary tract
nTd = nucleus of the descending trigeminal tract
NX = vagus nerve
s.l. = sulcus limitans
sm = somatic motor column
ss = somatic sensory column
Td = descending (spinal) trigeminal tract
VL = vagal lobe
vm = visceral motor column
VM = vagal motor nucleus
vs = visceral sensory column

INTRODUCTION

The vagus nerve is one of the most complex nerves in the body, conveying information to and from viscera as well as to and from cranial structures. In all vertebrates examined to date, the vagus nerve contains diverse populations of nerve fibers including those involved in visceromotor, branchiomotor, viscerosensory and cutaneous sensory activities. The visceromotor function comprises the preganglionic parasympathetic outflow from the lower medulla, while the branchiomotor system comprises the efferent innervation to striate muscles of the posterior branchial arches. Visceral sensory innervation includes both the gustatory sense as well as the sensory innervation of the gut and cardiorespiratory axis; the cutaneous sensory innervation includes the small division of the vagus that distributes to a small part of the outer ear or, in some fishes, to an area of skin overlying the gill covering.

This chapter presents an overview of the organization of vagal nerve nuclei in a variety of vertebrate species at different grades of organization. An attempt is made to emphasize common organizational principles rather than interspecies differences. The reader, however, should be wary in drawing generalizations based on an extremely limited number of species. As will be seen in the following discussions, vast differences in gross appearance of the vagal nuclei may be present even in closely related species. Yet despite these apparent differences, the underlying organizational plan, or so-called "bauplan," appears to be identical. A major goal of comparative neurobiology is the abstraction of organizational plans from examination of diverse species and the use of such abstractions in understanding the functional organization of the central nervous system.

FUNCTIONAL ORGANIZATION OF THE BRAIN

Functional Columns

Comparative neuroanatomists at the turn of the century (e.g., as described by Herrick[17] or Ariens Kappers, *et al.*[3]) discerned that the brainstem in virtually any vertebrate could be divided into four major longitudinal columns according to the nerve components terminating or originating therein (see Table 1, Figure 1). These four longitudinal subdivisions were also described as being related to the embryogenesis of the neural tube in that the function of each cell column is related to its place of origin along the ventricular surface of the neural tube. The neural tube is grossly divisible into an alar plate, lying dorsal to the sulcus limitans, and a basal plate situated ventral to this sulcus. Cell groups originating from the alar plate serve sensory functions while neurons generated from the basal plate serve motor functions (Figure 1). Somatic functions are performed by neurons generated at the dorsolateral and ventromedial portions of each half of the neural tube; visceral functions are carried out by neurons generated closest to the sulcus limitans. Since the vagus nerve contains components

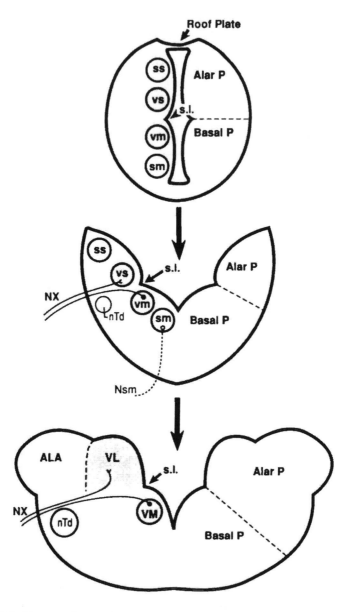

FIGURE 1. Schematic diagram of cross-sections through the medulla at different stages in the development of an idealized vertebrate. *Top*: Early neural tube stage. The sulcus limitans (s.l.) defines the boundary between alar and basal plates. The position of the four principal functional columns is indicated. *Middle*: Late neural tube stages. The roof plate widens and the rhombic lips spread laterally during development. The point of entry into the nervous system is shown for the vagus nerve (NX) and for a typical ventral (somatic motor) root such as the hypoglossal nerve. *Bottom*: The mature condition as shown for a vagally-advanced animal such as a catfish. The ALA (acousticolateral area) includes lateral line as well as acoustic and vestibular nuclei. In terrestrial vertebrates, this area contains only vestibular and auditory nuclei.

involved in three (somatic sensory, visceral sensory, visceral motor) of these four principal functions, vagal nerve nuclei are located in three of the four main zones. A confounding factor in this scheme is that in most vertebrates, although neurons are generated at the ventricular surface, the maturing neuroblasts migrate outward to collect into nuclei lying some distance from the ventricular surface. Thus the four longitudinal columns do not always maintain sharp boundaries.

TABLE 1
Major Functional Columns of the Brainstem

Sensory:

1. Somatic	Cutaneous	
	Proprioceptive	
2. Visceral	Gustatory	
	Cardiovascular, Gut	

Motor:

1. Somatic	Striate Muscles from somites	
2. Visceral	Striate Muscles from branchial arches (somitimeres)	
	Preganglionic autonomic	

The four main longitudinal columns[a] described in the classic literature of American comparative neuroanatomy and their vagal contributions are:

Somatic Sensory[b] — The vagus nerve provides cutaneous innervation to a small area of the skin in the vicinity of the caudal gill slits, operculum or outer ear. The fibers innervating this somatic sensory modality are believed to terminate in the spinal trigeminal nucleus.

Visceral Sensory — Although the visceral sensory components of the vagus nerve are functionally divisible into "special" (gustatory) and "general" (interoceptive) divisions, all visceral sensory fibers terminate within a single column in the medulla. The visceral sensory column lies in a periventricular position, just dorsal to the sulcus limitans. In terrestrial vertebrates, this column is represented by the nucleus of the solitary tract.

---

[a]The terminology used in this chapter reflects the historical usage of the terms "visceral" and "somatic" despite current doubts about their accuracy in terms of embryology. Historically, the term visceral has included structures derived from the visceral (branchial) arches in addition to structures relating to the coelomic cavity. Thus for the purposes of this chapter, the reader should not equate the term "visceral" with the modern idea of visceral in the sense of pertaining to autonomic functions or the coelomic cavity.

[b]Many authors during the first half of this century included the posterior lateral line nerve as a somatic sensory branch of the vagus nerve. Since the posterior lateral line nerve does not originate from vagal primordia, does not exit the skull along with branches of the vagus nerve and shares no functions with other branches of the vagus nerve, the lateral line nerves are not currently considered to be branches of the vagus but represent unique cranial nerves found in anamniote vertebrates.

Visceral Motor — The use of the term visceral in this context (in contradistinction to somatic) is confusing (see footnote a, previous page) since the term visceral then embraces both autonomic preganglionic neurons and alpha motoneurons that innervate striate muscle supposedly derived from branchial arches. Until recently,[c] anatomists believed that the vagally-innervated striate muscles were derived from visceral (branchial) arch muscle plates and so were considered nonsomitic.[36] Motoneurons innervating such musculature were considered *special* visceral efferent neurons as opposed to the *general* visceral efferent population which provides preganglionic parasympathetic innervation.

Special visceral — Striate muscles of the pharynx, and of derived pharyngeal structures such as the larynx, are innervated by the vagus nerve. In amniote vertebrates, the motoneurons that provide innervation to these organs lie in a migrated, ventrolaterally-situated motor nucleus referred to as n. ambiguus.

General visceral — The preganglionic parasympathetic population is largely collected into a compact nucleus, the dorsal motor nucleus of the vagus, which lies in a periventricular position, medially adjacent to the sulcus limitans. In most species, additional preganglionic parasympathetic neurons have migrated away from the ventricular surface and lie either in clusters or as scattered neurons within the ventrolateral tegmentum.

Somatic Motor — The vagus makes no contribution to this innervation.

Several recent findings in mammalian as well as non-mammalian vertebrates raise questions about the validity of this formulation. With regard to sensory nuclei, questions have been raised regarding exactly what vagal modality is represented in the spinal trigeminal nucleus and whether it is appropriate to consider this somatic. With regard to the motor nuclei, preganglionic parasympathetic neurons lie within the territory ascribed to the special visceral efferent column. Whether the parcellation of the afferent and efferent brainstem functions into the various nuclei is correct, or whether a reformulation of this concept is required must remain until further data are available.

Figure 2 shows the location of vagal sensory and motor nuclei in four vertebrate species typical of different grades of organization of the nervous system. Despite variation in the degree of migration and aggregation of cell masses in these different species, the relative positions of the various nuclei and major fiber tracts are consistent.

---

[c]Classically, the vagus nerve is described as innervating nonsomitic, branchiomeric muscles such as the intrinsic laryngeal muscles. Such muscles were believed to be derived from visceral (branchial) arch muscle plates. Recent work by Noden[34] indicates however that this formulation appears to be in error; some vagally-innervated muscles are derived from the rostralmost (occipital) somites.

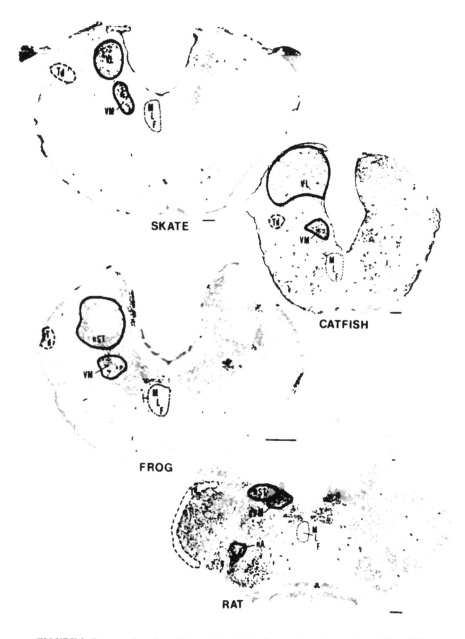

FIGURE 2. Cross-sections through the mid-medulla of several vertebrates selected from different vertebrate orders. The skate (*Raja*) is an elasmobranch; catfish (*Ictalurus*) is a teleost; the frog (*Rana*) is an amphibian; the rat (*Rattus*) is a mammal. The main vagal nuclei are outlined in each section; other important landmarks also are indicated. (Bar scale = 250 μm in each case.)

Variation in Gross Structure of Vagal Nuclei

Although the gross structure and organization of vagal nuclei is similar in amniote vertebrates, great variations can be found in vagal structures among the teleost fishes. Many fishes have independently evolved feeding specializations which involve elaboration of posterior branchial and pharyngeal structures. A concomitant elaboration of central vagal sensory and motor nuclei also occurs. For example, common carp (*Cyprinus carpio*) and the African fish, *Xenomystes,* have independently evolved pharyngeal modifications that appear to permit intraoral separation of food from substrate.[8,37] Both species have elaborate vagal lobes which contain sensory and motor elements representing portions of the viscerosensory and special visceromotor columns. Despite the gross re-arrangement of the vagal centers in these species, the essential topographic relations and connections of the vagal nuclei remain consistent.[12]

SENSORY ROOTS OF THE VAGUS NERVE AND ATTENDANT NUCLEI

General Somatic Sensory

In most vertebrates (but apparently not including skates; see Barry[6]), the vagus nerve contains a few sensory fibers that innervate cutaneous areas in a fashion similar to the trigeminal nerve or spinal dorsal roots. These general somatic sensory fibers of the vagus nerve enter the spinal (descending) trigeminal tract and terminate within a portion of the spinal trigeminal nucleus.[5,23,27,39] The presumption is that vagal fibers that enter the spinal trigeminal tract derive from ganglion cells that innervate skin overlying the operculum (in fishes), the tympanic membrane (in frogs) or the auricle (in mammals). Stuesse *et al.*[39] claim, however, that vagal fibers which innervate abdominal viscera also join the spinal trigeminal tract of the frogs they studied. In contrast, in domestic cats none of the coelomic visceral fibers project to the spinal trigeminal tract.

Visceral Sensory

The large majority of sensory nerve fibers in the vagus nerve serve visceral functions, including gustation. Essentially all of the viscerosensory fibers, whether gustatory or general visceral, terminate within the visceral sensory column. In most vertebrates, this column consists of the nucleus of the solitary tract and commissural nucleus of Cajal. In highly gustatory fishes, the equivalent nuclei are referred to as the facial, glossopharyngeal and vagal lobes, the general visceral nucleus, and the commissural nucleus of Cajal.[11,15,32] In the case of these fishes, the vagus nerve terminates only in the latter three structures; the facial lobe receives input from the facial (and possibly trigeminal[24]) nerve; the glossopharyngeal lobe receives input from the glossopharyngeal nerve.[20] The visceral lobes in such fish appear to be the primary sensory nuclei for gustation, with the general visceral afferents terminating in the general visceral and commissural nuclei.[32] This tendency toward separation of gustatory from general visceral modalities within the visceral sensory column appears to be a common feature of all extant vertebrates in which this question has been examined.[1,14,22,32]

Nucleus of the Solitary Tract

The solitary tract is a longitudinal bundle of poorly myelinated and unmyelinated axons which extends from the rostral medulla to the commissure of Cajal, lying just caudal to the obex. The axons of the solitary tract include both primary sensory fibers and higher order "association" fibers. In general, primary sensory fibers from cranial nerves VII (facial), IX (glossopharyngeal) and X (vagus) enter the solitary tract at their level of entrance into the brainstem. There is a tendency for the majority of sensory fibers from each cranial nerve to terminate within the solitary nucleus at, or somewhat caudal to, its level of entrance into the brainstem. Thus, the majority of vagal sensory fibers terminates in the posterior part of the nucleus of the solitary tract. This tendency should not, however, be construed as a hard and fast rule since in many vertebrates some vagal fibers ascend within the solitary tract to reach more rostral levels of the nucleus.

Vagal Lobe in Bony Fishes

Because many teleost fishes utilize chemosensory cues in locating and selecting food within the aquatic environment, the gustatory sense is generally better represented in this class as compared to other vertebrates. The gustatory specializations include elaborations of both an external (facial nerve-innervated) system and an intraoral (vagally innervated) system.[4] Elaboration of the vagal gustatory system apparently has evolved independently several times since diverse, unrelated teleosts exhibit vagal gustatory specialization. These include members of siluriformes,[4,9,15,20] cypriniformes,[15,29,31,33] gadiformes,[16,25] and osteoglossiformes.[8] Interestingly, the more recently evolved percimorph fishes appear to rely less on gustation than do their phylogenetically less derived relatives. Even in many percimorphs, however, vagal lobes are present rather than a diminutive nucleus of the solitary tract as occurs in most other vertebrates.

A range of sizes and degrees of differentiation occurs among even the highly gustatory fishes. A large, but simple vagal lobe can be found in ictalurid catfish (Figure 2 above). In this case one might imagine that the nucleus of the solitary tract has simply expanded in a medial and dorsal direction. The vagal lobe in these catfish is largely undifferentiated although some relatively subtle cytoarchitectonic patterns can be discerned.[10] Primary gustatory fibers terminate throughout the substance of the lobe.[9,20] Despite the lack of obvious cytodifferentiation, the vagal lobe of these catfish does maintain a diffuse representation of gustatory space. A crude orotopic map of the orobranchial cavity has been discerned by physiological methods.[20] A tendency toward a topographic representation of gustatory space may not be unique to fish[42] and

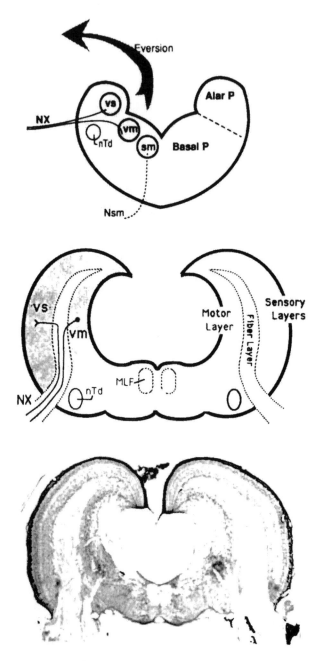

FIGURE 3. Schematic drawings showing the process by which eversion of the neural tube can produce the topological transformation required to produce a multilaminate vagal lobe containing both sensory and motor elements. Note that the essential topological relations between the vagal structures and other important features of the brainstem are maintained. Below: Cross section through the vagal lobe of a goldfish (*Carassius auratus*).

may be one organizing principle of the visceral sensory column. Indeed, the entire viscerosensory column appears to be organized into topographically-arranged functional domains.[1,21,32]

A very different type of vagal lobe can be found in some carps such as the goldfish.[12,15,32,33] In these fishes, the vagal lobe is a highly differentiated, laminated structure. The lobe contains not only cell populations functionally equivalent to those of the nucleus of the solitary tract, but also contains branchiomeric motoneurons classified as special visceral motor neurons (≡ n. ambiguus). Primary vagal sensory fibers terminate only in restricted layers of this structure[31] with a large part of the vagal lobe being devoted to interneuron systems.[12] Despite the derived juxtaposition of the primary gustatory nucleus and the branchiomotor neurons, a simple topological transformation will produce the arrangement of the vagal lobe from the basic vertebrate "bauplan" described above (see Figure 3).

Segregation of Functions Within the Visceral Sensory Column

As mentioned above, in all vertebrates in which the matter has been studied in detail, the gustatory portion of the visceral sensory column is separate from the portion devoted to general visceral activities. This is most obvious in fishes, but obtains in other vertebrates as well. Several lines of evidence indicate that even the general visceral portion of the visceral sensory column does not receive a homogeneous afferentation.

The general rule is one of specific organ system representation within the visceral sensory nuclei. In goldfish, the pharyngeal sensory input terminates in a structure separate from either the oral gustatory representation or the lower G.I. tract representation.[32] In pigeons,[21] the nucleus of the solitary tract can be divided into a lateral tier and a medial tier on the basis of connectivity and cytoarchitectonics. The lateral tier receives cardiopulmonary inputs while the medial tier receives G.I. tract afferentation. In general, Katz and Karten[21] concluded that input from each particular portion of the G.I. tract terminates in the part of the nucleus of the solitary tract adjacent to the vagal motor nuclei that innervate the same portion of the G.I. tract. Similarly, the nucleus of the solitary tract of rats is organized in an organotopic fashion. The rostral subnucleus receives gustatory inputs; intermediate and interstitial nuclei receive respiratory and airway inputs; and the medial portion of the NTS receives gastrointestinal inputs in an organotopically organized fashion.[1] Thus, at three different grades of vertebrate lineage, specificity and functional organization are the rule for visceral sensory organization.

MOTOR COLUMNS OF THE VAGUS NERVE

As described above, the motor functions of the vagus nerve can be divided into two groups. The so-called "special visceral" (called branchiomotor below) group innervates the striate branchiomeric muscles of the posterior branchial arches (#4 and caudalward = 2nd and caudalward gill arch); the general visceral group provides the preganglionic parasympathetic innervation to much of the head, thorax and upper abdomen. As classically described for amniote vertebrates, these two functions are separated into two nuclear groups, respectively the nucleus ambiguus and the dorsal motor nucleus of the vagus. This formulation is, however, flawed. In rats, for example, preganglionic parasympathetic neurons can be found within the nominal boundaries of the nucleus ambiguus.[7] The question can be asked, then, as to what is the basic organization of vagal motor nuclei throughout the vertebrate lineage? Are the functional distinctions of vagal motoneurons reflected in the underlying anatomical organization?

Separation of Branchiomotor and Parasympathetic Functions

Unfortunately, very few species have been examined within any class of non-mammalian vertebrates. Thus, at this point it is difficult to abstract a generalized pattern. For example, modern anatomical methods for distinguishing branchiomotor from general visceral efferent systems have been applied to only two species of bony fish,[20,32] two species of elasmobranch[6,44] and no agnathans.

Nonetheless, on the basis of this scant evidence, some broad generalizations may be drawn with the caveat that many more species need be studied. Among the teleostome vertebrates, the vagal motor complex is divisible into two major functional domains: the anteroventral portion of the vagal motor column innervates branchial muscles; the posterodorsal portion (termed the dorsal motor nucleus of the vagus in the following discussion) contains the bulk of the preganglionic parasympathetic neurons. A smaller, third portion of the vagal motor column may exist, consisting of preganglionic parasympathetic neurons that contribute to the branchial cardiac division of the vagus nerve.[44] This arrangement can be found most obviously in the dogfish, *Scyliorhinus*.[44] The branchiomotor neurons lie just medial to the sulcus limitans in the rostral medulla. The preganglionic parasympathetic neurons lie more posteriorly in a similar position. The branchial-cardiac neurons lie in the midmedulla, but in a migrated position roughly midway between the spinal trigeminal tract and the medial longitudinal fasciculus. This position is topologically similar to the position of the preganglionic parasympathetic neurons of the external formation of the nucleus ambiguus in rats.[7] A similar pattern of three separable vagal motor component nuclei can be found in goldfish.[32] With the exception of the cardiac neurons, the preganglionic parasympathetic neurons lie mostly caudal (and slightly medial) to the branchiomotor neurons. A population of cardiac neurons lies outside of the nominal boundaries of both the branchiomotor nucleus and the dorsal motor nucleus. A similar anteroposterior segregation of branchiomotor and dorsal motor nucleus neurons obtains in ictalurid catfish,[20] but the location of cardiac neurons is not known for this group.

Interestingly, in neither the dogfish nor the goldfish do the preganglionic parasympathetic (general visceral) neurons lie lateral to the branchiomotor nucleus as might be predicted on the basis of the classical descriptions of functional columns in the medulla.[17] Indeed, in goldfish, when the preganglionic parasympathetic and branchiomotor groups overlap in anteroposterior extent, it is the preganglionic parasympathetic neurons which lie more medially.[32] This arrangement, however, appears to be a derived condition, probably associated with the relatively gross enlargement of the vagal gustatory nuclei in this family.

On the basis of a recent study on hagfish,[28] an agnathan vertebrate, the branchiomotor and preganglionic parasympathetic vagal neurons may have been segregated, albeit grouped within a single vagal motor nucleus, early in the vertebrate lineage. In the hagfish, the dorsolateral population of vagal motor neurons has dendrites extending dorsally into the equivalent of the nucleus of the solitary tract; the ventromedially-situated motoneurons equivalent to nucleus ambiguus have dendrites extending into the lateral reticular formation. This dichotomous distribution of dendrites matches the difference in dendritic spread for neurons of the dorsal motor nucleus of the vagus and the nucleus ambiguus in other vertebrates. That is, preganglionic parasympathetic neurons have dendrites extending directly into the primary visceral sensory nucleus (nucleus of the solitary tract). In contrast, branchiomotor neurons have dendrites extending into the medullary lateral reticular formation (see Altschuler *et al.*, chapter 2 of this volume). Thus, in species in which the branchiomotor and general visceromotor populations overlap in anteroposterior extent, the general visceromotor neurons tend to be situated more dorsally or medially, i.e., closer to their input from the visceral sensory nucleus.

A substantial anteroposterior overlap of the branchiomotor and dorsal motor nucleus populations has been reported in the amphibia *Rana pipiens, R. catesbiana*,[39] *Xenopus*[38] and *Bufo japonica*.[35] Despite the overlap in anteroposterior extent, the two populations appear to remain segregated, at least in the two species examined most closely.[35,38] The preganglionic parasympathetic populations in these species lie medial and/or dorsal to the branchiomotor population. In the ranids studied, a population of cardiac neurons occurs somewhat separated from the main body of the dorsal motor nucleus neurons (see Figure 5 in Steusse *et al.*,[39] also Taylor *et al.*[41]) and may represent a population equivalent to the branchial-cardiac pool reported in dogfish.

In amniote vertebrates, the dorsal motor nucleus and branchiomotor nuclei are largely separated, the branchiomotor column being situated ventrolaterally and the dorsal motor nucleus retaining a periventricular position (e.g., Barbas-Henry and Lohman,[5] Leong *et al.*,[26] Katz and Karten[22]). Also, as a general tendency, preganglionic parasympathetic neurons that innervate the heart are distributed within the rostrolateral portion of the medullary tegmentum in the external formation of the nucleus ambiguus.[7] This may be analogous to the distribution of branchial-cardiac neurons in the same area in dogfish.[44] In some mammals, occasional non-cardiac preganglionic parasympathetic neurons also occur within this region of the medullary tegmentum (e.g., Weaver,[43] Takayama *et al.*[40]) although the majority of preganglionic neurons that innervate subdiaphragmatic viscera are confined to the dorsal motor nucleus.

A tentative hypothesis may be offered regarding the organization of the vagal motor nuclei in the vertebrate lineage. In the earliest vertebrates, branchiomotor and parasympathetic functions were segregated within the vagal motor complex with branchiomotor neurons forming the anteroventral part of the vagal motor column and preganglionic parasympathetic neurons forming the dorsal portion. During the course of phylogeny, the branchiomotor and preganglionic parasympathetic populations remained separate by virtue of a greater ventrolateral migration of the branchiomotor population. This ventriculofugal migration results in the situation found in amniotes.

Superimposed upon this general pattern of separation of branchial and preganglionic parasympathetic neurons is a tendency for a small population of preganglionic parasympathetic neurons to migrate ventrofugally to lie near the dendritic fields of the branchiomotor column. Even in species with periventricular branchiomotor somata, (e.g., present day catfish), the dendrites of these cells extend far into the ventrolateral reticular formation[32] (Figure 4), whereas parasympathetic neurons have relatively local dendritic ramifications. Thus descending branchial control information is transmitted through the ventrolateral medulla even in species with more dorsally-situated branchiomotor somata. It has proven to be biologically advantageous, perhaps because of facilitation of coordination between branchial (respiratory) and cardiac functions, for a population of cardiac preganglionic parasympathetic neurons to migrate ventriculofugally to assume a position within, or adjacent to the dendritic field of the branchiomotor neurons, (i.e., in the ventrolateral medullary reticular formation). This situation may be reflected in dogfish[44] and catfish (Kanwal and Finger, unpublished observations) where some cardiac neurons lie in a migrated (ventrolateral) position even though both branchiomotor and other preganglionic parasympathetic neurons retain the periventricular situation.

Segregation of Function within Branchiomotor Nuclei

In various species examined in detail at a variety of grades of organization, the general rule for the branchiomotor nuclei appears to be one of functional organization. That is, motoneurons innervating a particular muscle are grouped together within the vagal branchiomotor nucleus just as motor pools occur within the spinal cord.

For example, in goldfish[32] the palatal musculature is represented in a topographic fashion within the motor layer of the vagal lobe while the various pharyngeal muscles receive innervation from specific pools of branchiomotor neurons of the so-called lateral motor nucleus. Similarly, the n. ambiguus of the rat is organized in an organotopic fashion with strictly organized motor pools.[7] The degree of separation of motoneurons into discrete pools appears to be more related to the branchimotor repertoire of the animal than to phylogenetic position.

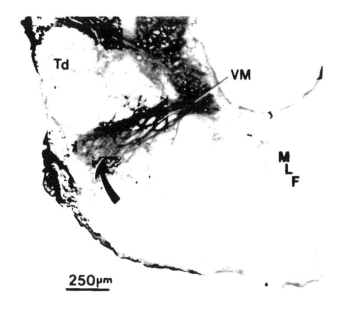

FIGURE 4. Photomicrograph of a cross section through the mid-medulla of an ictalurid catfish in which the vagus nerve was labeled with horseradish peroxidase. Note that despite the periventricular position of the vagal motor (n. ambiguus) somata (VM), the dendrites (arrow) of these branchiomotor cells extend into the ventrolateral medulla — into a site topologically equivalent to the position of the nucleus ambiguus in mammals (see Figure 2).

Segregation of Function within the Dorsal Motor Nucleus

The degree of organotopic separation of functions within the dorsal motor nucleus of the vagus appears dependent on the methodology and investigator as much as on the species chosen for investigation. Thus, a high degree of organ specificity is reported for pigeons[22] and for some mammals[1] but is reported lacking in other mammals such as the cat.[18,19] Even within a single species (rat), varying degrees of organization are reported. On the whole, one might intuitively expect some functional organization to this nucleus, but too few species have been studied in great enough detail to draw any firm conclusions regarding general phyletic patterns.

In the dogfish, Withington-Wray *et al.*[44] report that two distinct size-classes of neurons exist within the dorsal motor nucleus (dorsomedial and ventromedial vagal motor nuclei). The dorsomedial nucleus contains medium-sized cells while the ventromedial nucleus has large cells. These authors suggest that the ventromedial, large-celled group provides secretomotor innervation while the smaller, dorsomedial neurons provide innervation to the smooth muscle.

REFLEX CONNECTIONS

Despite superficial differences in the appearance of the vagal nuclei, a major organizational principle of the vagal system is that of organ-specific reflex connectivity. The general tendency toward organotopy may be seen in the organ-specific reflex systems which can be found throughout several grades of organization of contemporary vertebrates. In fish,[13,30] birds[2] and mammals[1] studied carefully to date, the primary vagal visceral sensory nuclei (e.g., vagal lobes or nucleus of the solitary tract) maintain specific, reflex type connections with the visceral motor nuclei (e.g., dorsal motor nucleus and nucleus ambiguus). For example, in catfish[30] and goldfish,[12,13] the vagal lobes and general visceral sensory nuclei project to the region of neuropil occupied by the dendrites of the nucleus ambiguus and to the dorsal motor nucleus of the vagus. Similarly, in pigeons, the nucleus of the solitary tract has reflex connections to the nucleus ambiguus and the dorsal motor nucleus.[2] Likewise in rats, the nucleus of the solitary tract projects to the nucleus ambiguus and dorsal motor nucleus. In the amniote vertebrates, the projection from the nucleus of the solitary tract to these two targets is organized organotopically. Thus for example, the projection to the vicinity of the ventrolateral part of the nucleus ambiguus arises chiefly from those areas of the nucleus of the solitary tract receiving cardiovascular or pulmonary inputs.[1,2] That preganglionic parasympathetic cardiac neurons also inhabit the vicinity of this solitary nucleus-target area cannot be overlooked.

Not all primary visceral sensory nuclei mediate reflex connections to the nucleus ambiguus and dorsal motor nucleus of the vagus. In catfish, for instance, such connections are restricted to vagal portions of the visceral sensory column while facial nerve visceral systems have connections to the medial reticular formation.[30] Furthermore, projections to the dorsal motor nucleus arise only from the non-gustatory components of the visceral sensory nuclei in goldfish; gustatory portions project to the branchiomotor neurons.[13] Thus the original distinction between special (gustatory) and general visceral sensory nuclei may have relevance to the type of reflex connections arising from the different primary sensory nuclei.

SUMMARY AND CONCLUSION

Although the detailed anatomy of the vagus nerve nuclei has been studied in only a handful of species, some generalizations may be offered regarding the organization of these structures. First, throughout the vertebrate lineage, the different functional components of the vagal nerve system originate or terminate in separable and largely consistent columns of the medulla. Sensory nuclei lie dorsal to the sulcus limitans while motor nuclei lie ventral to the sulcus.

Further, sensory nuclei are divisible into a somatic-type sensory nucleus, the spinal trigeminal nucleus, and a visceral sensory nucleus, the nucleus of the solitary tract or its equivalents. Within the visceral sensory column, gustatory inputs are segregated from general visceral ones; visceral inputs are organized into organ system domains.

Motor nuclei of the vagus nerve are separable into two major components: branchiomotor and preganglionic parasympathetic. This latter component may be further divided into migrated and non-migrated portions. The dendrites of the branchiomotor neurons generally are associated with the lateral reticular formation while those of the preganglionic parasympathetic neurons reach into the general visceral sensory nucleus. Finally, the overall organization of both the sensory and motor nuclei appears to be one of heterogeneity and topography rather than one of homogeneity and diffuseness. Specific vagal visceral reflex systems have been described for both anamniote and amniote vertebrates and thus may be the major organizational scheme underlying vagal nerve function.

REFERENCES

1. **Altschuler, S.M., Bao, X., Bieger, D., Hopkins, D.A., and Miselis, R.R.,** Viscerotopic representation of the upper alimentary tract in the rat: sensory ganglia and nuclei of the solitary and spinal trigeminal tracts, *J. Comp. Neurol.,* 283, 248-268, 1989.

2. **Arends, J.J.A., Wild, J.M., and Zeigler, H.P.,** Projections of the nucleus of the tractus solitarius in the pigeon (*Columba livia*), *J. Comp. Neurol.,* 278, 405-429, 1988.

3. **Ariens Kappers, C.U., Huber, G.C., and Crosby, E.C.,** *The Comparative Anatomy of the Nervous System of Vertebrates, Including Man,* Hafner Publishing Co., N.Y., 1967.

4. **Atema, J.,** Structure and function of the sense of taste in the catfish (*Ictalurus natalis*), *Brain Behav. Evol.,* 4, 273-294, 1971.

5. **Barbas-Henry, H.A., and Lohman, A.H.M.,** The motor nuclei and primary projections of the IXth, Xth, XIth, and XIIth cranial nerves in the monitor lizard, *Varanus exanthematicus,* *J. Comp. Neurol.,* 226, 565-579, 1984.

6. **Barry, M.A.,** Central connections of the IXth and Xth cranial nerves in the clearnose skate, *Brain Res.,* 425, 159-166, 1987.

7. **Bieger, D., and Hopkins, D.A.,** Viscerotopic representation of the upper alimentary tract in the medulla oblongata of the rat: the nucleus ambiguus, *J. Comp. Neurol.,* 262, 546-562, 1987.

8. **Braford, M. A. Jr.,** De gustibus non disputandum: a spiral center for taste in the brain of the teleost fish, *Heterotis niloticus, Science,* 232, 489-491, 1986.

9. **Finger, T.E.,** Gustatory pathways in the bullhead catfish. I. Connections of the anterior ganglion, *J. Comp. Neurol.,* 165, 513-526, 1976.

10. **Finger, T.E.,** Enkephalin-like immunoreactivity in the gustatory lobes and visceral nuclei in the brains of goldfish and catfish, *Neuroscience,* 6, 2747-2758, 1981.

11. **Finger, T.E.,** The gustatory system in teleost fish, in *Fish Neurobiology,* Northcutt, R.G., and Davis, R.E., Eds., University of Michigan Press, Ann Arbor, Michigan, 1983, 285-319.

12. **Finger, T.E.,** Sensorimotor mapping and oropharyngeal reflexes in goldfish, *Carassius auratus. Brain Behav. Evol.,* 31, 17-24, 1988.

13. **Finger, T.E.,** Specificity of gustatory and general visceral reflex systems in the brainstem of the goldfish, *Carassius auratus, Proc. Int. Symposium Olf. and Taste,* Graphic Communication System, Oslo, X, 277, 1990.

14. **Hamilton, R.B., and Norgren, R.,** Central projections of gustatory nerves, *J. Comp. Neurol.,* 222, 560-577, 1984.

15. **Herrick, C.J.,** Central gustatory paths in brains of bony fishes, *J. Comp. Neurol.,* 15, 375-456, 1905.

16. **Herrick, C.J.,** A study of the vagal lobes and funicular nuclei of the brain of the codfish, *J. Comp. Neurol.,* 17, 67-87, 1907.

17. Herrick, C.J., *An Introduction to Neurology, 3rd Edition,* W.B. Saunders, Philadelphia, 1922.

18. Kalia, M., and Mesulam, M.-M., Brainstem projections of sensory and motor components of the vagus complex in the cat. I. The cervical vagus and nodose ganglion, *J. Comp. Neurol.,* 193, 435-465, 1980.

19. Kalia, M., and Mesulam, M.-M., Brainstem projections of sensory and motor components of the vagus complex in the cat. II. Laryngeal, tracheobronchial, pulmonary, cardiac, and gastrointestinal branches, *J. Comp. Neurol.,* 193, 466-508, 1980.

20. Kanwal, J.S., and Caprio, J., Central projections of the glossopharyngeal and vagal nerves in the channel catfish, *Ictalurus punctatus:* clues to differential processing of visceral inputs, *J. Comp. Neurol.,* 264, 216-230, 1987.

21. Katz, D.M., and Karten, H.J., Visceral representation within the nucleus tractus solitarius in pigeon, *Columba livia, J. Comp. Neurol.,* 218, 42-73, 1983.

22. Katz, D.M., and Karten, H.J., Topographic representation of visceral target organs within the dorsal motor nucleus of the vagus nerve of the pigeon, *Columba livia, J. Comp. Neurol.,* 242, 397-414, 1985.

23. Kishida, R., Yoshimoto, M., Kusunoki, T., Goris, R.C., and Terashima, S., Vagal afferent C fibers projecting to the lateral descending trigeminal complex of crotaline snakes, *Exp. Brain Res.,* 53, 315-319, 1984.

24. Kiyohara, S., Houman, H., Yamashita, S., Caprio, J., and Marui, T., Morphological evidence for a direct projection of trigeminal nerve fibers to the primary gustatory center in the sea catfish, *Plotosus anguillaris, Brain Res.,* 379, 353-357, 1986.

25. Kotrschal, K., and Whitear, M., Chemosensory anterior dorsal fin in rocklings (*Gaidropsarus* and *Ciliata,* Teleostei, Gadidae): Somatotopic representation of the ramus recurrens facialis as revealed by transganglionic transport of HRP, *J. Comp. Neurol.,* 268, 109-120, 1988.

26. Leong, S.K., Tay, S.W., and Wong, W.C., The localization of vagal neurons in the terrapin (*Trionyx sinensis*) as revealed by the retrograde horseradish peroxidase method, *J. Autonom. Nerv. Sys.,* 11, 373-382, 1984.

27. Matesz, C., and Szekely, G., The motor column and sensory projections of the branchial cranial nerves in the frog, *J. Comp. Neurol.,* 178, 157-176, 1978.

28. Matsuda, H., Goris, R.C., and Kishida, R., Afferent and efferent projections of the glossopharyngeal-vagal nerve in the hagfish, *J. Comp. Neurol.,* 311, 520-530, 1991.

29. Mayser, P., Vergleichend anatomische Studien über das Gehirn der Knochenfische mit besonderer Beruksichtigung der Cyprinoiden, *Arch. Wiss. Zool.,* 36, 259-366, 1881.

30. Morita, Y., and Finger, T.E., Reflex connections of the facial and vagal gustatory systems in the brainstem of the bullhead catfish, *Ictalurus nebulosus, J. Comp. Neurol.,* 231, 547-558, 1985.

31. Morita, Y., and Finger, T.E., Topographic representation and laminar organization of the vagal gustatory system in the goldfish, *Carassius auratus, J. Comp. Neurol.,* 238, 187-201, 1985.

32. Morita, Y., and Finger, T.E., Topographic representation of the sensory and motor roots of the vagus nerve in the medulla of goldfish, *Carassius auratus, J. Comp. Neurol.,* 264, 231-249, 1987.

33. Morita, Y., Ito, H., and Masai, H., Central gustatory paths in the crucian carp, *Carassius carassius, J. Comp. Neurol.,* 191, 119-132, 1980.

34. Noden, D.M., Craniofacial Development: new views on old problems, *Anat. Rec.,* 208, 1-13, 1984.

35. Oka, Y., Takeuchi, H., Satou, M., and Ueda, K., Morphology and distribution of the preganglionic parasympathetic neurons of the facial, glossopharyngeal and vagus nerves in the Japanese toad: a cobaltic lysine study, *Brain Res.,* 400, 389-395, 1987.

36. Romer, A.S., *The Vertebrate Body, 4th Edition,* W.B. Saunders Co., Philadelphia, 1970.

37. Sibbing, F.A., Pharyngeal mastication and food transport in the carp (*Cyprinus carpio* L.): a cineradiographic and electromyographic study, *J. Morphol.,* 172, 223-258, 1982.

38. **Simpson, H.B., Tobias, M.L., and Kelley, D.B.,** Origin and identification of fibers in the cranial nerve IX-X complex of *Xenopus laevis*: lucifer yellow backfills *in vitro, J. Comp. Neurol.*, 244, 430-444, 1986.
39. **Stuesse, S.L., Cruce, W.L.R., and Powell, K.S.,** Organization within the cranial IX-X complex in ranid frogs: a horseradish peroxidase transport study, *J. Comp. Neurol.*, 222, 358-365, 1984.
40. **Takayama, K., Ishikawa, N., and Miura, M.,** Sites of origin and termination of gastric vagus preganglionic neurons: an HRP study in the rat, *J. Autonom. Nerv. Sys.*, 6, 211-223, 1982.
41. **Taylor, B., Finger, T.E., D'Arcy, G., and Roper, S.D.,** Accuracy of regeneration of vagal cardiac parasympathetic preganglionic axons after a nerve crush lesion, *J. Comp. Neurol.*, 221, 145-153, 1983.
42. **Travers, S.P., Pfaffmann, C., and Norgren, R.,** Convergence of lingual and palatal gustatory neural activity in the nucleus of the solitary tract, *Brain Res.*, 365, 305-320, 1986.
43. **Weaver, F.C.,** Localization of parasympathetic preganglionic cell bodies innervating the pancreas within the vagal nucleus and nucleus ambiguus of the rat brain stem: Evidence of dual innervation based on the retrograde axonal transport of horseradish peroxidase, *J. Auton. Nerv. Syst.*, 2, 61-69, 1980.
44. **Withington-Wray, D.J., Roberts, B.L., and Taylor, E.W.,** The topographical organization of the vagal motor column in the elasmobranch fish, *Scyliorhinus canicula*, L, *J. Comp. Neurol.*, 248, 95-104, 1986.

Chapter 2

VISCEROTOPIC REPRESENTATION OF THE ALIMENTARY TRACT IN THE DORSAL AND VENTRAL VAGAL COMPLEXES IN THE RAT

S.M. Altschuler, L. Rinaman and R.R. Miselis

TABLE OF CONTENTS

LIST OF ABBREVIATIONS

CT-HRP = cholera toxin horseradish peroxidase
DAB = 3,'3-diaminobenzidine tetrachloride
DMN = dorsal motor nucleus of the vagus nerve
lat DMN = lateral column of the DMN
med DMN = medial column of the DMN
NA = nucleus ambiguus
NA_c = compact formation of the NA
NA_{ex} = external formation of the NA
NA_l = loose formation of the NA
NA_{sc} = semicompact formation of the NA
NTS = nucleus tractus solitarii
NTS_{cen} = subnucleus centralis of NTS
NTS_{com} = commissural subnucleus of NTS
NTS_{gel} = subnucleus gelatinosus of NTS
NTS_{int} = intermediate subnucleus of the NTS
NTS_{is} = subnucleus interstitialis of NTS
NTS_{med} = medial subnucleus of NTS
PSPs = post synaptic potentials
PTI = paratrigeminal islands
TS = tractus solitarius
WGA-HRP = wheat germ agglutinin-horseradish peroxidase
VII = facial nucleus
IX = glossopharyngeal nerve
X = vagus nerve
XI = accessory nerve
XII = hypoglossal nucleus

INTRODUCTION

The neural control of the alimentary tract is dependent on input from the central and enteric nervous systems. Since a major source of central nervous system innervation to the gut is provided by the vagus nerve, considerable study has been devoted to determining the brainstem organization of vagal projections from the alimentary tract. The introduction of axoplasmic tracing technique has demonstrated a particularly strong visceral representation within the vagal motor nuclei (nucleus ambiguus (NA) and dorsal motor nucleus of the vagus nerve (DMN)) and sensory nucleus (nucleus tractus solitarii (NTS)).[8,19,24,25,42,43,44,45,77] Despite a plethora of neuroanatomical tracing studies over the last fifteen years, only recently has a precise viscerotopic organization for the alimentary tract been established within the dorsal and ventral vagal complex.[1,3,4,12,29,33,38,39,42,43,44,46,65,70,71,83,90] The formulation and acceptance of viscerotopic maps for vagally innervated structures has depended heavily on the development of new neuroanatomical tracers and injection strategies to control leakage and spread of the tracers from the injection site.

Over the last decade, our laboratory has studied the viscerotopic organization of the NA, NTS, and DMN in the rat using a sensitive retrograde and antegrade tracer, cholera toxin horseradish peroxidase (CT-HRP). This tracer, which we prepare in our lab (see Altschuler *et al.*[4] for detailed methods of synthesis) is created by the covalent conjugation of HRP to CT. We have found this tracer to be more effective than free HRP and equally effective to the wheat germ agglutinin conjugate of HRP in labeling afferent terminal fields.[1,4,83] Additionally, this tracer is especially effective in labeling distal dendritic processes of retrogradely labeled neurons.[3,4,7,69,70,83] The superior labeling seen with this tracer is derived from its ligand affinities for the superficial carbohydrate residues (GM1 gangliosides) of plasma membranes and intracellular transport mechanisms.

The receptor binding properties of CT-HRP have allowed us to use a very dilute concentration (range 0.20-0.45% as determined by Lowry or Bradford assays[15,54]) of the tracer in our studies without sacrificing the quality of afferent terminal, neuronal, or dendritic labeling. Recently, we have found this tracer to be very effective in ultrastructural neural tracing studies[69] as well. The initial low protein concentration of the tracer has aided in controlling spread from the injection site and spurious labeling of adjacent structures. The small quantities of tracer that leak from the injection site have been easily diluted with serial saline washes to concentration levels inadequate for binding. Additional details concerning our injection strategies and methods to control spread can be found in our prior published reports.[1,3,4,69,70,83]

This chapter will focus on our current knowledge of the viscerotopic organization of sensory and motor projections from the alimentary tract in the ventral and dorsal vagal complexes of the rat. A precise understanding of the organization of these vagal nuclei provides a framework for further investigations directed at determining the connectivity of these brainstem areas with higher levels of the visceral neural axis and the neuromodulation of their output. The sections on the NA and DMN will also describe the dendritic architecture of retrogradely labeled motoneurons, including synaptic relationships to afferent terminals, providing an anatomical basis for the most complete analysis of possible afferent interactions with these motor nuclei and motoneuronal interactions within the nucleus.

VENTRAL VAGAL COMPLEX

Nucleus Ambiguus (NA)

The NA, located in the ventrolateral medulla, is comprised of a continuum of rostrocaudally aligned subdivisions that begin rostrally at the level of the facial nucleus and extend caudally to the spinal medullary junction.[12] These subdivisions have been designated as the compact (NA_c), semicompact (NA_{sc}), loose (NA_l), and external (NA_{ex}) formations (Figures 1 and 2). The dorsal division of the NA is comprised of the NA_c, NA_{sc}, and NA_l and is the source of special visceral efferents innervating the striated muscle of the upper gastrointestinal and respiratory tracts (branchiomeric musculature). Subdivisions of the dorsal division are readily discernible by their different cellular densities when the medulla is sectioned in the sagittal plane[3,12] (Figure 2). The NA_{ex}, which comprises the ventral division of the NA, lies ventral and lateral to the dorsal division and is the source of general visceral efferents innervating the thoracic viscera. In the rat, the heart receives significant innervation from motoneurons located within the NA_{ex}.[12,27] It should also be emphasized that the dorsal division of the NA is no longer considered to be a source (DMN is only source) of general visceral efferent innervation to abdominal viscera.[3,12,83] The dorsal and ventral divisions constitute the NA of classical descriptions.[12]

The viscerotopic organization of the NA discussed in this section is derived from studies primarily performed in the rat where direct intramuscular injections of the tracer into different parts of the upper alimentary tract were performed.[3,12] Tracer injections into all parts (cervical, thoracic and subdiaphragmatic) of the esophagus showed neuronal labeling limited to the NA_c, while in contrast, injections of soft palate, pharynx and cricothyroid muscle, resulted in retrograde neuronal labeling limited to the NA_{sc} (Figure 3). Within each formation a distinct pattern of cell labeling and dendritic projections was found for each structure injected.[3] In contrast to the precise viscerotopic organization developed for the NA_c and NA_{sc}, limited information is presently available concerning the organization of the NA_l.

Although the esophagus of the rat (and striated portions in other mammals[40,50,51,62,90]) derives its vagal motor innervation from the NA_c, the population of motoneurons projecting to different levels of the esophagus is not entirely homogenous. Utilizing fluorescent dyes as tracers, Beiger and Hopkins[12] have demonstrated that separate populations of neurons innervate the different levels of the esophagus. The cervical esophagus has the most restricted repre-

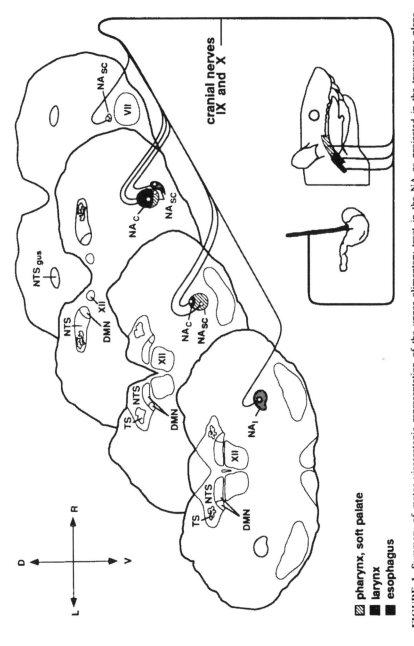

FIGURE 1. Summary of motor viscerotopic representation of the upper alimentary tract in the NA as projected in the transverse plane. Motoneurons innervating the striated muscle of the upper alimentary tract are located within the three subdivisions (NA$_c$, NA$_{sc}$, NA$_i$) of the dorsal division of the NA.

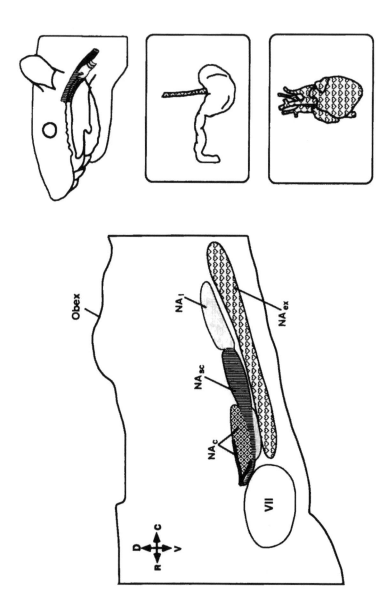

FIGURE 2. Summary of the motor viscerotopic representation of the upper alimentary tract in the NA as projected in the sagittal plane. The NA is comprised of the two major subdivisions (dorsal and ventral) that begin at the level of the VII and extend caudally to the spinal-medullary junction. The dorsal division is comprised of the NA_c, NA_{sc}, and NA_i, and the ventral division of the NA_{ex}. Each subdivision has a precise viscerotopic organization and is characterized by a different cellular density.

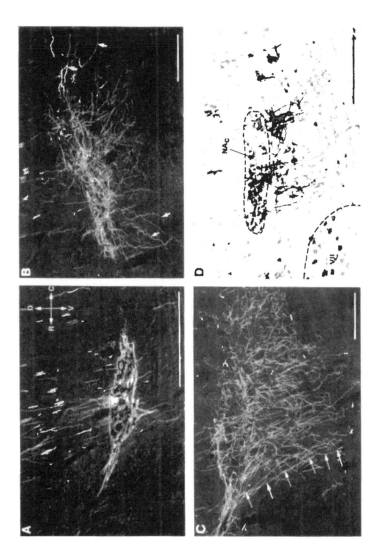

FIGURE 3 (A-D). A-D are darkfield photomicrographs of sagittal sections through the NA following injection of CT-HRP into the subdiaphragmatic esophagus. In A, motoneuronal labeling is restricted to the NA_c. Photomicrographs B-D demonstrate unique distributions of motoneuronal labeling in the NA_{sc} for each structure (soft palate, pharynx, and cricothyroid muscle) injected with CT-HRP. The arrows in B and C indicate extranuclear dendritic projections. (Calibration bars in A and D = 500 μm and B and C =250 μm; R=rostral, C=caudal, D=dorsal, V=ventral.)

sentation; its motoneurons are limited to the most rostral and dorsal aspects of the NA_c[3,12] (Figures 2 and 4). Motoneurons projecting to the thoracic and subdiaphragmatic esophagus, in contrast, are located throughout the entire rostrocaudal and mediolateral extent of the NA_c (Figures 2 and 3). Although the rostrocaudal distribution of labeled cells overlaps considerably following injection of the thoracic and subdiaphragmatic esophagus, a more rostral level of maximal cell labeling is found after injection of the thoracic esophagus.[3] These findings suggest that a crude rostrocaudal organotopy exists within the NA_c corresponding to rostrocaudal positioning along the esophagus.

The NA_{sc} lies immediately lateral and ventrocaudal to NA_c and is the source of motoneurons projecting to the palatopharyngeal area of the alimentary tract and the cricothyroid muscle[3,12] (Figures 2-3). Motoneuronal pools projecting to soft palate, pharynx and cricothyroid muscle in the rat have distinct topographical distributions within the NA_{sc}[3] (Figure 3). In the rat, the motoneurons innervating the cricothyroid muscle are displaced from those motoneurons innervating intrinsic laryngeal musculature (located in the loose formation[12]) and occupy an area within the NA_{sc} that is generally more rostral and lateral to those motoneurons projecting to the soft palate and pharynx. The distributions of soft palate and pharyngeal motoneurons overlap to some extent; however, within the caudal NA_{sc}, soft palate motoneurons are preferentially located more caudal and dorsal to pharyngeal motoneurons.[3] Beiger and Hopkins[12] have further evaluated the representation of the pharyngeal musculature utilizing fluorescent dyes. Motoneurons projecting to the thyopharyngeal muscle were limited to the more rostral portion of the NA_{sc} while those projecting to the hypopharyngeal muscle were distributed over the entire NA_{sc}.

A prominent characteristic of both the NA_c and the NA_{sc} is the extensive bundling of dendrites within the confines of the nucleus[3,12] (Figure 5). These dendritic bundles are oriented primarily in rostrocaudal direction and are evident following sectioning of the medulla in either the horizontal or sagittal plane.[3] Utilizing CT-HRP as our tracer, we have been able to demonstrate intranuclear bundling of dendrites following direct intramuscular injection of the tracer into the soft palate, pharynx, and all levels of esophagus. Intranuclear bundling of dendrites is only lacking following injection of the cricothyroid muscle. Beiger and Hopkins[12] have demonstrated a similar intranuclear dendritic architecture following injection of free HRP into the supranodosal vagus and wheat germ agglutinin (WGA)-HRP injection into the esophagus.

The NA_{sc} is also the site of origin of ventrolateral and dorsomedial oriented dendritic bundles. The bundles were demonstrated following injection of CT-HRP in the soft palate and pharynx and sectioning the medulla in the transverse plane[3] (Figure 6). These bundles differ from longitudinal dendritic bundles in a number of ways. Motoneuron dendrites contributing to these bundles are limited to the same rostrocaudal plane and do not extend rostrocaudally throughout the nucleus. Additionally, these bundles are not confined entirely to the NA_{sc}, but actually penetrate the adjacent reticular formation (Figure 6).

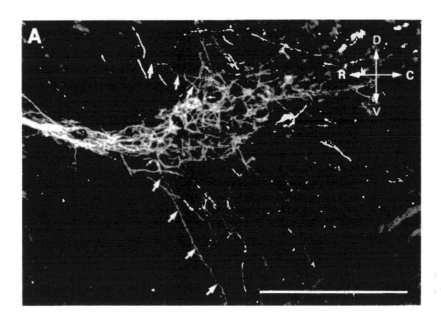

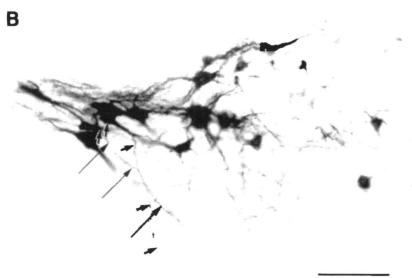

FIGURE 4 (A-B). A is a darkfield photomicrograph of a sagittal section following injection of CT-HRP into the cervical esophagus. Motoneuronal labeling is restricted to the rostral and dorsal portions of the NA$_c$. B is a brightfield photomicrograph at higher magnification of a sagittal section 80 μm medial to the section in A. The different sets of arrows in A and B indicate extranuclear dendritic projections whose origin could be traced to cell bodies located in the NA$_{sc}$. (Calibration bar in A = 500 μm and in B = 125 μm; R=rostral, C=caudal, D=dorsal, V=ventral.)

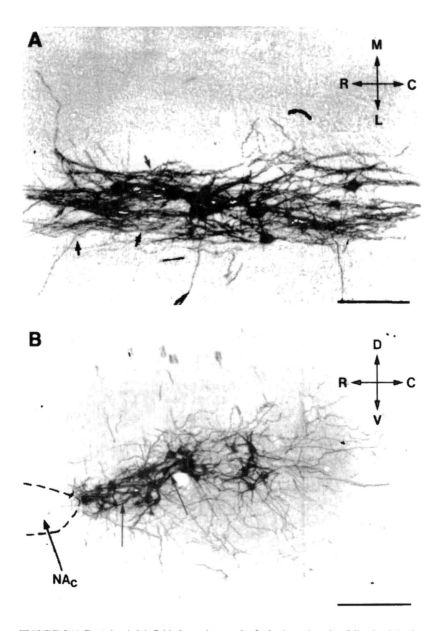

FIGURE 5 (A-B). A is a brightfield photomicrograph of a horizontal section following injection of CT-HRP into the thoracic esophagus. B is a brightfield photomicrograph of a sagittal section following injection of tracer into the soft palate. Note the intranuclear dendrites form bundles (arrows) that run primary in a rostrocaudal direction and are confined to the boundaries of the NA$_c$ and NA$_{sc}$ respectively in A and B. (Calibration bar in A = 125 μm and in B = 250 μm; R=rostral, C=caudal, D=dorsal, V=ventral, M=medial, L=lateral.)

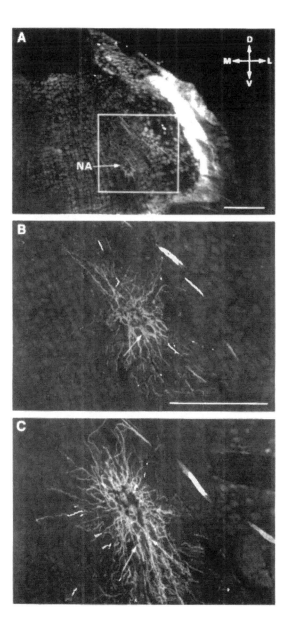

FIGURE 6 (A-C). A is a low power darkfield photomicrograph of the NA in the transverse plane following injection of CT-HRP into the subdiaphragmatic esophagus. The box outlined in A is a comparable region appearing at higher magnification in B and C. B and C are darkfield photomicrographs following injection of tracer into the soft palate and the pharynx, respectively. The arrows in B and C indicate dendritic bundles projecting into the adjacent reticular formation. In A there is an absence of extranuclear dendrites and in B and C there are extensive extranuclear dendrites. (Calibration Bars in A and B = 500 µm. B and C are at the same magnification; M=medial, L=lateral, D=dorsal, V=ventral.)

Dendritic bundles have been postulated to serve as networks for the generation of complex motor events where a synchronization of motoneuronal activity is required.[48,72,78,79,80,81,82] The extensive longitudinal bundling of dendrites found in the NA, one of the major motor nuclei involved in swallowing,[56,57] suggests a role for these structures in maintaining a precise sequence of muscle activation through the rostrocaudal integration of motoneuronal activity during the swallowing motor sequence. In contrast, transverse dendritic bundles may provide a mechanism for localized modification of motor output without affecting the sequence of muscle activation.

The existence of extranuclear dendrites of NA motoneurons was first demonstrated by Shapiro and Miselis[83] utilizing CT-HRP as the neural tracer. Following the injection of the cricothyroid muscle with this tracer, extensive radiating dendritic projections were demonstrated penetrating the adjacent reticular formation. The penetration of the adjacent reticular formation by dendritic projections originating from motoneurons located in the NA_{sc} has also been found following injection of free HRP into the supranodosal vagus nerve.[12] In our most recent studies utilizing CT-HRP,[3] we have also been able to demonstrate extranuclear dendritic projections originating from the NA_c as well as the NA_{sc} (Figures 3,4,6). Motoneurons within the NA_c projecting to the cervical esophagus were found to have extranuclear dendrites penetrating the adjacent reticular formation in a distribution that was unique when compared to adjacent structures (Figure 4). These dendrites may be responsible for coordinating the action of the upper esophageal sphincter with musculature active during the buccopharyngeal phase of swallowing. In the rat, the upper esophageal sphincter and the cricothyroid muscle are subject to a simultaneous early inhibition during swallowing.[5] Although the motoneuronal pools projecting to these muscles are located in different areas of the NA, a portion of their dendritic projections penetrates the same area of the adjacent reticular formation, providing a basis to receive the same inhibitory input.[3] In contrast to cervical esophageal motoneurons, the dendrites of thoracic and subdiaphragmatic esophageal motoneurons were confined to the NA_c (Figures 3 and 5).

The extranuclear dendritic fields, when reconstructed from either serial sagittal or horizontal sections, were found to be more extensive for the musculature represented in the NA_{sc} than for the cervical esophagus[3] (Figure 7). Based on the size of the dendritic fields, the potential for modulation by multiple central afferents would appear to be greater for musculature represented within the NA_{sc}. The potential dendritic-afferent contacts may provide an anatomical substrate for the musculature represented in the NA_{sc} to participate in major functional motor behaviors (swallowing, respiration, phonation[6,14,56]). Since the esophagus is essentially limited to one primary motor function, peristalsis, which endures comparatively less modulation once initiated, it is not unexpected that motoneurons projecting to this structure receive afferent projections from limited areas of the brainstem, the subnucleus centralis of the NTS (NTS_{cen}).[11,21,22,73,84]

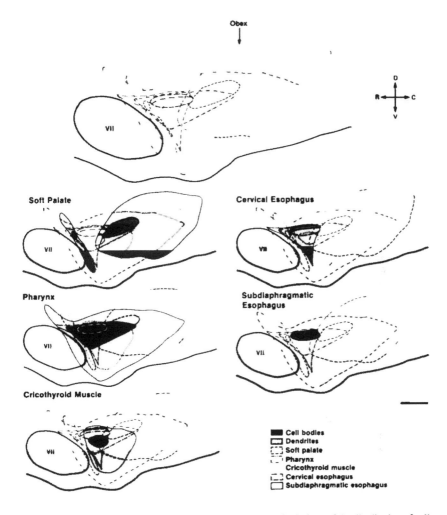

FIGURE 7. Summary diagrammatic representation in the sagittal plane of the distribution of cell bodies and extranuclear dendrites in the NA following injection of intramuscular injection of CT-HRP into different regions of the upper alimentary tract. (Used with permission from Altschuler, S.M., X. Bao, and R.R. Miselis, Dendritic architecture of nucleus ambiguus motoneurons projecting to the upper alimentary tract in the rat, *J. Comp. Neurol.* 309, 402-414, 1991.)

DORSAL VAGAL COMPLEX

Dorsal Motor Nucleus of the Vagus Nerve (DMN)

The DMN is considered the source of general visceral efferent fibers that make synaptic contact with postganglionic neurons located in the myenteric plexus of the bowel wall.[4,9,18,47] The smooth muscle of the gastrointestinal tract in turn receives its motor innervation from neurons located within the myenteric plexus indicating that no direct contacts exist between vagal fibers originating in the DMN and the smooth muscle of the gastrointestinal tract. In the rat where the entire esophagus consists of striated muscle, motoneurons of the DMN begin their innervation of the alimentary canal at the level of the stomach and continue to innervate the gastrointestinal tract as far caudal as the descending colon. Innervation of the esophagus by DMN motoneurons occurs in those mammals where a portion of the esophagus consists of smooth muscle (cat for example[61]).

The right and left DMN contribute efferent axons respectively to the right and left cervical vagal nerves. These nerves cross above the diaphragm and then enter the abdominal cavity where they have been designated as the left and right subdiaphragmatic vagus nerves, respectively. The left or dorsal subdiaphragmatic vagus further divides into the celiac and left gastric nerves, while the right or ventral subdiaphragmatic vagus divides into the hepatic, accessory celiac and right gastric nerves.[64]

The ability to easily apply neuroanatomical tracers to either vagal nerve branches or directly to the different abdominal viscera has led to the development of organizational maps of the DMN based on both injection strategies. Although these two injection strategies have often provided conflicting results regarding DMN organization, more recent studies utilizing adequate measures to control tracer spread have yielded results where vagal branch-organization topology can be correlated with viscerotopic representation within the DMN.[4,28,64,70,83]

The studies of Fox and Powley[28] and Norgren and Smith,[64] where tracers were applied directly to the branches of the subdiaphragmatic vagus, provided conclusive evidence that the DMN is organized mediolaterally with respect to these branches. Motoneurons located within large medial columns of the right and left DMN contribute efferent axons to the left and right gastric nerves, respectively. The celiac and accessory celiac nerves are made up of axons of motoneurons located in smaller lateral columns of the right and left DMN. The representation of the hepatic branch consists of a few scattered neurons located within the left medial DMN.

Our laboratory's initial studies with CT-HRP, where the representation of the stomach and pancreas in DMN was investigated utilizing direct intramuscular injection of the tracer, demonstrated localized retrograde labeling of motoneurons bilaterally within the medial columns of the DMN[70,83] (Figures 8 and 9). These results suggested to us that motoneurons innervating specific abdominal viscera are localized within either the medial or lateral bilaterally symmetrical columns.

This concept has been supported by our recent experiments where the representation of the small and large intestines within the DMN has been investigated using the same tracer and injection strategies. These studies demonstrated a significant representation for cecum that was localized to the two lateral columns of the DMN (Figures 8 and 9) in a rostrocaudal distribution conforming to the pattern of DMN labeling seen after application of tracer to

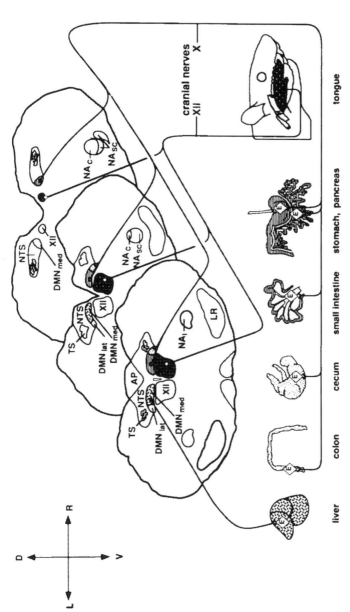

FIGURE 8. Summary of motor viscerotopic representation of the alimentary tract in the DMN as projected in the transverse plane. A mediolateral organization within the DMN exists corresponding to the rostrocaudal positioning along the alimentary canal. DMN motoneurons projecting to enteric neurons within the stomach, pancreas and duodenum are limited to the medial columns bilaterally. Motoneurons projecting to liver originate within left medial DMN. Those motoneurons projecting to the jejunum, ileum, cecum and colon are located within the lateral columns of the DMN (D=dorsal, V=ventral, L=left, R=right).

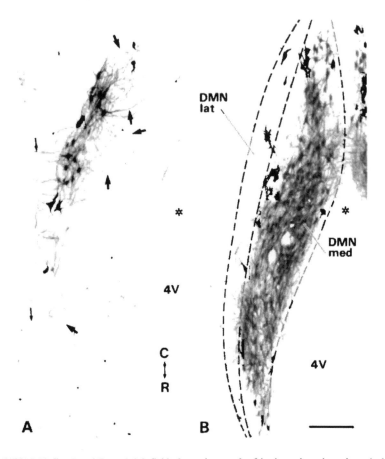

FIGURE 9 (A-B). A and B are brightfield photomicrograph of horizontal sections through the DMN following injection of CT-HRP into the cecum and stomach, respectively. A distinct topographical organization of motoneuronal labeling exists within the DMN such that gastric motoneurons are found within med DMN and cecal motoneurons are found within the lat DMN. Dendrites are indicated by thick arrows and axons by thin arrows. The level of the obex is indicated by an asterisk in each photomicrograph. (Calibration bar =250 μm; C=caudal, R=rostral. Used with permission from Altschuler, S.M., D.A. Ferenci, R.B. Lynn, and R.R. Miselis, Representation of the cecum in lateral dorsal motor nucleus of the vagus nerve and commissural subnucleus of the nucleus tractus solitarii in rat, *J. Comp. Neurol.* 304, 261-274,1991.)

the celiac and accessory celiac branches of the vagus nerve.[4,28,64] Although the representations of the stomach and the cecum dominate the medial and lateral columns respectively, other areas of the bowel have a sparse representation localized to either the medial or lateral columns.

Motoneurons innervating the duodenum were limited to the medial columns, while the jejunum, ileum and ascending colon receive motor innervation from the lateral columns.[4] In very recent investigations, we have demonstrated that motoneurons located in the lateral columns of the DMN provide innervation to the ascending, transverse and descending portions of the colon through the celiac and accessory celiac branches of the vagus (unpublished observation). DMN innervation to the level of the descending colon has been confirmed by the presence of labeled vagal fibers in this area of the bowel following the injection of either ^{3}H-leucine or the fluorescent carbocyanine dye DiI into the DMN.[9,18] These anatomical studies support a mediolateral organization within the DMN corresponding to rostrocaudal positioning along the alimentary canal with the stomach, duodenum, pancreas and liver represented in medial columns and the more distal areas of the small bowel, cecum, and colon represented in the lateral columns (Figure 8). This organizational scheme has been corroborated by recent electrophysiological studies in the rat[10] and appears similar to that previously described for the cat DMN by Satomi *et al.*[74] Additionally, evidence is now emerging that a more precise viscerotopic organization for the stomach exists within the medial column of the DMN. Recent studies in the cat and rat have demonstrated that the antrum/pylorus is represented most medially, the fundus most laterally, and the body of the stomach diffusely throughout the mediolateral extent of this column.[2,65,66,83]

The use of CT-HRP in visceral tract tracing studies provided the first demonstration that DMN motoneurons have both extensive intranuclear and extranuclear dendritic arborizations.[4,69,70,83] Within the confines of DMN, motoneurons located in both the medial and lateral columns exhibit similar dendritic architectonics. The majority of dendrites of gastric and cecal motoneurons projects primarily in a rostrocaudal direction within the confines of the medial and lateral column, respectively[4,83] (Figure 9). Additionally, at all rostrocaudal levels, a portion of each column's motoneuron dendritic arbors penetrates the adjacent column (Figure 10). The dendritic architecture of DMN motoneurons appears to provide for the coordination of efferent activity both throughout the rostrocaudal extent of the cell column and between columns.

The NTS is the major extranuclear site of termination of DMN motoneuron dendrites. The course of penetration and sites of termination within the NTS of these dendritic projections vary according to their column of origin (Figure 10). Dendrites of gastric and cecal motoneurons exit the DMN in trajectories that are essentially perpendicular to each other and terminate in areas of the NTS that overlap the central terminal field of their respective primary sensory neurons[4] (Figure 10). This anatomical arrangement of DMN motoneuron dendrites and sensory afferent terminals within the NTS would support the existence of organ specific monosynaptic interactions between these anatomical structures. The existence of synaptic contacts between labeled sensory afferent terminals and motoneuron dendrites has been demonstrated at the ultrastructural level in the subnucleus gelatinosus (NTS$_{gel}$, gastric afferent terminal field) of the NTS following injection of CT-HRP into the stomach or its application to the cervical vagus[69] (see section on *Synaptic Connectivity Between Vagal Sensory Afferents and Vagal Motoneurons*). It is quite conceivable that the majority of peripheral sensory afferent-dendritic contacts in the NTS occur on an organ specific basis, as it has been demonstrated that the extranuclear dendrites of

Cecum   Stomach

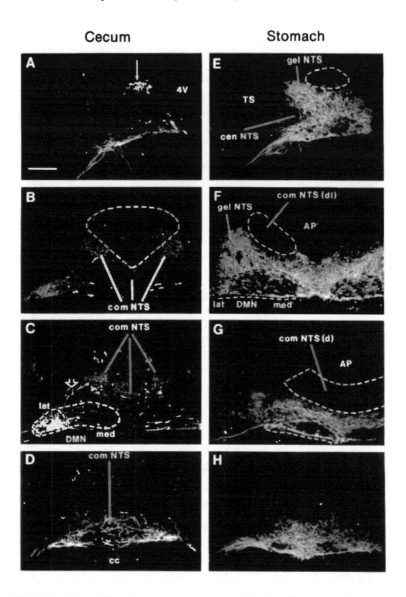

FIGURE 10 (A-H). A-D and E-H are series of darkfield photomicrographs at four different rostrocaudal levels through the dorsal vagal complex following injection of CT-HRP into the cecum and stomach, respectively. The areas of afferent terminal labeling and motoneuronal labeling appear topographically distinct at each rostrocaudal level for the cecum and stomach. Note in A, a small area of cecal terminal labeling (arrow) lying dorsomedial to NTS$_{gel}$ which is the site of stomach afferent terminal labeling. In E and F dendrites of stomach projecting motoneurons appear to encircle but not penetrate the area of cecal afferent terminals within the NTS$_{com}$ (area enclosed by broken line). The arrow in C indicates a dendrite from a cecal projecting motoneuron that projects and terminates within the NTS$_{com}$ (cecal afferent terminal field). (Calibration bar = 250 μm; all photomicrographs are at the same magnification. Used with permission from Altschuler, S.M., D.A. Ferenci, R.B. Lynn, and R.R. Miselis, Representation of the cecum in lateral dorsal motor nucleus of the vagus nerve and commissural subnucleus of the nucleus tractus solitarii in rat, *J. Comp. Neurol.* 304, 261-274,1991.)

gastric and cecal motoneurons encircle or avoid the afferent terminal field of the other respective organ[4] (Figure 10). Additionally, gastric motoneuron dendrites also avoid and encircle the esophageal afferent terminal field in the NTS_{cen}[4] (Figure 10).

Nucleus Tractus Solitarii (NTS)

The NTS is the first synaptic site for afferent projections from peripheral structures conveyed through cranial nerves V (minor component), VII, IX and X. The organization of afferent terminal fields within the NTS is broadly based on the sensory modality they subserve. The most obvious and first organizational scheme formulated for the NTS was its division into a rostral-lateral gustatory half and caudal-medial visceral half.[34] This scheme, which was based on the incubation of whole nerve branches with free HRP, has been fine tuned by studies that have provided information on organ specific representation within the NTS. The topographical representation of the alimentary tract within the NTS has been extensively studied by organ specific injections of neuroanatomical tracers and will be the focus of the discussion in this section.

Afferent information from the alimentary tract is conveyed to the NTS primarily through the IXth and Xth cranial nerves. The cell bodies of vagal and glossopharyngeal afferent nerve fibers are located within a fused ganglionic mass that is comprised of the multiple ganglia of these nerves.[1,4] Within this fused ganglionic mass, sensory neurons projecting to the soft palate and pharynx are located superiorly, and those projecting to the esophagus, stomach, pancreas, and small and large bowel are located inferiorly, indicating a crude viscerotopic organization exists corresponding to rostrocaudal positioning along the alimentary tract[1,4,70] (and unpublished results) (Figure 11).

In the rat, direct intramuscular injections of HRP conjugates into different areas of the alimentary tract result in afferent terminal labeling confined to the NTS, paratrigeminal islands and the spinal trigeminal nucleus. Labeling within the trigeminal complex is restricted to injections of the soft palate, pharynx, and larynx and may represent the terminal field of general somatic afferents conveyed through glossopharyngeal nerve.[1] These results are not presented.

The NTS of the rat is a complex nucleus made up of multiple subnuclei that have different cell morphology, packing density, intensity of Nissl staining, neuropeptide content and connectivity. Afferents from the gastrointestinal tract project primarily to the medial division of the NTS (area medial to tractus solitarius (TS)) and terminate with a viscerotopic organization in distinct subnuclei. The NTS subnuclei associated with the alimentary tract include gelatinosus (gel), centralis (cen), commissuralis (com), medialis (med), interstialis (is), and intermedialis (int) (Figure 12).

When the distributions of alimentary tract afferents are reconstructed in the horizontal plane (Figure 13), the major organizational feature apparent is a rostrocaudal segregation of terminal fields corresponding to rostrocaudal positioning along the alimentary tract.[1,4,70,83] The soft palate is represented most

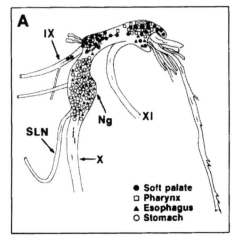

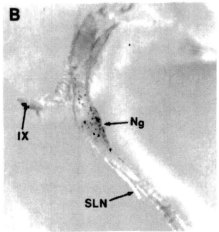

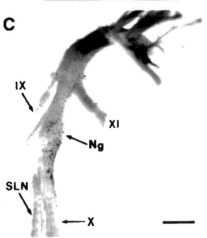

FIGURE 11 (A-C). A is summary diagrammatic representation of the distribution of sensory neuron labeling within the ganglia of the IX and X nerve following injection of tracer into various sites of the alimentary tract. The stomach has the greatest representation of all areas surveyed of the alimentary tract. The topographical distribution of labeled neurons following injection of the small bowel, cecum, colon and pancreas is similar to that found after injection of the stomach. B and C are photomicrograph of ganglionic labeling following injection of tracer into the cecum and stomach. Note that ganglionic labeling is limited to the Ng. (Calibration bar=1mm; B and C are at the same magnification.)

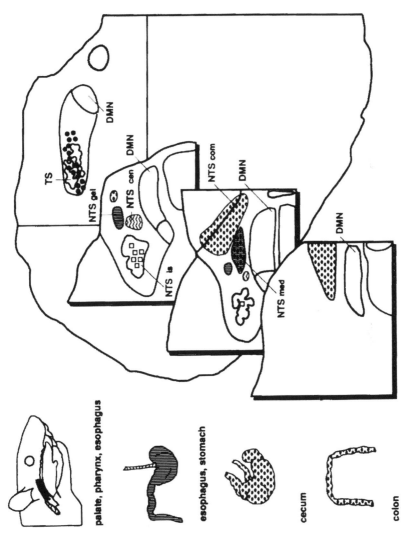

FIGURE 12. Summary of the sensory viscerotopic representation (afferent terminal fields) of the alimentary tract in the NTS as projected in the transverse plane.

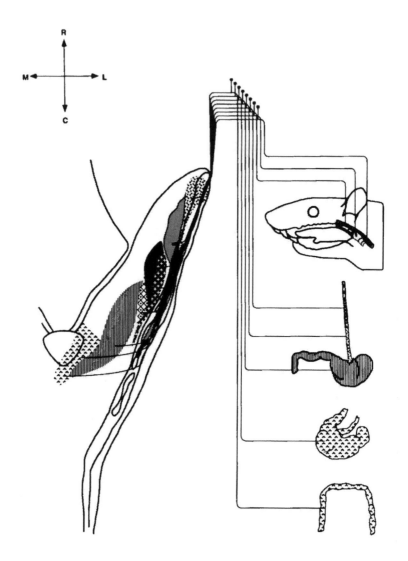

FIGURE 13. Summary of the sensory viscerotopic representation (afferent terminal fields) of the alimentary tract in the NTS as projected in the horizontal plane. The NTS is characterized by a rostrocaudal segregation of afferent terminal fields corresponding to rostrocaudal positioning along the alimentary tract.

rostrally in the NTS. Prominent labeling is present in the NTS_{is} with less dense labeling extending medially into the NTS_{int} and rostral NTS_{med}. A portion of palatal afferents terminates rostrally in the lateral division of the NTS (area lateral to TS), supporting the presence of gustatory receptors in this structure (Figure 14). The NTS_{is} and NTS_{int} represent sites within the NTS where the terminal fields of the soft palate, pharynx, and larynx overlap (Figures 12-14).

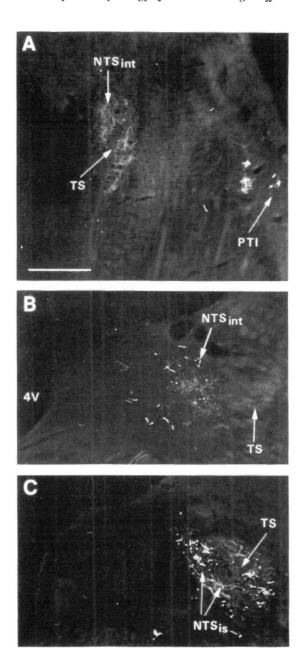

FIGURE 14 (A-C). A is a darkfield photomicrograph of a horizontal section through the NTS following injection of CT-HRP into the soft palate. B and C are darkfield photomicrographs of transverse sections through the NTS following injection of tracer into the pharynx and larynx, respectively. Note in A, terminal labeling is present both medial and lateral to the TS and in the PTI. For the pharynx and larynx terminal labeling is found primarily in the NTS_{is} and NTS_{int}. (Calibration bar = 250 μm; all photomicrographs are at the same magnification.)

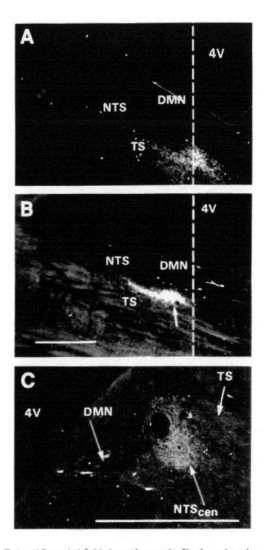

FIGURE 15 A-C. A and B are darkfield photomicrograph of horizontal sections through the dorsal vagal complex following injection of CT-HRP into the cervical (A) and subdiaphragmatic esophagus (B). Terminal labeling is limited to NTS_cen in both cases, however, terminal labeling following cervical esophageal injection extends further rostrally. C is a darkfield photomicrograph of a transverse section through the medulla at the rostrocaudal level indicated by the arrow in B following injection of tracer into the subdiaphragmatic esophagus. (Calibration bars in B and C = 500 μm; A and B are at the same magnification.)

Within the NTS_{is} and NTS_{int}, however, soft palate afferents are represented most rostrally, laryngeal afferents most caudally, and pharyngeal afferents intermediate to those of the soft palate and larynx (Figure 13).

Afferents from the esophagus, stomach and cecum terminate caudal and medial to palatal and pharyngeal afferents. The distribution of afferents from these structures demonstrates very little overlap in comparison to palatal and pharyngeal afferents. Esophageal afferents terminate entirely within the NTS_{cen}, distributing throughout the entire rostrocaudal extent of this subnucleus (Figure 15). The terminal fields of the cervical, thoracic and subdiaphragmatic esophagus show considerable overlap in their rostrocaudal distribution within the subnucleus. However, a crude topographical organization does appear to exist since injection of the cervical, thoracic and subdiaphragmatic esophagus results respectively in the heaviest labeling within the rostral, middle and caudal portions of the NTS_{cen} (Figures 13 and 15).

The most dense concentration of gastric afferents within the NTS is found within the NTS_{gel}, which is located dorsomedial to the NTS_{cen} (Figure 10). Gastric afferents also penetrate sites within the NTS_{med} and NTS_{com}, resulting in a more caudal distribution than esophageal afferents (Figures 10 and 13). Cecal afferents project most prominently to the dorsolateral portion of the NTS_{com}, with less prominent extensions rostrally in the periventricular portions of the NTS (an area dorsal and medial to the NTS_{gel}) and caudally into NTS_{med} and ventromedial portion of the NTS_{com} (Figure 10). Although both gastric and cecal afferents are found in the NTS_{com} and NTS_{med}, there is no overlap in the distributions of their terminal fields.

The pancreas and small intestines represent viscera where direct injection of the CT-HRP into the structure has failed to result in afferent terminal labeling within the NTS.[4,70] This result may be a reflection of a lower density of vagal afferent fibers within these structures or their inaccessibility to the tracer using our current injection strategies.

Synaptic Connectivity Between Vagal Sensory Afferents and Vagal Motoneurons

Vagal efferent fibers have a continuous low-frequency spontaneous discharge that is modulated by sensory inputs.[23,32,87] Acute ipsilateral vagotomy causes cessation of the spontaneous activity of efferent fibers in the vagus nerve, demonstrating that some degree of vagal afferent input is necessary for the ongoing activity of vagal motoneurons. A dominant feature of vagal efferent responses to sensory stimulation is the relatively small degree of central processing that occurs.[13] In the *in vitro* slice preparation, stimulation of vagal sensory fibers leads to short-latency alterations in the electrical activity of vagal motoneurons.[17,89] Interestingly, one class of vagal motoneuronal response to afferent stimulation originates as postsynaptic unitary dendritic spikes in the distal dendrites of the motoneurons.[89] The codistribution of vagal gastric sensory terminals and the dendrites of vagal gastric motoneurons in the NTS_{gel} suggests it as a likely site for monosynaptic gastric vago-vagal contacts.[83]

We examined the ultrastructure of gastric vagal motoneurons and gastric vagal sensory afferents in the dorsal vagal complex of rats to determine whether monosynaptic contacts exist between them.[69] CT-HRP was injected into the stomach wall to retrogradely label the somata and the full dendritic tree of gastric vagal motoneurons and to anterogradely (transganglionically) label the central terminals of gastric vagal sensory neurons.

Electron microscopic examination of DAB-processed tissue revealed particulate reaction product concentrated in multivesicular bodies, lipofuscin granules, and the smooth endoplasmic reticulum of labeled neurons and their dendrites in the DMN. Reaction product was also observed in axons within and lateral to the DMN. In general, only two to four synaptic boutons contacted the perikarya of labeled DMN neurons in a given thin section, although up to seven axosomatic synaptic contacts were sometimes observed. Synapses on labeled neurons were both symmetrical and asymmetrical, but the asymmetrical type was most common. Labeled dendrites in the DMN ranged from 200 nm to 5 μm in diameter and were heavily invested with synaptic inputs from a variety of morphologically distinct types of axon terminals. Synapses made on labeled dendrites were also primarily asymmetrical.

Labeling was infrequently observed in axon terminals in the DMN, supporting previous work in rat, cat and monkey which reported sensory afferents to be rare in the DMN.[20,52,55,60,63] The DAB reaction product in labeled terminals was characteristically sequestered in small vesicles ranging in diameter from 20 to 40 nm. Labeled terminals were morphologically identical to those in the NTS (see description below) and generally formed asymmetrical synapses with unlabeled dendrites 1 μm or smaller in diameter. The asymmetrical type of synapse correlates with an excitatory function,[26,49,58,67,68] consistent with evidence that primary sensory neurons form only excitatory synapses in the central nervous system. Labeled sensory terminals were never observed presynaptic to cell bodies. In exceedingly rare instances, labeled terminals were presynaptic to labeled dendrites within DMN confines, supporting a previous report.[60]

Electron-dense label in the NTS was located in dendrites, axons and axon terminals. Labeled terminals exhibited a homogeneously dense axoplasm containing dark mitochondria, lucent spherical vesicles averaging 40 nm in diameter, and occasional dense core vesicles of larger caliber. Large labeled dendrites were commonly observed entering the NTS from the underlying DMN. The diameters of labeled dendrites in the NTS ranged from 200 nm to 4 μm, their average size decreasing with increasing distance from the DMN. In many instances, labeled dendrites possessed spinous processes. In the NTS, medial to and below the NTS$_{gel}$, labeled dendrites were frequently sectioned in the longitudinal plane. Individual dendrites in these areas received numerous synaptic contacts from a variety of terminal types. Although labeled terminals were present in these areas, those that formed synapses were always presynaptic to unlabeled dendrites and spines.

Within the NTS$_{gel}$, the majority of labeled dendrites were of small caliber (less than 2 μm) and were generally sectioned transversely or obliquely; longitudinally-sectioned labeled dendrites were rarely observed. As in the other areas of the NTS discussed above, labeled dendrites were postsynaptic to a variety of morphologically distinct types of axon terminals. In addition, labeled sensory

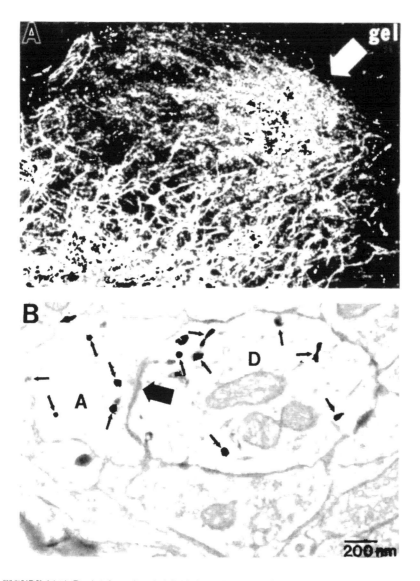

FIGURE 16 (A-B). A (*above*) is a darkfield photomicrograph of a transverse section through the dorsal vagal complex following injection of CT-HRP into the stomach wall. Prominent dendritic projections are seen extending into the NTS$_{gel}$ where they overlap with gastric sensory afferent terminals. B (*below*) is an EM photomicrograph demonstrating CT-HRP label in the NTS$_{gel}$ (small arrows point to DAB reaction product). A labeled gastric sensory afferent terminal (A) is demonstrated forming a synapse (large arrow) with a labeled gastric motoneuron dendrite (D). These monosynaptic contact were found almost exclusively within the NTS$_{gel}$.

afferents in the NTS$_{gel}$ were frequently observed forming asymmetrical synaptic contacts with labeled dendrites and dendritic spines (Figure 16).

The observation that vago-vagal monosynaptic contacts are located almost exclusively on distal motoneuronal dendrites in the NTS$_{gel}$ supports the idea that there may be a distinct organization of synaptic endings on the dendritic tree of vagal motoneurons. Even synapses made on the most distal portion of a dendrite can contribute effectively to somatic depolarization.[89] Although unitary post synaptic potentials (PSPs) generated by terminals synapsing on a neuron's distal dendrites may be of smaller amplitude when recorded at the soma than PSPs generated at more proximal locations, the spines that are present on vagal motoneuronal dendrites create irregular geometries that may cause higher local potentials for a given synaptic current. Distal synapses could have important consequences for dendritic integration, since the potential created within a dendrite could markedly change the driving force for other nearby PSPs. The peak amplitude of PSPs generated in dendrites quickly attenuates toward the soma, but the high transmission coefficient in the distal direction would lead to marked distal dendritic depolarization, and therefore significantly reduce the driving force for all distally-located PSPs on the same dendritic branch.

CONCLUSIONS

Given the complexity of the ventral and dorsal vagal complexes and the number of visceral systems represented within them, a key question is how the microcircuitry and biochemical organization of these areas allows for the processing of afferent information they receive and the orchestration of appropriate autonomic responses. The form of the vagal motoneuron's dendritic tree expresses the cell's receptive field and provides some insight into its role in the nervous system. Vagal motoneurons within the dorsal vagal complex have widespread dendrites which ramify rostrocaudally within both the DMN and the NTS, enabling them to receive input from fibers of diverse origin. In a similar vein, vagal motoneurons located within the NA_{sc} have extensive extranuclear dendrites that penetrate the ventrolateral reticular formation, an area previously shown to receive central afferent projections from different areas of the brainstem.[30,36,53,73,88]

A number of different brain areas including the medial frontal cortex, insular cortex, central nucleus of the amygdala, paraventricular nucleus of the hypothalamus, lateral hypothalamic area, nucleus raphe obscuras, ventral medulla and dorsal vagal complex (intrinsic connections, and nodose ganglion[75,76]) have the potential to influence vagal motor activity by virtue of their connectivity with the dorsal vagal complex, and they all may be important in the central control of normal digestive processes as well as in producing the gastric changes seen during stress, emotional upset and fear.[16,59,85,86] At this time, however, only a subset has been experimentally implicated in these gastric processes. Electrical stimulation of many of the above mentioned brain areas alters gastric motor activity through central, vagally-dependent mechanisms.[31,35,37,41,86] These brain nuclei are part of the so-called "visceral neuraxis," a name reflecting the potentially integral role of its components in the regulation of autonomic activity.

ACKNOWLEDGMENTS

The authors would like to thank S. Green for her technical assistance and J. Giordano for her assistance in the preparation of the manuscript. This research was supported by NIH grants DK-01747 (S.M.A) and GM-27739 (R.R.M), NIMH Grant 17168 (L.R.), Office of Naval Research Fellowship (L.R.), and E.I. du Pont de Nemours and Co. (L.R.).

REFERENCES

1. **Altschuler, S.M., Bao, X., Bieger, D., Hopkins, D.A., and Miselis, R.R.** Viscerotopic representation of the upper alimentary tract in the rat: Sensory ganglia and nuclei of the solitary and spinal trigeminal tracts, *J. Comp. Neurol.*, 283, 248-268, 1989.

2. **Altschuler, S.M., Miselis, R.R., Moran, T.H., McHugh, P.R., and Schwartz, G.J.**, Topographical distribution of the proximal and distal stomach in the dorsal motor nucleus in rat, *Soc. Neurosci. Abstr.*, 16, Part 1, 864, 1990.

3. **Altschuler, S.M., Bao, X., and Miselis, R.R.**, Dendritic architecture of nucleus ambiguus motoneurons projecting to the upper alimentary tract in the rat, *J. Comp. Neurol.*, 309, 402-414, 1991.

4. **Altschuler, S.M., Ferenci, D.A., Lynn, R.B., and Miselis, R.R.**, Representation of the cecum in lateral dorsal motor nucleus of the vagus nerve and commissural subnucleus of the nucleus tractus solitarii in rat, *J. Comp. Neurol.*, 304, 261-274, 1991.

5. **Andrew, B.L.**, The nervous control of the cervical oesophagus of the rat during swallowing, *J. Physiol. (Lond.)*, 134 ,729-740, 1956.

6. **Arnold, G.E.**, Physiology and pathology of the cricothyroid muscle, *Laryngoscope* ,71, 687-752, 1961.

7. **Bao, X., Altschuler, S.M., and Miselis, R.R.**, Topographical arrangement and dendritic architecture of hypoglossal motoneurons in the rat, *Soc. Neurosci. Abstr.*, 14, Part 1, 338, 1988.

8. **Beckstead, R.M., and Norgren, R.**, An autoradiographic examination of the central distribution of the trigeminal, facial, glossopharyngeal, and vagal nerves in the monkey, *J. Comp. Neurol.*, 184, 455-472, 1979.

9. **Berthoud, H.-R., Jedrzejewska, A., and Powley, T.L.**, Simultaneous labeling of vagal innervation of the gut and afferent projections from the visceral forebrain with DiI injected into the dorsal vagal complex in the rat, *J. Comp. Neurol.*, 301, 65-79, 1990.

10. **Berthoud, H.-R., Carlson, N.R., and Powley, T.L.**, Topography of efferent vagal innervation of the rat gastrointestinal tract, *Am. J. Physiol. Regul. Integr. Comp. Physiol.*, 260, R200-R207, 1991.

11. **Bieger, D.**, Muscarinic activation of rhombencephalic neurones controlling oesophageal peristalsis in the rat, *Neuropharmacology* 23(12A), 1451-1464, 1984.

12. **Bieger, D., and Hopkins, D.A.**, Viscerotopic representation of the upper alimentary tract in the medulla oblongata in the rat: the nucleus ambiguus. *J. Comp. Neurol.*, 262, 546-562, 1987.

13. **Blackshaw, L.A., Grundy, D., and Scratcherd, T.**, Involvement of gastrointestinal mechano- and intestinal chemoreceptors in vagal reflexes: and electrophysiological study, *J. Auton. Nerv. Syst.*, 18, 225-234, 1987.

14. **Bosma, J.F., and Fletcher, S.**, The upper pharynx; a review. Part II, *Physiology. Ann. Otol. Rhinol. Laryngol.*, 71, 134-157, 1962.

15. **Bradford, M.M.**, A rapid and sensitive method for the quantitation of microgram quantities of protein utilizing the principle of protein-dye binding, *Ann. Biochem.*, 72, 248-254, 1976.

16. **Carlson, A.J.**, Contribution to the physiology of the stomach.-I. The character of the movements of the empty stomach in man, *Am. J. Physiol.*, 31, 151-192, 1912.

17. **Champagnat, J., Denavit-Saubie, M., Grant, K., and Shen, K.F.,** Organization of synaptic transmission in the mammalian solitary complex, studied in vitro, *J. Physiol.*, 381, 551-573, 1986.

18. **Connors, N.A., Sullivan, J.M., and Kubb, K.S.,** An autoradiographic study of the distribution of fibers from the dorsal motor nucleus of the vagus to the digestive tube of the rat, *Acta Anat.*, 115, 266-271, 1983.

19. **Contreras, R.J., Beckstead, R.M., and Norgren, R.,** The central projections of the trigeminal, facial, glossopharyngeal and vagus nerves: an autoradiographic study in the rat, *J. Auton. Nerv. Syst.*, 6, 303-322, 1982.

20. **Cottle, M.,** Degeneration studies of primary afferents of the IXth and Xth cranial nerves in the cat, *J. Comp. Neurol.*, 122, 329-343, 1964.

21. **Cunningham, E.T., and Sawchenko, P.E.,** A circumscribed projection from the nucleus of the solitary tract to the nucleus ambiguus in the rat: anatomical evidence for somatostatin-28-immunoreactive interneurons subserving reflex control of esophageal motility, *J. Neurosci.*, 9, 1668-1682, 1989.

22. **Cunningham, E.T., and Sawchenko, P.E.,** Central neural control of esophageal motility: a review, *Dysphagia*, 5, 35-51, 1990.

23. **Davison, J.S., and Grundy, D.,** Modulation of single vagal efferent fibre discharge by gastrointestinal afferents in the rat, *J. Physiol. (Lond.)*, 284, 6-82, 1978.

24. **Dennison, S.J., Merritt, V.E., Aprison, M.H., and Felten, D.L.,** Redefinition of the location of the dorsal (motor) nucleus of the vagus in the rat, *Brain Res. Bull.*, 6, 77-81, 1981.

25. **Dennison, S.J., O'Connor, B.L., Aprison, M.H., Merritt, V.E., and Felten, D.L.,** Viscerotopic localization of preganglionic parasympathetic cell bodies of origin of the anterior and posterior subdiaphragmatic vagus nerves, *J. Comp. Neurol.*, 197, 259-269, 1981.

26. **Eccles, J.C.,** *The Physiology of Synapses*, New York, Academic Press, 1964.

27. **Escardo, J.A., Schwaber, J.S., Paton, J.F.R., and Miselis, R.R.,** Rostro-caudal topography of cardiac vagal innervation in the rat, *Soc. Neurosci. Abstr.*, 17, Part 2, 993, 1991.

28. **Fox, E.A., and Powley, T.L.,** Longitudinal columnar organization within the dorsal motor nucleus represents separate branches of the abdominal vagus, *Brain Res.*, 341, 269-282, 1985.

29. **Fryscak, R., Zenker, W., and Kantner, D.,** Afferent and efferent innervation of the rat esophagus. A tracing study with horseradish peroxidase and nuclear yellow, *Anat. Embryol.*, 170, 63-70, 1984.

30. **Fulwiler, C.E., and Saper, C.B.,** Subnuclear organization of the efferent connections of the parabrachial nucleus in the rat, *Brain Res. Rev.*, 7, 229-259, 1984.

31. **Grijalva, C.V., Tache, Y., Gunion, M.W., Walsh, J.H., and Geiselman, P.J.,** Amygdaloid lesions attenuate neurogenic gastric mucosal erosions but do not alter gastric secretory changes induced by intracisternal bombesin, *Brain Res. Bull.*, 16, 55-61, 1986.

32. **Grundy, D., Hutson, D., and Scratcherd, T.,** A permissive role for the vagus nerves in the genesis of antro-antral reflexes in the anesthetized ferret, *J. Physiol.*, 381, 377-384, 1986.

33. **Gwyn, D.G., Leslie, R.A., and Hopkins, D.A.,** Gastric afferents to the nucleus of the solitary tract in the cat, *Neurosci. Lett.*, 14, 13-17, 1979.

34. **Hamilton, R.B., and Norgren, R.,** Central projections of gustatory nerves in the rat, *J. Comp. Neurol.*, 222, 560-577, 1984.

35. **Henke, P.G.,** The centomedial amygdala and gastric pathology in rats, *Physiol. Behav.*, 25, 107-112, 1980.

36. **Herbert, H., Moga, M.M., and Saper, C.B.,** Connections of the parabrachial nucleus with the nucleus of the solitary tract and the medullary reticular formation in the rat, *J. Comp. Neurol.*, 29, :540-580, 1990.

37. **Hermann, G.E., McCann, M.J., and Rogers, R.C.,** Activation of the bed nucleus of the stria terminalis increases gastric motility in the rat, *J. Auton. Nerv. Syst.*, 30, 123-128, 1990.

38. **Hinrichsen, C.F.L., and Ryan, A.T.,** Localization of laryngeal motoneurons in the rat: Morphological evidence for dual innervation, *Exp. Neurol.*, 74, 341-355, 1981.

39. **Holstege, G., Graveland, G., Bijker-Biemond, C., and Schuddeboom, I.,** Location of motoneurons innervating soft palate, pharynx and upper esophagus. Anatomical evidence for a possible swallowing center in the pontine reticular formation, *Brain Behav. Evol.,* 23, 47-62, 1983.

40. **Hudson, L.C., and Cummings, J.F.,** The origins of innervation of the esophagus of the dog, *Brain Res.,* 326, 125-136, 1985.

41. **Hurley-Gius, K.M., and Neafsey, E.J.,** The medial frontal cortex and gastric motility: microstimulation results and their possible significance for the overall pattern of organization of rat frontal and parietal cortex, *Brain Res.,* 365, 241-248, 1986.

42. **Kalia, M.,** Brain stem localization of vagal preganglionic neurons, *J. Auton. Nerv. Syst.,* 3, 451-481, 1981.

43. **Kalia, M., and Mesulam, M-M.,** Brain stem projections of sensory and motor components of the vagus complex in the cat: II.Laryngeal, tracheobronchial, pulmonary, cardiac, and gastrointestinal branches, *J. Comp. Neurol.,* 193, 467-508, 1980.

44. **Kalia, M., and Mesulam, M.-M.,** Brain stem projections of sensory and motor components of the vagus complex in the cat: The cervical vagus and nodose ganglion, *J. Comp. Neurol.,* 193, 435-465, 1980.

45. **Kalia, M., and Sullivan, J.M.,** Brainstem projections of sensory and motor components of the vagus nerve in the rat, *J. Comp. Neurol.,* 211, 248-264, 1982.

46. **Katz, D.M., and Karten, H.J.,** Visceral representation within the nucleus of the tractus solitarius in the pigeon, Columba livia, *J. Comp. Neurol.,* 218, 42-73,1983.

47. **Kirshgessner, A.L. and Gershon, M.D.,** Identification of vagal efferent fibers and putative target neurons in the enteric nervous system of the rat, *J. Comp. Neurol.,* 285, 38-53, 1989.

48. **Kriebel, M.E., Bennett, M.V., Waxman, S.G., and Pappas, G.D.,** Oculomotor neurons in fish: Electrotonic coupling and multiple sites of impulse initiation, *Science,* 166, 520-524, 1969.

49. **Landis, D.M.D.,** Membrane and cytoplasmic structure at synaptic junctions in the mammalian central nervous system, *J. Electron Microsc. Tech.,* 10, 129-151, 1988.

50. **Lawn, A.M.,** The nucleus ambiguus of the rabbit, *J. Comp. Neurol.,* 127, 307-320, 1966.

51. **Lawn, A.M.,** The localization, in the nucleus ambiguus of the rabbit, of the cells of origin of motor fibers in the glossopharyngeal nerve and various branches of the vagus nerve by means of retrograde degeneration, *J. Comp. Neurol.,* 127, 293-306,1966.

52. **Leslie, R.A., Gwyn, D.G., and Hopkins, D.A.,** The central distribution of the cervical vagus nerve and gastric afferent and efferent projections in the rat, *Brain Res. Bull.,* 8, 37-43, 1982.

53. **Loewy, A.D., and Burton, H.,** Nuclei of the solitary tract: Efferent projections to the lower brain stem and spinal cord of the cat, *J. Comp. Neurol.,* 181, 421-450, 1978

54. **Lowry, O.H., Rosebrough, N.J., Farr, A.L., and Randall, R.J.,** Protein measurement with the folin phenol reagent, *J. Biol. Chem.,* 193, 265-275, 1951.

55. **Mclean, J.H., and Hopkins, D.A.,** Ultrastructure of the dorsal motor nucleus of the vagus nerve in monkey with a comparison of synaptology in monkey and cat, *J. Comp. Neurol.,* 231, 162-174, 1985.

56. **Miller, A.J.,** Deglutition, *Physiological reviews,* 62(1), 129-184, 1982.

57. **Miller, A.J.,** Neurophysiological basis of swallowing, *Dysphagia,* 1, 91-100, 1986.

58. **Milner, T.A., Morrison, S.F., Abate, C., and Reis, D.J.,** Phenylethanolamine N-methyltransferase-containing terminals synapse directly on sympathetic preganglionic neurons in the rat, *Brain Res.,* 448, 205-222, 1988.

59. **Mittleman, B., and Wolff, H.,** Emotions and gastroduodenal function: experimental studies on patients with gastritis, duodenitis, and peptic ulcer, *Psychosom. Med.,* 4, 5-61, 1942.

60. **Neuhuber, W.L., and Sandoz, P.A.,** Vagal primary afferent terminals in the dorsal motor nucleus of the rat: are they making monosynaptic contacts on preganglionic efferent neurons? *Neurosci. Lett.,* 69, 126-130, 1986.

61. **Niel, J.P., Gonella, J., and Roman, C.,** Localisation par la technique de marquage a la peroxydase des corps cellulaires des neurons ortho et parasympathiques innervant le sphincter oesphgien inferieur du chat, *J. Physiol. (Paris),* 76, 591-599, 1980.

62. Nomura, S., and Mizuno, N., Central distribution of efferent and afferent components of the cervical branches of the vagus nerve, *Anat. Embryol.*, 166, 1-18, 1983.
63. Norgren, R., Projections from the nucleus of the solitary tract in the rat, *Neuroscience*, 3, 207-218, 1978.
64. Norgren, R., and Smith, G.P., Central distribution of subdiaphragmatic vagal, branches in the rat, *J. Comp. Neurol.*, 273,207-223, 1988.
65. Okumura, T., and Namiki, M., Vagal motor neurons innervating the stomach are site-specifically organized in the dorsal motor nucleus of the vagus nerve in rats, *J. Auton. Nerv. Syst.*, 29, 157-162, 1990.
66. Pagani, F.D., Norman, W.P., and Gillis, R.A., Medullary parasympathetic projections innervate specific sites in the feline stomach, *Gastroenterology*, 95, 277-288, 1988.
67. Peters, A., Synaptic specificity in the cerebral cortex, in *Synaptic Function*, Edelman, G.M., Gall, W.E., and Cowan, W.M., eds., New York, Wiley and Sons, 1987, 373-397.
68. Pickel, V.M., Joh, T.H., and Chan, J., Substance P in the rat nucleus accumbens: ultrastructural localization in axon terminals and their relation to dopaminergic afferents, *Brain Res.*, 444, 247-264, 1988.
69. Rinaman, L., Card, J.P., Schwaber, J.S., and Miselis, R.R., Ultrastructural demonstration of a gastric monosynaptic vagal circuit in the nucleus of the solitary tract in rat, *J. Neurosci.*, 9, 1985-1996.
70. Rinaman, L., and Miselis, R.R., The organization of vagal innervation of rat pancreas using cholera toxin-horseradish peroxidase conjugate, *J. Auton. Nerv. Syst.*, 21, 109-125, 1987.
71. Rogers, R.C., and Hermann, G.E., Central connections of the hepatic branch of the vagus nerve: a horseradish peroxidase histochemical study, *J. Auton. Nerv. Syst.*, 7, 165-174, 1983.
72. Roney, K.J., Scheibel, A.B., and Shaw, G.L., Dendritic bundles: survey of anatomical experiments and physiological theories, *Brain Res. Rev.*, 1, 225-271, 1979.
73. Ross, C.A., Ruggiero, D.A., and Reis, D.J., Projections from the nucleus tractus solitarii to the rostral ventrolateral medulla, *J. Comp. Neurol.*, 242, 511-534, 1985.
74. Satomi, H., Yamamoto, T., Ise, H., and Takatama, H., Origins of the parasympathetic preganglionic fibers to the cat intestine as demonstrated by the horseradish peroxidase method, *Brain Res.*, 151, 571-578, 1978.
75. Sawchenko, P.E., Central connections of the sensory and motor nuclei of the vagus nerve, in *Vagal Nerve Function: Behavioral and Methodological Considerations*, Kral, J.G., Powley, T.L., and Brooks, C.McC., eds., Amsterdam, Elsevier Science Publishers, 1983, 13-26.
76. Sawchenko, P.E., Cunningham, E.T., Jr., and Levin, M.C., Anatomic and biochemical specificity in central autonomic pathways, in *Organization of the Autonomic Nervous System: Central and Peripheral Mechanisms*, Ciriello, J., Calaresu, F.R., Renaud, L.P., and Polosa, C., eds., New York, Alan R. Liss, Inc., 1987, 267-281.
77. Scharoun, S.L., Barone, F.C., Wayner, M.J., and Jones, S.M., Vagal and gastric connections to the central nervous system determined by the transport of horseradish peroxidase, *Brain Res. Bull.*, 13, 573-583, 1984.
78. Scheibel, M.E., and Scheibel, A.B., Organization of spinal motoneurons dendrites in bundles, *Exp. Neurol.*, 28, 106-112, 1970
79. Scheibel, M.E. and Scheibel, A.B., Developmental relationship between spinal motoneuron dendrite bundles and patterned activity in the hind limb of cats, *Exp. Neurol.* 29, 328-335, 1970.
80. Scheibel, M.E., and Scheibel, A.B., Developmental relationship between spinal motoneuron dendrite bundles and patterned activity in the forelimb of cats, *Exp. Neurol.*, 30, 367-373, 1971.
81. Scheibel, M.E. and Scheibel, A.B., Dendrite bundles as sites for central programs: an hypothesis, *Intern. J. Neuroscience*, 6, 195-202, 1973.
82. Schoenen, J., Dendritic organization of the human spinal cord: the motoneurons, *J. Comp. Neurol.*, 211, 226-247, 1982.

83. **Shapiro, R.E., and Miselis, R.R.,** The central organization of the vagus nerve innervating the stomach of the rat, *J. Comp. Neurol.*, 238, 473-488, 1985.

84. **Stuesse, S.L., and Fish, S.E.,** Projections to the Cardioinhibitory region of the nucleus ambiguus of rat, *J. Comp. Neurol.*, 229, 271-278, 1984.

85. **Tache, Y.,** The peptidergic brain-gut axis: influence on gastric ulcer formation, *Chron. Int.*, 4, 11-17, 1987.

86. **Tache, Y.,** Central nervous system regulation of gastric acid secretion, in *Physiology of the Gastrointestinal Tract,* Johnson, L.R., ed, New York, Raven Press, 1987, 911-928.

87. **Tonoue, T., Nishimura, H., Tokushige, K., and Seino, K.,** Thyrotropin-releasing hormone-induced changes in electroencephalographic and vagal activity in the cross-circulated brain of the rat, *Brain Res.*, 378, 394-397, 1986.

88. **Van Bockstaele, E.J., Pieribone, V.A., and Aston-Jones, G.,** Diverse afferents converge on the nucleus paragigantocellularis in the rat ventrolateral medulla: Retrograde and anterograde tracing studies, *J. Comp. Neurol.*, 290, 561-584, 1989.

89. **Yarom, Y., Sugimori, M., and Llinas, R.,** Ion currents and firing patterns of mammalian vagal motoneurons in vitro, *Neuroscience*, 16, 719-737, 1985.

90. **Yoshida, Y., Miyazaki, T., Hirano, M., Shin, T., Totoki, T., and Kanaseki, T.,** Localization of efferent neurons innervating the pharyngeal constrictor muscles and the cervical esophagus muscle in the cat by means of the horseradish peroxidase method, *Neurosci. Lett.*, 22, 91-95, 1981.

Chapter 3

THE DORSAL VAGAL COMPLEX FORMS A SENSORY-MOTOR LATTICE: THE CIRCUITRY OF GASTROINTESTINAL REFLEXES

T.L. Powley, H.-R. Berthoud, E.A. Fox and W. Laughton

TABLE OF CONTENTS

INTRODUCTION

In a treatise on vagal afferents, it is instructive to consider vagal efferents. Vagal afferents provide the central nervous system with the information required to initiate gastrointestinal reflexes, but they do not organize these responses in isolation. The afferent traffic must be integrated in a manner that addresses the appropriate motor outflow to the alimentary canal. These reflex circuits, organized in the medulla, also provide the substrate by which convergent inputs from the forebrain and rest of the central nervous system exercise control over the gastrointestinal processes.

Analysis of the neural circuits responsible for the myriad vagal reflexes has been only modestly successful. For example, how enterogastric, hepatopancreatic, gastrocolic, or the various cephalic reflexes are effected selectively by the vagal brainstem nuclei is not clear. In particular, the structural substrates responsible for differentiating and executing individual gastrointestinal functions have not been clearly identified.

In the medulla, only limited anatomical segregation of functional units has been suggested by the numerous neuroanatomical and neurophysiological mapping studies that have been reported. Examined individually, neither the NST (the nucleus of the solitary tract, the primary afferent relay nucleus) nor the dmnX (dorsal motor nucleus of the vagus, the vagal preganglionic motor nucleus) appears to be organized into tightly partitioned subnuclei with distinctly different neuronal populations. Such partitioning might suggest that individual functional patterns are generated in discrete anatomical elements within that subnucleus. Rather, each of these nuclei appears to be composed of relatively unspecialized neurons organized into broad, partially overlapping zones corresponding to different nerve branches (not individual viscera) and thus to constitute an equally broad topography which might be considered quasi-viscerotopic. This same conclusion has been reached through examinations of the distributions of afferent terminals (examples: Norgren and Smith,[62] Torvik[82]) and the pools of preganglionics innervating a particular target.[21] A complementary conclusion is suggested by an examination of the maps of neurotransmitters and neuropeptides[17,32,42] in these regions. Furthermore, both the NST and dmnX exhibit characteristics of the reticular formation, including an "isodendritic" dendritic architecture.[16,22,74,81,88] At first look, this organization in the dorsal vagal complex reminds one of Nauta's pedagogical characterization of the reticular formation as "making no engineering sense."

In this review, we propose that there is in fact a morphological organization in the vagal trigone capable of generating much of the apparent specificity of the gastrointestinal reflexes and that it is the sensory-motor lattice formed by the NST and the dmnX complexed into a single unit. While neither nucleus alone is organized in a punctate manner that could easily provide the specificity of the separate vagal reflexes, the NST and dmnX, considered together as the dorsal vagal complex, do evidence a striking plan which is theoretically capable of generating the functional specificity. This plan might even satisfy the requirements of Nauta's hypothetical engineer baffled by reticular formation architecture.

Specifically, three sets of observations suggest the basis of the lattice organization of the vagal trigone: (1) Viewed from a perspective dorsal to the medulla, the pattern of projections of alimentary canal primary afferents in the NST is a series of terminal fields forming transversely disposed bands or patches corresponding to different nerves and nerve branches and thus to different receptor surfaces. (2) The pools of abdominal preganglionic neurons in the dmnX consist of longitudinally running columns of cells corresponding to different branches of the abdominal vagus. (3) The dmnX cells and the overlying portion of the NST are welded together. That is, they are effectively fused because (a) the sensory and motor nuclei have a common horizontal boundary; (b) the two nuclei evidence some intermingling of their neurons; (c) the NST has substantial second—or higher—order projections into the dmnX; (d) some dendrites of the motor neurons reach dorsally into the sensory nucleus, and (e) some dendrites of NST neurons may reach into the neuropil of the dmnX.

Before fully considering the evidence for the lattice hypothesis, the evidence for each of these three observations will be considered separately. The formulation of this lattice hypothesis and the evidence for it were briefly summarized before,[66,67] but the idea and its evidence are examined more fully below.

THE ELEMENTS OF THE SENSORY-MOTOR LATTICE FOR DIGESTIVE REFLEXES

The Nucleus of the Solitary Tract (NST)

The NST is the central relay nucleus for first-order parasympathetic sensory inputs from most of the gastrointestinal tract. It receives the visceral afferents from the entire alimentary receptor sheet beginning with the tongue and oral cavity and running through the esophagus, stomach, duodenum, and the rest of the small intestine as well as the large bowel.[2,26,62] It also receives afferent inputs from other organs of digestion such as the liver[1,40,77] and perhaps the pancreas.[56,76] In effect, then, the NST serves as the primary sensory station for most major gastrointestinal reflexes. Further, the NST receives inputs from trigeminal and spinal sympathetic afferents as well.[49]

The NST lies in a horizontal plane (in tetrapods) in the dorsal medulla oblongata. It is a paired, bilaterally symmetrical structure that is fused caudally on the midline (the commissural subnucleus), where the medulla is closed, and is unfused rostrally, where it lies off the midline and under the floor of the fourth ventricle. From a dorsal perspective the NST has the appearance of a "Y" with its two arms pointing rostrally (see Figure 1).

Degeneration[82] and tracer[2,33,62] studies have established that there is a rough rostral-caudal somatotopy representing the alimentary canal in NST. Taking the

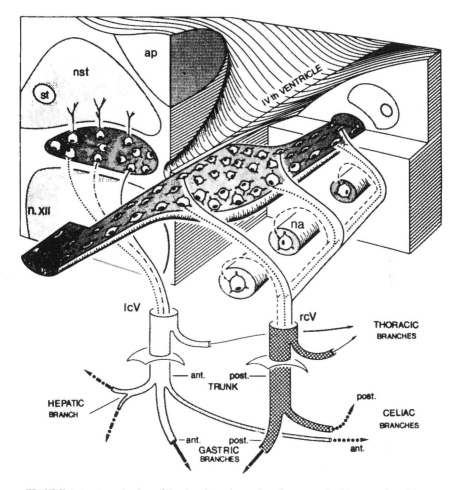

FIGURE 1. A schematic view of the dorsal vagal complex of the medulla oblongata viewed from a caudal and lateral (right) perspective and the abdominal vagal trunks with their respective branches. The dorsal motor nucleus can be seen in a horizontal orientation on the right side of the brainstem and a frontal perspective on the left side of the brainstem. Corresponding to one of the cytoarchitectonic differences that has been observed, the medial (gastric) cell columns on either side are indicated with smaller perikarya, and the lateral (celiac) cell columns are indicated with larger somata. This view and the different lines of symbols used for groups of axons illustrate that each column of perikarya in the dmnX gives rise to a separate branch of the subdiaphragmatic vagus. The nucleus ambiguus, which innervates supradiaphragmatic and striated tissues, is also illustrated on the right side where it is positioned ventrolaterally and parallel to the dmnX, its common location in mammals. (Other abbreviations: ap = area postrema; lcV = left cervical vagus; na = nucleus ambiguus; nst = nucleus of the solitary tract; n.XII = hypoglossal nucleus; rcV = right cervical vagus; st = solitary tract.)

different branches of the cranial nerves as indices of different parts of the sensory sheet, the rostral pole of the nucleus receives the afferents from the oral cavity, including those of taste. The caudal commissural part of the nucleus receives the afferents from the abdominal viscera, with the middle rostrocaudal levels of the nucleus receiving the sensory fibers arising from the pharynx, larynx and esophagus. Discrete nerve branches are read into successively more caudal terminal fields or bands. Beginning rostrally and moving caudally, these branches include the chorda tympani (of the facial nerve), lingual-tonsillar (glossopharyngeal), pharyngeal (glossopharyngeal), superior laryngeal (vagal), recurrent laryngeal (vagal), hepatic (vagal), gastric (vagal), and celiac (vagal) branches (see the schematic summary in Figure 2). Although other areas of the NST also receive pulmonary and cardiovascular afferents, the present review is limited to the alimentary tract and the organs of digestion.

The Dorsal Motor Nucleus of the Vagus (dmnX)

The dmnX constitutes the preganglionic parasympathetic "final common path" for central nervous system control over both secretory and smooth muscle responses of the alimentary canal. It also contains some preganglionics innervating pulmonary,[31] and in some species perhaps cardiovascular, tissues as well, although again, the present review is restricted to the gastrointestinal tract. The striated musculature of the upper alimentary canal is innervated by the nucleus ambiguus.[9]

Viewed from above, the dmnX closely replicates the shape of the NST (see Figure 1). The motor nucleus lies immediately ventral to, and in register with, the NST. From a perspective that reveals the horizontal pattern of the dmnX, the nucleus appears as a paired, bilaterally symmetrical structure consisting of a longitudinally elongated, spindle-shaped aggregate of cells on either side of the midline. Like the NST, the dmnX has the overall profile of a figure "Y" in the horizontal plane. Caudally, the dmnX spindles are fused on the midline in a position immediately dorsal and dorsolateral to the central canal. Rostrally, as the fourth ventricle opens, each half nucleus swings slightly laterally to maintain a position just ventral and ventromedial to the corresponding side of the NST. The dimensions of the dmnX spindles on either side are such that, in many species, including the rat, the largest concentrations of motorneurons occur at the mid-longitudinal level of the area postrema or the obex, while a smaller number of somata are located in either tapering pole of the spindle (see Figures 1 and 2). Viewed from the frontal perspective, all but the most caudal dmnX is flattened in the dorsal-ventral dimension. The flattening gives the nucleus in either hemimedulla an ovoid shape more rostrally and a plano–convex lens shape somewhat more caudally.

Recently we and others have accumulated evidence indicating that the dmnX is composed of a series of longitudinally arrayed columnar subnuclei, each corresponding to one of the distinct branches of the abdominal vagus. In particular, the rat (which has five primary abdominal branches[71,73]) has five major columns.[21] Four are distinct groupings of cells organized as paired, symmetrical distributions that in composite form the general profile of the dmnX (see Figure 1). These subnuclei consist of a medial column of cells

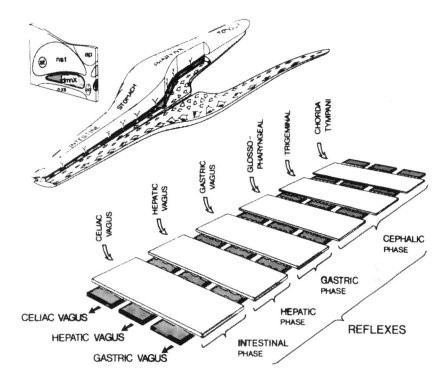

FIGURE 2. A schematic summary illustrating the structural basis of the sensory-motor lattice hypothesis. The dorsal vagal complex in the upper left part of the figure, as in Figure 1, is viewed from a dorsal caudal and lateral (right) perspective. This horizontal view shows the dmnX [the more ventral nucleus (shaded) with different sized cells illustrating the separate columns] on both left and right sides of the brainstem, with the NST (more dorsal unshaded nucleus) represented only on the left side of the brain. A corresponding frontal view of a section through the left side of the vagal trigone region is included in the upper left corner of the figure. The lower right half of the panel illustrates the formal idea of a lattice in which the longitudinally arrayed columns of the dmnX are orthogonal to the incoming afferent terminals of the several nerve branches projecting to the NST. This formal lattice sketch illustrates branches supplying the afferents on the left side, with the corresponding reflexes labeled on the right side. The afferent inputs are also translated into a rough or quasi-viscerotopic map and expressed in terms of organs on the dorsal surface of the nucleus of the solitary tract in the sketch in the upper left half of the figure. (Inset panel abbreviations: ap = area postrema; na = nucleus ambiguus; nst = nucleus of the solitary tract; n.XII = hypoglossal nucleus; st = solitary tract.)

forming the medial half or more of the nucleus on either side (left dmnX corresponds to the ventral gastric branch; right dmnX to the dorsal gastric) and a lateral column forming the lateral pole of the nucleus throughout most of its length on either side (left dmnX contains the column of the accessory celiac branch; right dmnX contains the column of the celiac branch). The fifth column of cells, corresponding to the branch with the fewest efferents (i.e., the hepatic, which has less than 10% of the number of efferent axons that the gastric branch does), is less coherent. Whereas the first four columns of cells are spatially discrete, this hepatic grouping is found within the medial gastric branch column on the left dmnX. Details of this organization based on retrograde tracer mapping with True Blue are given in Fox and Powley[21] and Powley *et al.*[68]

Several of the individual elements of this organization have been substantiated with other techniques and, in some cases, in other species. Norgren and Smith,[62] as well as Powley *et al.*,[67,70] have identified the same columnar pattern for the several branches in the rat with horseradish peroxidase (HRP). Other retrograde tracer studies have documented the same medial columnar pattern of the gastric branches in both rat[18,81] and cat.[64,89] Further, Ferenci *et al.*[19] have shown that the lateral cell columns are labeled after cholera toxin horseradish peroxidase injections into the cecum, thus confirming again that the celiac branch efferents (the celiacs carry the innervation of the cecum[5,12]) originate in the lateral columns. Martin *et al.*,[48] using HRP injections into the ileum, also illustrated that the celiac columns innervate the small intestine, and Satomi *et al.*[79] obtained a similar pattern with HRP injections into the cat intestine.[a]

Additionally, albeit indirectly, a number of reports have suggested on cytoarchitectonic criteria the type of intranuclear pattern described above and in Figure 1. Such cytoarchitectonic evidence for the columnar pattern includes studies on the camel and llama,[85] mouse,[69] rabbit,[37] rat[22,44] and whale.[29] A survey of specimens of a number of additional species (including the chimpanzee, human, manatee, pig, polar bear, and zebra, as well as llama and camel) again provided some evidence for cytoarchitectonic differentiation of the various longitudinal columns (Powley, unpublished data). In a recent analysis of dendritic patterns of preganglionic neurons in the dmnX, we have also observed that the lateral celiac and medial gastric columns are distinguished not only in terms of size of their somata but also by having significantly different dendritic fields measured in terms of extent and amount of branching.[22,24]

Unit recording has also established that the efferents innervating the stomach (i.e., forestomach, sheep) are found in a coherent longitudinal column on either side of the dmnX.[27] An electrophysiological study of the dog[3] is consistent with the suggestion that different branches map onto spatially discrete columns insofar as a given vertical penetration of the recording microelectrode tended to repeatedly encounter efferent units projecting through the same abdominal branch.

Functional analyses also suggest the same columnar organization of the dmnX. Recently, Laughton and Powley[41] completed an experiment mapping,

---

[a] A variety of other studies have injected retrograde tracers into individual viscera and also reported labeled cells throughout the longitudinal extent of the dmnX. Many of these organ-injection studies have been plagued by (at least some) spread or leakage of tracer from the injection site to surrounding tissues, which has blurred the medial/lateral separation of columns, although these experiments also at least tend to support the longitudinal organization of the dmnX (for discussion and references, see Fox and Powley[23]).

through the use of semi-microelectrode stimulation, the spatial organization of dmnX preganglionic neurons that control gastric acid, insulin, and glucagon secretion. We found a general correspondence to the columnar pattern described above, insofar as each of the three vagal secretory responses was represented symmetrically on either side of the midline and could be elicited throughout the longitudinal extent of the nucleus, with some differences in the medial-to-lateral displacement of the "centers-of-gravity" of the different responses. Similarly, in an earlier and complementary experiment employing punctate electrical stimulation, Pagani *et al.*[65] (cats) identified a longitudinal zone within the dmnX on either side of the medulla that was responsible for gastric motility.

Finally, an additional set of observations also underscores this longitudinal plan of the separate pools of gastrointestinal efferents found in the dmnX. Since the basic longitudinal plan in the nucleus is a representation of the five major and *primary* branches separating from the abdominal vagal trunks, we investigated the question of whether within a single column in the dmnX the more distal "secondary" branches arising from the corresponding main vagal branch might map onto a finer and more discrete spatial plan (and, if so, of what topography). By separately labeling the two readily identifiable secondary branches originating from the anterior gastric branch, we found that the column of dmnX motorneurons associated with the anterior gastric branch was composed of two finer, spatially distinct longitudinal subcolumns.[67] Particularly relevant in the present context is the fact that, although the major column could be decomposed into subcolumns consisting of relatively small populations of cells, even these finer subcolumns run the full longitudinal extent of the dmnX (see also Ewart *et al.*,[18] Okumura and Namiki[63] and Pagani *et al.*[64]). A similar point is made by a closer look at the hepatic branch column. Although this column consists of only a very few motor neurons, it too runs the full rostrocaudal extent of the dmnX.

Interconnections between the NST and the dmnX

In effect, the NST and the dmnX are fused together. This point needs some emphasis, because the extent of the weld traditionally seems to have been underestimated. At least two conventions probably contribute to this underestimation. First, the two nuclei are most commonly viewed or represented in their least extensive dimension, i.e., in coronal sections (see left hemimedulla in Figure 1 and inset of Figure 2). From these frontal sections, it is hard to appreciate the fact that the two nuclei are in such tight register throughout their extensive horizontal and sagittal spans. Second, the two nuclei are most commonly illustrated with staining protocols that typically stain cell bodies indiscriminately. These stains do not describe the ramifications of interpenetrating dendrites and axons in a common neuropil. Furthermore, without selective labeling of some type, any intermingled cells (e.g., those dmnX cells ectopically displaced in the NST or NST cells situated among dmnX neurons) are unlikely to be detected.

In spite of this tendency to underestimate the extent of NST-dmnX overlap, it is nonetheless clear that the two areas do articulate extensively and directly. A subset of central terminals of primary vagal afferents have been shown to synapse directly onto neurons within the dmnX as well as the NST.[13,57] Further, in the case of the dendrites, the dorsally distributed processes of preganglionics receive direct monosynaptic connections from first order gastric afferents within the subnucleus gelatinosis region of the NST.[75] Anterograde tracing studies have also established that second-order neurons with their somata in the NST, at least those in the more caudal parts of the NST, produce a significant projection into the dmnX as well as into other relay nuclei of the brainstem.[15,60,78] It is also the case that when NST or dmnX neurons are either selectively labeled with retrograde tracers[22,24] or identified electrophysiologically,[13] a minority of those at the interface between the two nuclei can be considered ectopic or intermingling cases.

THE VAGAL TRIGONE AS A SENSORY-MOTOR LATTICE — THE HYPOTHESIS

To recapitulate, structural and functional analyses of the separate vagal nuclei have suggested that neither the NST nor the dmnX is tightly compartmentalized in a manner that might serve independently as a structural substrate for the observed specificity or selectivity in digestive reflexes. A consideration of the two nuclei as a unit, however, suggests a new perspective. The predominantly transverse organization of the terminal fields and second-order neurons found in the NST and the longitudinal organization of the dmnX are crossed at right angles. The fact that these sensory and motor architectures are oriented orthogonally and are effectively fused means that the system has the spatial characteristic of a lattice.

The features of this organization might account for some of the individuation of the alimentary reflexes. The crossed organization provides an efficient plan for complexing the various receptor sheets or afferent inputs to the several different vagal responses. In fact, if one starts from the premise that the NST consists of bands or patches of afferent terminal endings and the dmnX consists of columns of preganglionic motorneurons, then arraying the bands and columns as a right-angle grid would provide a network with a very high—indeed the highest that the elements will theoretically yield—spatial resolution. Each intersecting node could potentially serve as a module which organizes reflex arcs of a particular type. Intersecting arrays have been recognized as a frequently encountered neural solution for optimizing feature analysis in sensory systems and for effecting complex, highly specific selection strategies in both sensory-motor and sensory-sensory systems. The same strategy of crossing vectors of information is employed in numerous neural models of analysis and detection (for discussions of these and related issues, confer, for example to Bullock,[11] Glassman,[25] and Sejnowski[80]). Of course, other types of networks or neural matrices (even random distributions) might employ long projections that would accomplish the same outcome, but the lattice also makes good engineering sense in terms of its efficiency. Any other solution for addressing all relevant sensory inputs to the appropriate preganglionic outputs would increase the length and complexity of the "wiring."

In a sense the specific geometries of the nuclei involved almost ensure that the system works—at least in some measure—as a lattice of these intersecting patterns. Both the NST and the dmnX are quite long (e.g., > 4 mm for the rat, > 8 mm for the cat, and 10 mm for the human). In general, dendrites are almost universally confined to maximum radius of 500 microns with respect to the soma (see discussion of this issue in Kaas[30]), and the actual value is even less in the vagal trigone. Dendrites of the NST radiate from the perikaryon probably less than 200 microns on average;[13,16,46,88] dendrites of the dmnX radiate an average of less than 300 microns[22,24,59,81] Thus, one would expect that many of the strongest local NST-dmnX interactions would occur within the radius of one of the intersections or modules. Certainly dmnX dendrites receiving monosynaptic inputs from primary sensory neurons would be found within such an intersection. Interneurons and long rostrocaudal projections from the NST might well span greater longitudinal distances, but one might still expect a substantial amount of processing at the level of the individual intersections.

Finally, there are important qualifications to the lattice idea that should be made explicit. It should be emphasized that the somatotopy that has been identified in both the NST as well as the dmnX are based on nerve branches and/or organ injections, not specified functions or particular (sub)modalities. Any individual branch carries a variety of submodalities of afferent and efferent information. Thus, a node or a module in the lattice architecture may provide only a partial specification of the given response. Within the lattice intersection that would represent gastro-gastric reflexes, for example, one might be able to find a number of different reflexes involving chemical, mechanical, or nocioceptive inputs and secretory, motility, or accommodation responses. Differentiation among such a family of reflexes within one of the modular levels of the lattice must involve more fine-grained anatomical specializations (perhaps akin to the striosomes found in the striatum), chemical codes or, of course, a combination of both.

Furthermore, the branch topography does not involve a one-for-one code of organs. While in some cases the branches appear to be a relatively good index of the innervated organ, if not the specific function, in other cases the particular organ or function of interest may be distributed across the branches in a complex pattern. For example, we have recently found that vagally controlled pancreatic insulin secretion is expressed over the gastric and hepatic branches of the abdominal vagus but not the two celiac branches[6,8] (see also the discussion in Laughton and Powley[41]), whereas proximal duodenal motility is distributed among all three sets of vagal branches.[5,12] The same holds true on the sensory side. Gustation, for example, is represented by at least three branches projecting to the NST.[61] Such an organization also seems reflected in the complex sorting and distribution of fibers in the vagal trunks and their derivative branches.[72,73]

IMPLICATIONS AND TESTS OF THE LATTICE MODEL

The functional implications—as well as one kind of test—of the proposed lattice organization can be considered with an example. Recall that in our microstimulation study of the dmnX (employing over 200 stimulation sites), we found that gastric acid secretion could be elicited along the rostrocaudal extent of the nucleus. We observed similar patterns for both pancreatic insulin and glucagon secretion.[41] At face value, these observations might be taken to suggest that gastric acid secretion (as well as both insulin and glucagon) is not mediated by a well-defined, spatially discrete subnucleus within the dmnX. Considered in conjunction with the two ideas reviewed above, however, the observation is compatible with the argument that there is a highly organized topographic network within the system. The two sets of observations are (a) that the acid secretion is influenced by a variety of inputs and involves several separate and largely independent phases such as the cephalic, gastric, and intestinal phases, and (b) that at different points along their lengths, the gastric branch columns in the dmnX (in either hemimedulla) lie immediately in contact with the NST terminal fields corresponding to the oropharynx, gastric and intestinal inputs. In effect, the rostral-to-caudal dispersion of preganglionics influencing gastric acid secretion through the major extent of the medulla, a pattern that might be construed as lacking localization, seems to be a highly organized system for bringing a given effector response under the control of the different sensory bands arranged in the NST. While this stimulation experiment constitutes some of the original evidence for the hypothesis and should not be considered an a *posteriori* test, it does suggest how other mapping experiments measuring other responses might be used to evaluate one aspect of the lattice proposition. Even though vagal branches are organized longitudinally, in theory a particular response organized within a column might only be found in, for example, the caudal pole of the longitudinal spindle. If most preganglionic response modalities were not distributed longitudinally like those examined so far (namely, pancreatic insulin secretion, pancreatic glucagon secretion, gastric acid secretion, and gastric motility), it would impeach the idea that the vagal trigone is a lattice vis-a-vis functional responses.

A second class of tests or predictions follows directly from the implications just considered. It would predict that although a given vagal response might be elicited from the full length of the dmnX (but not from the full medial-to-lateral limits), the identical responses would in fact be engaged by different inputs mapped into the overlying regions of the NST. Gastric secretion elicited from the rostral dmnX would be controlled by cephalic stimuli. Similar secretion elicited from the caudal dmnX would be controlled by afferents originating in gastric or intestinal fields. Selective damage to the rostral dmnX or the efferent fascicles originating from that site should selectively disable the vagal reflexes with oral triggers, while similar selective surgeries in the caudal dmnX should compromise the gastric or intestinal phases of vagal reflexes. Neither type of partial damage should entirely eliminate an effector organ response type—only particular sensory-motor or sensory-secretory combinations. Similarly, selective damage to some of the intersections of one of the sensory bands in the NST should block some stimulus-driven vagal motor responses, namely those to the corresponding class of inputs, while sparing others to the same class of inputs. It should, for example, be possible to eliminate gastro-gastric reflexes while sparing gastro-colonic reflexes. Although we do not know of any experiments which have investigated and established such a double dissociation, and since there is as yet no test of the idea based on blocking, there are data generally consistent with the lattice hypothesis. For example, in an earlier study,[7] we observed that rats with selective NST lesions which presumably (on the basis of anatomical reconstructions) would have blocked vagal reflexes with a gastric afferent limb (e.g., gastro-pancreatic reflexes) did in fact spare other reflexes with the same efferent limb (i.e., oro-pancreatic or, more specifically, cephalic insulin release).

Comparative physiology offers a third means of evaluating the explanatory power of the lattice idea. From the previous considerations, one would predict that not all intersects would play equally important roles in the physiology of an animal. The intestinal phases of gastric physiology might be more important in some species, while cephalic responses might be more prominent in others. Carnivores and hindgut fermenters might specialize quite different vagal reflexes. If so, then one might expect to find differences in cell numbers, packing densities, or the proportion of the vagal trigone area occupied by the corresponding lattice intersection (i.e., one would expect "coordinate transformations"). Certainly, among mammals there are significant differences in the shape, longitudinal level of maximal cell number, and profiles of the rostral and caudal tails of the dmnX spindles[38,84,85] (also Powley, unpublished data) that would yield face validity to this idea. In the case of the rat, for example, the medial dmnX columns associated with the gastric branches have more preganglionics (in either absolute or relative terms) rostrally under the oral NST fields, while the lateral cell columns associated with the celiac branch columns are more concentrated caudally.[21,62,70] Such an organization suggests that the rat should have proportionately more cephalic phase reflexes mediated by the gastric branches and more intestinal phase responses in the celiac branches (which innervate the intestine).[5,12,19] Cross-species differences or specializations have not yet been systematically compared with the present lattice idea, and the relevant comparative physiology may still be too sketchy, but the idea is empirically testable. (For additional examples, see below.)

These explicit comparisons of disparate species can also be viewed in a different, complementary light. Some of the difficulties in understanding the dmnX organization probably stem from the differences in profiles of the dmnX in different species at different levels and planes of section (see below). This variability or apparent absence of order seems to reinforce the supposition that the dmnX was not precisely organized. In contrast, the columnar organization taken together with the proposal that different axial levels of the nucleus will be hypertrophied or hypotrophied (perhaps even eliminated) depending on the gastrointestinal specializations of the particular species, can potentially incorporate variability into what we propose is a universal architecture of the dorsal vagal complex. While this chapter concentrates on the motor side of the lattice, clearly the same regional variations in development of the subnuclei and underlying regularity would also be expected in the different NST nodes of the lattice.

RECONCILING OBJECTIONS AND POTENTIAL INCONSISTENCIES

The lattice hypothesis is predicated on three major aspects of vagal organization which include the transversely arrayed map of the NST, the longitudinally arrayed columns of the dmnX, and the local organization of the neuropil that welds the two nuclei together. Fundamental revision of any of these cornerstones would constitute a major challenge to the proposal. In this regard, a substantial consensus seems to exist concerning the accuracy of the first and third ideas. The second, the columnar organization of the dmnX, is a recently established concept, however, and thus it is less clear that there is yet a consensus on this point. Certainly various alternative formulations have been suggested. Because the organization of the dmnX has been a controversial issue, some of the alternative views need to be considered.

Classical Models of dmnX Organization

One alternative proposal of dmnX organization merits a thorough examination. It is—or at least historically has been—the most widely held expectation concerning dmnX organization. It is also at least superficially incompatible with the columnar plan described above. This alternative plan is based on two separate assumptions. The first is that the dmnX is compartmentalized into frontal subunits that are distributed as a chain along the longitudinal axis (that, in effect, the dmnX organization is parallel to, rather than at right angles to, the NST organization). The second presupposition is that there should be a viscus-by-viscus order or viscerotopic representation in the dmnX.

These two assumptions dominated the experimental analyses of the dmnX for over a century. In 1955, when Mitchell and Warwick[50] published their widely-used summary of well over 100 years of analyses of dmnX organization, virtually all of the earlier work was framed in terms of a search for a viscerotopy compartmentalized along the longitudinal axis. No consensus favoring any one version of such a topography had developed by that time. In fact, the proposed ideas were mutually contradictory, with inverted visceral topographies, partially inverted topographies, normal or noninverted topographies and no viscerotopy, all being claimed. Subsequently, none of these plans has found wide support either. Surprisingly though, in the first century or more of work, medial-to-lateral possibilities such as the parallel columnar organization were not entertained; neither, for that matter, were dorsal-to-ventral organizational options considered. The issue of possible topographies was reduced to the restricted question of whether or not there was (and, if so, then what kind of) a viscerotopy along the axial dimension. In our view, the observations that were originally interpreted in terms of a rostral-caudal plan are equally consistent with the longitudinal columnar organization that we and others have characterized in the last few years. These observations are examined below after a reconsideration of the history of the problem.

The presupposition that any topography in the dmnX would be organized as a chain of transverse subnuclei arrayed along a longitudinal axis seems to have developed from at least three independent ideas and/or sets of observations. First, the dmnX has long been recognized as a condensation of cells in the more extensive general visceral efferent column that includes the rostral salivatory nuclei associated with the glossopharyngeal and facial nerves.[4,14,39,58] In early attempts to map the dmnX, there seems to have been a widely held, if tacit, extrapolation from this *inter*nuclear organization to an *intra*nuclear plan: i.e., if the general visceral efferent column is organized into specialized compartments along the neuroaxis, then it would be reasonable to expect further compartmentalization along the same axis. The equally tenable (or equally tenuous, depending on point of view) extrapolation that the pervasive columnar organization of the medulla (e.g., general visceral motor, special somatic motor, etc.) might be replicated at the intranuclear level was apparently overlooked.

The second set of observations that reinforced the original preoccupation with a rostral-to-caudal viscerotopy was experimental. Some of the initial, and frequently cited, experimental attempts to identify the rostral-caudal intranuclear organization were interpreted as support for the idea of an inverted viscerotopy on the longitudinal axis.[47,51,52] These experiments are relevant here not because they are directly contradictory to the recent observations on a columnar organization, but because they cemented early expectations about dmnX organization. Even with the issues about adequacy of the experiments and other specifics set aside, the results of these experiments are not, strictly speaking, in conflict with the longitudinal columnar representation of the GI tract. Molhant and Malone did not examine topographic representation of the organs of the alimentary canal. In fact, they treated the alimentary canal as one "organ" or unit and attempted to compare its representation with that of other units (e.g., the respiratory tree, the cardiovascular system). This lack of relevance should be underscored because the same considerations apply to most other early or classical claims of viscerotopy. Although the issue of topography in the dmnX has been widely discussed without qualifications, it has meant different things in the early and recent discussions.

Early Comparative Descriptions of the Vagal Trigone

A third group of experimental results was (we believe) prematurely forced into this same mold. A number of studies have taken a comparative approach and a correlative analysis to make inferences about the rostral-to-caudal assumption. The prototype here is the provocative series of papers by Vermeulen,[84,85,86,87] who compared the longitudinal spindle-shaped profiles of the dmnX in a variety of ruminants and nonruminants and correlated the shape and size of the nucleus with the elaboration of the ruminant stomach. Since the belly of the spindle (the greatest concentration of cells) tended to be shifted somewhat rostrally and the oral pole of the dmnX was correspondingly somewhat larger in ruminants (see also Kitchell *et al.*[38]), Vermeulen suggested that the stomach area might be found in the rostral dmnX. Such experiments clearly do not demonstrate that all gastric cells are in the rostral pole of the nucleus or that no other types of gastrointestinal preganglionics (e.g., neurons innervating the pancreas) are also in the rostral pole. In retrospect, the Vermeulen correlations can be as easily explained as a relative hypertrophy of a given set of intersections in a lattice organization (see the earlier discussion of these intersections). Nonetheless, these correlative comparative analyses have been subsumed by and used as foundational evidence for the widely held rostral-to-caudal paradigm.

The hold of the rostral-to-caudal model on thinking in this area can be appreciated by a re-examination of an even more influential paper on dmnX viscerotopy. After reviewing the literature prior to 1955, Mitchell and Warwick[50] approached the issue empirically by sectioning the trunks and branches of the vagus at different levels in rhesus monkeys and mapping patterns of chromatolysis in the dmnX. After sectioning the anterior abdominal vagus, the investigators obtained chromatolysis through the longitudinal extent of the dmnX, with a somewhat greater concentration of chromatolytic cells in the rostral pole. Furthermore, unaffected cells were found throughout the longitudinal extent of the dmnX (see their Figure 5). In fact, their results are consistent with the longitudinal columnar patterns of the preganglionics already described, and the points just raised regarding the Molhant, Malone and Vermeulen experiments are again relevant here. Nonetheless, the investigators (we assume at least in part because of the rostral-to-caudal presupposition) construed their results in terms of an inverted viscerotopy. "Incomplete" was adopted as a qualifier in explicit recognition of the fact that cells projecting into the abdomen were found throughout the axial dimension of the nucleus.

A Sampling Bias

There is another relatively prevalent analysis performed on the dmnX which has occasionally been interpreted (overinterpreted we believe) as evidence for a rostral-to-caudal compartmentalization of visceral representation within the nucleus. Results of tracer experiments and stimulation studies have often been expressed in terms of the frontal level of the medulla yielding the largest or best response (e.g., the largest number of labeled cells or the greatest physiological response are found at the level of the obex; for examples, see Pagani *et al.*[65] and Yoshida *et al.*[90]). Recall, however, that the dmnX is typically roughly spindle-shaped (see Figures 1 and 2). Unless cell counts or response magnitudes are corrected by the overall cell number and cell density at different levels of the neuroaxis, any conclusions about viscerotopy will be heavily biased. All effects will be more easily observed at the level containing the most cells. Indeed, it is instructive to note that, given the spindle-shaped distribution of preganglionics, this "level-of-best-response" sampling procedure would obtain the same outcome from (at least) three totally different and incompatible possible dmnX organizations. Whether the hypothetical dmnX organization were random with preganglionics completely intermingled without any topographic pattern, or whether the dmnX were organized as longitudinal columns as in fact it is, or whether the dmnX were organized in parallel with the NST patches with the function of interest represented at the frontal level containing the largest number of dmnX neurons, the same conclusion would be drawn. The sampling strategy would suggest that the function of interest was localized at just that level with the greatest number of cells. Not surprisingly, then, this is the conclusion that has consistently emerged in experiments employing the level-of-best-response sampling strategy.

Non-mammalian and Specialized dmnXs

Comparative neuroanatomy has been the source of another set of observations that may have complicated the task of identifying the general organization plan of the dmnX and hence that has implications for the lattice hypothesis. Basically this additional source of complications is the fact that some species have considerably more complex dmnXs. By way of review, recall that we have proposed that gastrointestinal reflexes are realized by this lattice structure in which preganglionic fibers in the abdominal vagal branches originate from the longitudinal columnar subnuclei in the dmnX. Recall also that we have suggested this organization is not peculiar to rodents but is in fact the vertebrate Bauplan. A point we did not emphasize earlier, however, is that the rat is probably a particularly useful species for examining the fundamental aspects of the organization. It is a fortuitous experimental model because its dmnX is nearly exclusively specialized for the gastrointestinal tract. Of the approximately 10,000 neurons in the rat dmnX,[44] nearly 7,500 project to the subdiaphragmatic viscera[21,70] (see also Lu and Sakai[45]). Much of the residual population in the rat dmnX is probably comprised of interneurons and preganglionics which distribute through the supradiaphragmatic recurrent laryngeal[45] and pulmonary branches of the vagus.[31] Like those innervating the gut, the preganglionics innervating the pulmonary fields are also apparently distributed longitudinally.[31] It should also be stressed however that the rat is not idiosyncratic in these organizational respects. It is a good model for most mammalian species including man, dog, cat, monkey, guinea pig, porpoise, camel, and buffalo.

However, some other species—specifically some non-mammalian species—have more complex dorsal motor nuclei with proportionally more motor neurons in the region committed to innervating tissues other than those of the gastrointestinal tract. For example in fish, amphibians, and reptiles the neurons homologous to those of the mammalian nucleus ambiguus are typically not situated ventrolaterally as they are in mammals. Much or all of this special visceral motor or branchiomeric homolog appears not to migrate ventrolaterally but rather to remain complexed with the general visceral motor homolog of the dmnX.

Another factor which expands the dmnX in some species is the fact that animals with smooth muscle esophagi also have a pool of preganglionics in the dmnX that innervate this additional tissue. Avian species with their smooth muscle upper alimentary tract, including their often highly developed crops, are paramount cases in point. As the recent experiments of Katz and Karten[34,36] have nicely demonstrated, these more rostral structures in the bird are associated with their own dmnX subnuclei as well. A full discussion of the organization of these additional and extensive pools of preganglionics in the avian dmnX involves the issue of whether they are organized into (hypertrophic) nodes in a lattice structure and is beyond the scope of the present review. However, it is relevant to observe that abdominal branches in the bird, which are treated as a unit in Katz and Karten's work,[36] appear to be organized as a longitudinal column running rostrocaudally in the medulla.[b]

We think that the existing observations on the organization of the dmnX can be reconciled with the columnar representation of gastrointestinal efferents described earlier. Many of the alternative interpretations which might be, and in some cases have been, construed as inconsistent have focused on more global organ-system organizational plans and are not strictly relevant. Still other alternatives are drawn from species where the dorsal vagal motor complex includes special visceral motor neurons and/or substantial numbers of preganglionics innervating other smooth muscle organs or organ-systems that might make the dmnX plan superficially more complex. Making allowances for such species specializations and also making allowances for the various degrees of hypertrophy and hypotrophy at the different lattice intersections discussed earlier, we suggest that the fundamental Bauplan of the dorsal vagal complex includes the lattice organization of alimentary canal afferents with the gastrointestinal preganglionics we have reviewed in this chapter.

---

[b]The rat esophagus is basically striated and represented in the nucleus ambiguus. However, there is a minor internal smooth muscle coat. This layer is innervated by preganglionics that appear to be sprinkled longitudinally, if sparsely, through the dmnX (see Altschuler et al.[2]).

EXTENSIONS OF THE LATTICE HYPOTHESIS

The area postrema should be considered an element in the vagal lattice. As one of the circumventricular organs, the area postrema serves to transduce inputs not obviously represented in the afferent supply to the NST. Lying outside the blood-brain barrier, the area postrema has access to hormonal and metabolic stimuli in the blood as well as access to humoral factors in the cerebrospinal fluid. In effect, the area postrema constitutes the vagal trigone's window on the fluxes of circulating hormones, peptides, and metabolites that have the potential to (and in several cases have been shown to) modulate the expression of the digestive reflexes.

Anatomically, the area postrema is positioned immediately dorsomedially to the NST/dmnX complex at the level of the calamus scriptorius, or roughly at the level of a coronal plane passed through a midlongitudinal point of the vagal complex (see Figures 1 and 2). Structurally, the area postrema is welded into the NST-dmnX lattice by similar types of connectivities and neuropil interactions already described for the NST and dmnX. In addition to its humoral inputs, the area postrema receives afferents that travel through the solitary tract.[43] Further, this circumventricular organ contains scattered neurons that project to the NST and at least indirectly to the dmnX.[53,81]

More functionally, the area postrema might be considered the equivalent of one of the broad bands of the NST. Two analogies, in addition to the connections outlined above, support this conclusion. First, the area postrema integrates the information of another independent "receptor sheet" into the vagal trigone. Secondly, like the other transversely arrayed bands of afferent terminations within the NST, the area postrema has a relatively restricted rostrocaudal extent and is largely distributed in a thick coronal "band." (Others, such as Norgren and Smith,[62] have also suggested that the area postrema should be considered a subunit of the NST.)

A specific example may help clarify this idea and also amplify one of the types of predictions made in the previous section. In the rat, the species that has been most exhaustively examined, the "belly" of the spindle shaped dmnX lies immediately subjacent to the area postrema. At these frontal planes, the dmnX reaches its maximum width and contains the greatest percentage of its neurons (Figure 1). Other species with similar peaks include man, rabbit, dog, and cat. A general inference would be that, in these species, a correspondingly large percentage of preganglionic neurons are influenced by the humoral factors transduced by the area postrema (as well as by sensory influences of the immediately adjacent NST). A more specific version of this idea may be more easily translated into specific experimental tests. The dmnX increases in cross-sectional area so dramatically at this level because the medial columns associated with the gastric branches are enlarged at this level.[21,70] In contrast, the columns associated with the hepatic and celiac branches of the vagus remain relatively constant in size along the axial dimension and do not hypertrophy at this level. The net effect of this pattern is that, for example, the celiac and gastric columns each occupy roughly half of the dmnX in the caudal part of the nucleus, but at the level of the area postrema, the expansion of the gastric column changes the ratio from roughly one-to-one to five-to-one. A functional inference that could be evaluated experimentally is that, compared to those of the gastric branch responses, the motor and secretory responses mediated by the two celiac branches are less heavily modulated by the types of humoral and hormonal signals seen by the area postrema and, in contrast, proportionately more engaged by afferent traffic in the more caudal commissural NST.

Another extension of the lattice proposal would be to make it more explicitly three-dimensional. For the sake of simplicity our description so far has been largely two-dimensional. Referring to the NST fields as bands obviously oversimplifies what is actually a much richer and more complex assemblage of subnuclei. Different afferent terminations within the NST are in some cases more dorsally located and in other cases more ventrally located; what we have called bands or patches do not have regular and rigidly geometric profiles.[2,35,62,82,88] To the extent that the vagal trigone mechanisms of the GI reflexes can be understood as a sensory-motor lattice, it may also be of heuristic value to consider these substrates as embedded in a three-dimensional architecture that includes the different "laminae" or dorso-ventral zones within the trigone. Furthermore, tracer analyses of descending forebrain and diencephalic projections to the trigone have suggested that different inputs terminate in different layers of the NST. For example, van der Kooy *et al.*[83] have reported that prefrontal cortical projections terminate in dorsal layers of the NST, while descending subcortical projections end in a more ventral zone just above the dmnX.

Another case of comparative neuroanatomy adds considerable prima facie support to both the basic idea of the lattice organization of the vagal complex and the extensions, including a series of laminae in the third dimension. The hypertrophic vagal systems seen in a number of fish form quite literally a three-dimensional lattice and suggest that such a plan may inhere in the NST/dmnX complex of other vertebrate species with less fully developed or more cryptic vagal systems (see Nieuwenhuys and Meek[58]). Many fish have extraordinarily developed vagal lobes. These lobes are typically homologized with the NST. In the more developed fish these lobes become as precisely and rigidly multilaminate (up to 15 layers!) as the mammalian cerebral cortex.[10,20,28,58] In a functional vein, Finger[20] has offered the provocative idea that this laminar architecture of the fish NST may serve as a neural network for identifying or sorting food from gravel. Extending this example, it has also recently been reported that the area postrema can also take on a similar and equally precise laminar pattern in some fish.[54] Although experimental interest has typically focused on the afferent elements, it is also accepted that the vagal motorneurons of these fish form a plate or very regular deep layers underlying, and in register with, the extraordinary sensory plates. Golgi profiles have even suggested that some of these motor neurons send dendrites up into the overlying sensory fields.[55]

Finally, and by way of brief summary, a last set of extensions, or areas in which extensions are needed, concerns different levels of organization and the need to develop a more comprehensive understanding of alimentary reflexes. We have proposed that the vagal trigone with its lattice organization contains the basic architecture or warp and woof responsible for organizing individual gastrointestinal reflexes. We have already indicated in the earlier section, however, that within an individual node in the lattice architecture, considerable additional selectivity must obtain to account for the individual elemental vagal reflexes. In addition to such an *intra*modular organization or addressing, there must also be an extensive *inter*modular organization that is as yet only dimly envisioned.

Although little certitude yet exists concerning even the precise categories needed, most investigators would probably accept the idea that individual gastrointestinal reflexes are normally organized into different classes (and perhaps hierarchies) of coordinated reflexes. Some situations or stimuli might serve to provide a global activation of the parasympathetic outflow. Others might serve to address anatomically distributed ensembles of neurons with shared functional modes (e.g., all lattice modules or vagal preganglionics that influence glucose availability). Still others might selectively address one organ and not another while others might serve to organize complex responses into a coordinated functional unit (e.g., emesis or general GI motility). In order to develop an adequate understanding of alimentary reflexes, it will be necessary to extend our understanding of the organization and addressing in dorsal vagal complex to include an explanation of how functional sets or mosaics of reflexes are coordinated at the inter- as well as intramodular levels within the general lattice architecture found in the vagal trigone.

REFERENCES

1. **Adachi, A.,** Projection of the hepatic vagal nerve in the medulla oblongata, *J. Auton. Nerv. Syst.*, 10, 287-293, 1984.
2. **Altschuler, S.M., Bao, X., Bieger, D., Hopkins, D.A., and Miselis, R.R.,** Viscerotopic representation of the upper alimentary tract in the rat: Sensory ganglia and nuclei of the solitary and spinal trigeminal tracts, *J. Comp. Neurol.*, 283, 248-268, 1989.
3. **Andrews, P.L.R., Fussey, I.V., and Scratcherd, T.,** The spontaneous discharge in abdominal vagal efferents in the dog and ferret, *Pflugers Arch.*, 387, 55-60, 1980.
4. **Ariens Kappers, C.U., Huber, G.C., and Crosby, E.C.,** *The Comparative Anatomy of the Nervous System of Vertebrates, Including Man,* Hafner, New York, 1967.
5. **Berthoud, H.-R., Carlson, N.R., and Powley, T.L.,** Topography of efferent vagal innervation of the rat gastrointestinal tract, *Am. J. Physiol.*, 260, R200-R207, 1991.
6. **Berthoud, H.-R., Fox, E.A., and Powley, T.L.,** Localization of vagal preganglionics that stimulate insulin and glucagon secretion, *Am. J. Physiol.*, 258, R160-R168, 1990.
7. **Berthoud, H.-R., and Powley, T.L.,** Altered plasma insulin and glucose after obesity-producing bipiperidyl brain lesions, *Am. J. Physiol.*, 248, R46-R53, 1985.
8. **Berthoud, H.-R., and Powley, T.L.,** Identification of vagal preganglionics that mediate cephalic phase insulin response, *Am. J. Physiol.*, 258, R523-R530, 1990.

9. **Bieger, D., and Hopkins, D.A.,** Viscerotopic representation of the upper alimentary tract in the medulla oblongata in the rat: The nucleus ambiguus, *J. Comp. Neurol.*, 262, 546-562, 1987.

10. **Braford, M.R.,** *De gustibus non est disputandum:* A spiral center for taste in the brain of the teleost fish, *Heterotis niloticus, Science*, 232, 489-491, 1986.

11. **Bullock, T.H.,** Some principles in the brain analysis of important signals: Mapping and stimulus recognition, *Brain Behav. Evol.*, 28, 145-156, 1986.

12. **Carlson, N., Berthoud, H.-R., and Powley, T.L.,** Viscerotopic organization of abdominal vagal branches as determined by induced motility responses, *Neurosci. Abstr.*, 15, 264, 1989.

13. **Champagnat, J., Denavit-Saubie, M., Grant, K., and Shen, K.F.,** Organization of synaptic transmission in the mammalian solitary complex, studied *in vitro, J. Physiol.*, 381, 551-573, 1986.

14. **Contreras, R.J., Gomez, M.M., and Norgren, R.,** Central origins of cranial nerve parasympathetic neurons in the rat, *J. Comp. Neurol.*, 190, 373-394, 1980.

15. **Cunningham, E.T. Jr., and Sawchenko, P.E.,** Local projections from the medial part of the nucleus of the solitary tract in rat, *Neurosci. Abstr.*, 12, 1055, 1986.

16. **Davis, B.J., and Jang, T.,** A Golgi analysis of the gustatory zone of the nucleus of the solitary tract in the adult hamster, *J. Comp. Neurol.*, 278, 388-396, 1988.

17. **Diz, D.I., Barnes, K.L., and Ferrario, C.M.,** Functional characteristics of neuropeptides in the dorsal medulla oblongata and vagus nerve, *Fed. Proc.*, 46, 30-35, 1987.

18. **Ewart, W.R., Jones, M.V., and King, B.F.,** Central origin of vagal nerve fibres innervating the fundus and corpus of the stomach in rat, *J. Auton. Nerv. Syst.*, 25, 219-231, 1988.

19. **Ferenci, D.A., Altschuler, S.M., and Miselis, R.R.,** Representation of cecum in lateral dorsal motor nucleus and commissural subnucleus of the nucleus tractus solitarius in rat, *Soc. Neurosci. Abst.*, 15, 264, 1989.

20. **Finger, T.E.,** Sensorimotor mapping and oropharyngeal reflexes in goldfish, *Carassius auratus, Brain Behav. Evol.*, 31, 17-24, 1988.

21. **Fox, E.A., and Powley, T.L.,** Longitudinal columnar organization within the dorsal motor nucleus represents separate branches of the abdominal vagus, *Brain Res.*, 341, 269-282, 1985.

22. **Fox, E.A., and Powley, T.L.,** Dendritic morphology of functionally identified neurons in the dorsal motor nucleus of the vagus, *Neurosci. Abstr.*, 15, 662, 1989.

23. **Fox, E.A., and Powley, T.L.,** False-positive artifacts of tracer strategies distort autonomic connectivity maps, *Br. Res. Rev.*, 14, 53-77, 1989.

24. **Fox, E.A., and Powley, T.L.,** The morphology of identified preganglionic neurons in the dorsal motor nucleus of the vagus, *J. Comp. Neurol.*, in press.

25. **Glassman, R.B.,** Parsimony in neural representations: Generalization of a model of spatial orientation ability, *Physiol. Psychol.*, 13, 43-47, 1985.

26. **Hamilton, R.B., and Norgren, R.,** Central projections of gustatory nerves in the rat, *J. Comp. Neurol.*, 222, 560-577, 1984.

27. **Harding, R., and Leek, B.F.,** The locations and activities of medullary neurons associated with ruminant forestomach motility, *J. Physiol.*, 219, 587-610, 1971.

28. **Herrick, C.J.,** A study of the vagal lobes and funicular nuclei of the brain of the codfish, *J. Comp. Neurol.*, 17, 67-87, 1907.

29. **Jansen, J., and Osen, K.K.,** Morphogenesis and morphology of the brainstem nuclei of cetacea. II. The nuclei of the accessory, vagal, and glossopharyngeal nerves in baleen whales, *J. Hirnforsch.*, 1, 53-87, 1984.

30. **Kaas, J.H.,** The segregation of function in the nervous system: Why do sensory systems have so many subdivisions? *Contributions to Sensory Physiology*, 7, 201-240, 1982.

31. **Kalia, M.,** Organization of central control of airways, *Annu. Rev. Physiol.*, 49, 595-609, 1987.

32. **Kalia, M., Fuxe, K., Hokfelt, T., Johansson, O., Lang, R., Ganten, D., Cuello, C., and Terenius, L.,** Distribution of neuropeptide immunoreactive nerve terminals within the subnuclei of the nucleus of the tractus solitarius of the rat, *J. Comp. Neurol.*, 222, 409-444, 1984.

33. **Kalia, M., and Sullivan, J.M.,** Brainstem projections of sensory and motor components of the vagus nerve in the rat, *J. Comp. Neurol.*, 211, 248-264, 1982.

34. **Katz, D.M., and Karten, H.J.,** Subnuclear organization of the dorsal motor nucleus of the vagus nerve in the pigeon, *Columba livia, J. Comp. Neurol.,* 217, 31-46, 1983.

35. **Katz, D.M., and Karten, H.J.,** Visceral representation within the nucleus of the tractus solitarius in the pigeon, *Columba livia, J. Comp. Neurol.,* 218, 42-73, 1983.

36. **Katz, D.M., and Karten, H.J.,** Topographic representation of visceral target organs within the dorsal motor nucleus of the vagus nerve of the pigeon, *Columba livia, J. Comp. Neurol.,* 242, 397-414, 1985.

37. **Kimmel, D.L.,** Differentiation of the bulbar motor nuclei and the coincident development of associated root fibers in the rabbit, *J. Comp. Neurol.,* 72, 83-148, 1940.

38. **Kitchell, R.L., Stromberg, M.W., and Davis, L.H.,** Comparative study of the dorsal motor nucleus of the vagus nerve, *Am. J. Vet. Res.,* 38, 37-49, 1977.

39. **Kuhlenbeck, H.,** *The Central Nervous System of Vertebrates,* S. Karger, New York, 1967.

40. **Laughton, W.B., Campfield, L.A., and Nelson, D.O.,** Hepatic portal and gastric afferent processing in nucleus of the solitary tract of the rat, *Soc. Neurosci. Abst.,* 13, 385, 1987.

41. **Laughton, W.B., and Powley, T.L.,** Localization of efferent function in the dorsal motor nucleus of the vagus, *Am. J. Physiol.,* 252, R13-R25, 1987.

42. **Leslie, R.A.,** Neuroactive substances in the dorsal vagal complex of the medulla oblongata: Nucleus of the tractus solitarius, area postrema, and dorsal motor nucleus of the vagus, *Neurochem. Int.,* 7, 191-211, 1985.

43. **Leslie, R.A., and Gwyn, D.G.,** Neuronal connections of the area postrema, *Fed. Proc.,* 43, 2941-2943, 1984.

44. **Lu, Y.L., and Sakai, H.,** Cytoarchitectonic study on the dorsal motor nucleus of the rat vagus, *Okajimas Folia Anat. Jpn.,* 61, 221-234, 1984.

45. **Lu, Y.L., and Sakai, H.,** Localization of the neurons of origin of efferent fibers in the glossopharyngeal, vagus and accessory nerves in the rat by means of retrograde degeneration and horseradish peroxidase methods, *Okajimas Folia Anat. Jpn.,* 61, 287-310, 1984.

46. **Maley, B., Mullett, T., and Elde, R.,** The nucleus tractus solitarii of the cat: A comparison of Golgi impregnated neurons with methionine- enkephalin- and substance P-immunoreactive neurons, *J. Comp. Neurol.,* 217, 405-417, 1983.

47. **Malone, E.F.,** The nucleus cardiacus nervi vagi and the three distinct types of nerve cells which innervate the three different types of muscle, *Am. J. Anat.,* 151, 121-129, 1913-1914.

48. **Martin, K., Kong, T.H., Renehan, W., Schurr, A., Dong, W., Zhang, X., and Fogel, R.,** Identification and function of brain stem neurons regulating rat ileal water absorption, *Am. J. Physiol.,* 257, G266-G273, 1989.

49. **Menetrey, D., and Basbaum, A.I.,** Spinal and trigeminal projections to the nucleus of the solitary tract: A possible substrate for somatovisceral and viscerovisceral reflex activation, *J. Comp. Neurol.,* 255, 439-450, 1987.

50. **Mitchell, G.A.G., and Warwick, R.,** The dorsal vagal nucleus, *Acta Anat.,* 25, 371-395, 1955.

51. **Molhant, M.,** Le noyau ventral du vague et le noyau ambiguu, *Nevraxe,* 12, 225-317, 1911.

52. **Molhant, M.,** Les connexions anatomiques et la valeur fonctionelle du noyau dorsal du vague, *Nevraxe,* 11, 137-234, 1910-1911.

53. **Morest, D.K.,** Experimental study of the projections of the nucleus of the tractus solitarius and the area postrema in the cat, *J. Comp. Neurol.,* 130, 277-300, 1967.

54. **Morita, Y., and Finger, T.E.,** Area postrema of the goldfish, Carassius auratus: Ultrastructure, fiber connections, and immunocytochemistry, *J. Comp. Neurol.,* 256, 104-116, 1987.

55. **Morita, Y., Murakami, T., and Ito, H.,** Cytoarchitecture and topographic projections of the gustatory centers in a teleost, *Carassius carassius, J. Comp. Neurol.,* 218, 378-394, 1983.

56. **Neuhuber, W.L.,** Vagal afferent fibers almost exclusively innervate islets in the rat pancreas as demonstrated by anterograde tracing, *J. Auton. Nerv. Syst.,* 29, 13-18, 1989.

57. **Neuhuber, W.L., and Sandoz, P.A.,** Vagal primary afferent terminals in the dorsal motor nucleus of the rat: Are they making monosynaptic contacts on preganglionic efferent neurons? *Neurosci. Lett.,* 69, 126-130, 1986.

58. **Nieuwenhuys, R., and Meek, J.,** Constructional principles of the brain stem in anamniotes, with emphasis on actinopterygian fishes, in *Fortschritt der Zoologie, Band 30. Vertebrate Morphology,* Duncker/Fleischer, Ed., Gustav Fischer Verlag, Stuttgart, 1985, 515-528.

59. **Nitzan, R., Segev, I., and Yarom, Y.,** Voltage behavior along the irregular dendritic structure of morphologically and physiologically characterized vagal motoneurons in the guinea pig, *J. Neurol.,* 63, 333-346, 1990.

60. **Norgren, R.,** Projections from the nucleus of the solitary tract in the rat, *Neuroscience,* 3, 207-218, 1978.

61. **Norgren, R.,** Central neural mechanisms of taste, in *Handbook of Physiology - The Nervous System III,* Darian-Smith, I., Ed., Am. Physiol. Soc., Bethesda, 1984, 1087-1128.

62. **Norgren, R., and Smith, G.P.,** Central distribution of subdiaphragmatic vagal branches in the rat, *J. Comp. Neurol.,* 273, 207-223, 1988.

63. **Okumura, T., and Namiki, M.,** Vagal motor neurons innervating the stomach are site-specifically organized in the dorsal motor nucleus of the vagus nerve in rats, *J. Auton. Nerv. Syst.,* 29, 157-162, 1990.

64. **Pagani, F.D., Norman, W.P., and Gillis, R.A.,** Medullary parasympathetic projections innervate specific sites in the feline stomach, *Gastroenterology,* 95, 277-288, 1988.

65. **Pagani, F.D., Norman, W.P., Kasbekar, D.K., and Gillis, R.A.,** Localization of sites within dorsal motor nucleus of vagus that affect gastric motility, *Am. J. Physiol.,* 249, G73-G84, 1985.

66. **Powley, T.L., and Berthoud, H.-R.,** Neuroanatomical bases of cephalic phase reflexes, in *Chemical Senses: Appetite and Nutrition, Vol. 4,* Friedman, M.I., et al., Eds., Marcel Dekker, Inc., New York, 1991.

67. **Powley, T.L., Fox, E.A., Baronowsky, E., Keller, D.L., Berthoud, H.-R.,** Longitudinal column of gastric branch neurons in the dorsal motor nucleus of the vagus is composed of subcolumns corresponding to distal divisions of gastric branch, *Soc. Neurosci. Abstr.,* 13, 386, 1987.

68. **Powley, T.L., Fox, E.A., and Berthoud, H.-R.,** Retrograde tracer technique for assessment of selective and total subdiaphragmatic vagotomies, *Am. J. Physiol.,* 253, R361-R370, 1987.

69. **Powley, T.L., and Prechtl, J.C.,** Gold thioglucose selectively damages dorsal vagal nuclei, *Brain Res.,* 367, 192-200, 1986.

70. **Powley, T.L., Wang, F.B., and Baronowsky, E.,** 3-D digital atlas of the dorsal motor nucleus of the vagus, *Neurosci. Abstr.,* 15, 264, 1989.

71. **Prechtl, J.C., and Powley, T.L.,** Organization and distribution of the rat subdiaphragmatic vagus and associated paraganglia, *J. Comp. Neurol.,* 235, 182-195, 1985.

72. **Prechtl, J.C., and Powley, T.L.,** A light and electron microscopic examination of the vagal hepatic branch of the rat, *Anat. Embryol.,* 176, 115-126, 1987.

73. **Prechtl, J.C., and Powley, T.L.,** The fiber composition of the abdominal vagus of the rat, *Anat. Embryol.,* 181, 101-115, 1990.

74. **Ramon-Moliner, E.,** The morphology of dendrites, in *The Structure and Function of Nervous Tissue, Vol. 1,* Bourne, G.E., Ed., Academic Press, N.Y., 1968, 205-267.

75. **Rinaman, L., Card, J.P., Schwaber, J.S., and Miselis, R.R.,** Ultrastructural demonstration of a gastric monosynaptic vagal circuit in the nucleus of the solitary tract in rat, *J. Neurosci.,* 9, 1985-1996, 1989.

76. **Rinaman, L., and Miselis, R.R.,** The organization of vagal innervation of rat pancreas using cholera toxin-horseradish peroxidase conjugate, *J. Auton. Nerv. Syst.,* 21, 109-125, 1987.

77. **Rogers, R.C., and Hermann, G.E.,** Central connections of the hepatic branch of the vagus nerve: A horseradish peroxidase histochemical study, *J. Auton. Nerv. Syst.,* 7,165-174, 1983.

78. **Rogers, R.C., Kita, H., Butcher, L.L., and Novin, D.,** Afferent projections to the dorsal motor nucleus of the vagus, *Brain Res. Bull.,* 5, 365-373, 1980.

79. **Satomi, H., Yamamoto, T., Ise, H., and Takatama, H.,** Origins of the parasympathetic preganglionic fibers to the cat intestine as demonstrated by the horseradish peroxidase method, *Brain Res.,* 151, 571-578, 1978.

80. **Sejnowski, T.J.,** Computational models and the development of topographic projections, *TINS*, 10, 304-305, 1987.
81. **Shapiro, R.E., and Miselis, R.R.,** The central organization of the vagus nerve innervating the stomach of the rat, *J. Comp. Neurol.*, 238, 473-488, 1985.
82. **Torvik, A.,** Afferent connections to the sensory trigeminal nuclei, the nucleus of the solitary tract and adjacent structures: An experimental study in the rat, *J. Comp. Neurol.*, 106, 51-142, 1956.
83. **van der Kooy, D., Koda, L.Y., McGinty, J.F., Gerfen, C.R., and Bloom, F.E.,** The organization of projections from the cortex, amygdala, and hypothalamus to the nucleus of the solitary tract in rat, *J. Comp. Neurol.*, 224, 1-24, 1984.
84. **Vermeulen, H.A.,** Note on the size of the dorsal motor nucleus of the Xth nerve in regard to the development of the stomach, *Proc. Royal Acad. Amsterdam*, 16, 305-311, 1913.
85. **Vermeulen, H.A.,** The vagus area in camelidae, *Proc. Royal Acad. Amsterdam*, 17, 1119-1134, 1915.
86. **Vermeulen, H.A.,** The vagus-area in Camelopardalus Giraffe, *Proc. Royal Acad. Amsterdam*, 18, 647-670, 1915.
87. **Vermeulen, H.A.,** On the vagus and hypoglossus area of *Phocaena communis, Proc. Royal Acad. Amsterdam*, 18, 965-980, 1916.
88. **Whitehead, M.C.,** Neuronal architecture of the nucleus of the solitary tract in the hamster, *J. Comp. Neurol.*, 276, 547-572, 1988.
89. **Yamamoto, T., Satomi, H., Ise, H., and Takahashi, K.,** Evidence of the dual innervation of the cat stomach by the vagal dorsal motor and medial solitary nuclei as demonstrated by the horseradish peroxidase method, *Brain Res.*, 122, 125-131, 1977.
90. **Yoshida, J., Polley, E.H., Nyhus, L.M., and Donahue, P.E.,** Brain stem topography of vagus nerve to the greater curvature of the stomach, *J. Surg. Res.*, 46, 60-69, 1989.

Chapter 4

CENTRAL CONNECTIONS OF THE NUCLEI OF THE VAGUS NERVE

R.A. Leslie, D.J.M. Reynolds and I.N.C. Lawes

TABLE OF CONTENTS

LIST OF ABBREVIATIONS

ACE = central nucleus of the amygdala
AP = area postrema
BNSTL = lateral bed nucleus of the stria terminalis
CFS = cerebrospinal fluid
DMX = dorsal motor nucleus of the vagus nerve
DVC = dorsal vagal complex
HRP = horseradish peroxidase
LH = lateral hypothalamic nucleus
NA = nucleus ambiguus
NTS = nucleus of the solitary tract
PBN = nucleus parabrachialis
PHA-L = *Phaseolus vulgaris* leukoagglutinin
PVH = paraventricular hypothalamic nucleus
SNG = subnucleus gelatinosus

INTRODUCTION

The vagus nerve, as its name implies, is the largest and most extensively ramifying nerve of the autonomic nervous system; it is involved in conveying information to and from most of the viscera of the thorax and abdomen as well as many structures of the head and neck. It is a "mixed nerve" in that it consists of both visceral and somatic afferent fibers and parasympathetic and branchial efferents. The major terminal field of afferent fibers of this nerve occurs in the nucleus of the solitary tract (NTS), although some of its fibers project to other caudal brainstem nuclei such as the nucleus of the spinal tract of the trigeminal nerve, the area postrema (AP), and the dorsal motor nucleus of the vagus nerve (DMX). Because of their close anatomical association in the dorsomedial portion of the caudal rhombencephalon, the NTS, AP and DMX are often referred to collectively as the dorsal vagal complex (DVC). Together, these nuclei constitute the major afferent and efferent nuclei of the vagus. It should be emphasized, however, that the nucleus ambiguus (NA) in a more ventral position in this brainstem region is the other important efferent (or "ventral motor") nucleus of the vagus nerve.

Because it is such a large and noticeable macroscopic structure, early anatomists were able to use gross dissection techniques to map the peripheral distribution of branches of the vagus nerve with much accuracy. It was not until the relatively recent advent of light microscopic nerve fiber tracing techniques, however, that much more was discovered about the details of peripheral and central projection sites of this nerve.

A large number of studies have emerged in recent years that have used modern neuroanatomical methods to elucidate the central projection sites and neurons of origin of the afferent and efferent fibers of the vagus nerve, respectively. Other studies have been aimed at examining the central connections of these target nuclei in order to determine which brain regions modulate the information flowing into and out of them. This chapter will review the literature pertaining to the latter question and will speculate on how the vagus nerve can interact with other brain nuclei to effect coordinated control of so many visceral structures. Furthermore, the central vagal connections will be discussed in an evolutionary context, and the functional implications of this will be explored.

TECHNICAL CONSIDERATIONS

Brodal[9] outlined some of the different neuroanatomical techniques that have been developed to study the connectivity of discrete elements of the central nervous system. The first major technical advance depended upon the introduction of new histological techniques that were useful in visualizing either neuronal cell bodies or fibers under the light microscope. These included stains such as hematoxylin which is commonly used for routine histological examinations of many tissue types, Weigert's stain for myelin sheathes, Golgi's methods which stain entire neurons (used so effectively by Ramon y Cajal), and the various Nissl stains which stain the Nissl bodies of neuronal somata (i.e., the rough endoplasmic reticulum within the cell).

A large step forward was made when methods were developed to trace the extent of long fiber connections in the central nervous system. For many years such methods were based upon degeneration of fibers after experimental lesions were made of the fiber tract or cell bodies or, conversely, by looking for atrophic changes in the cell bodies after fiber tract lesion. Thus, terminal fields of fiber tracts could be examined by making use of stains that recognize deteriorating myelin sheaths (e.g., the Marchi method) or terminal boutons. Silver impregnation methods such as that developed by Glees and elaborated by Nauta and Gygax and Fink and Heimer have proved to be very useful in this regard and are still occasionally in use. These methods do have some serious disadvantages, however, such as the length of time needed to perform some of them (it is not unusual for such methods to take many weeks after the initial experimental lesion to yield a useful result). Furthermore, lesions will interrupt fibers of passage as well as fibers intrinsic to the pathway of interest. This problem is still not completely overcome by more modern methods. The original techniques also have limited sensitivity; for example, some will not detect unmyelinated fibers at all. Slight alterations in some of the techniques will delimit only subpopulations of axons, for example, only those of a certain diameter, therefore one must be careful in attempting any quantification of fiber numbers in case the tract of interest contains a heterogeneous population of axons.

More recent methods rely on axonal transport of radiolabeled amino acids or peptides or of histochemically-defined enzymes after their injection into brain nuclear regions or target sites of fiber tracts, respectively. In the first case, autoradiography can be performed on tissue sections taken from the suspected terminal field region of the brain after enough time has passed since the injection for orthograde transport of the amino acid to the bouton region.[57] In the second case, the enzyme (the common one used is horseradish peroxidase or HRP) is transported retrogradely from the terminal boutons to the cell bodies.[21] More sensitive histochemical procedures have revealed that orthograde transport of HRP or other molecules also occurs and can be used instead of the autoradiographic procedure to trace pathways.[31] Several modifications of these techniques have been developed in recent years to increase the sensitivity and decrease the "fiber of passage problem" of these newer methods. One big problem concerned the amount of tracer spread from the injection site. It is difficult to limit the spread of the injected tracer to the neurons or target tissues of interest. One way to approach this problem has been to link a lectin molecule (such as wheatgerm agglutinin) to the HRP molecule to ensure that the amount of extracellular spread of the tracer is not too extensive. Another recent modification of the HRP technique involves the use of cholera toxin-conjugated HRP[38,62] which has the advantage that the entire dendritic tree of a retrogradely labeled neuron is filled with the tracer.

THE AREA POSTREMA (AP)—
AN IMPORTANT VAGAL SENSORY NUCLEUS

In a gross and microscopic study of the calamus region of the human medulla oblongata, Wilson[65] described a "gentle prominence" of grey matter in the AP of Retzius[36] on the caudal floor of the fourth ventricle of the brain. He commented upon its atypical vascularity and "loose and open texture," and illustrated neurons within the region. For this reason he termed this brain region the "nucleus postremus." For many years, however, there was uncertainty about whether this brain stem region actually contained neuronal cell bodies and could therefore be considered a brain nucleus. Wislocki and Putnam[67] believed the human AP contained neuronal somata but could find none in any of their animal preparations. A later study by King[18] identified multipolar cells in the AP of the cat, but he was unable to identify these as neuronal and considered that they might be developing astrocytes. As late as the 1950s some investigators denied the presence of neurons within the AP of subhuman species (e.g., Wislocki and LeDuc[66]). The relatively late realization that the AP is a neuronal structure (a "true brain nucleus") probably accounts for the lack of popularity of the term nucleus postremus, and the term area postrema is thus now universally used. The neurons of the AP have now been shown to be small, averaging only about 12 μm in diameter, and relatively devoid of Nissl substance. They are particularly resistant to Golgi staining methods as are their immediate neighbors in the subnucleus gelatinosus (SNG)[55] of the NTS. In fact, their morphology is remarkably similar to that of the neurons in the SNG (see Klara and Brizzee[19] and Leslie *et al.*[26]). Furthermore, the AP, like the SNG, appears to receive vagal afferent fibers which are mainly of gastric origin.[16] Thus the two main sensory nuclei of the vagus, the NTS and the AP, should probably be considered together in a discussion of the central connections of the vagus.

The one outstanding difference between the two main sensory vagal nuclei is the fact that the AP has a weak blood-brain diffusion barrier (it "lies outside the blood-brain barrier") and thus may be influenced directly by blood- or CSF-borne humoral elements. Despite this dramatic difference, as mentioned above, the two brain areas are remarkably similar in most other respects. In fact, the AP could be considered a portion of the NTS with a unique vascular system. It appears to have at least as much in common with the NTS as it does with other circumventricular organs.[25]

CENTRAL CONNECTIONS OF THE
VAGAL SENSORY NUCLEI

The first thing one notices when reviewing the literature on this subject is the large number of structures of the central nervous system that receive direct projections from the NTS (see Table 1). The NTS appears to be a central sorting station for a vast amount of sensory information coming into it from the cervical, thoracic and abdominal viscera. Like several other small brainstem nuclei (such as the locus coeruleus) the NTS then sends out a large ramifying network of fibers to many different regions of the brain. It also receives a reasonably large amount of direct reciprocal information from these sites, but, unlike the efferent information from it, much of this afferent information appears to pass through at least one synapse on the way to the nucleus (see below).

TABLE 1
Central Connections of the Nucleus of the Solitary Tract

Input to the Nucleus of the Solitary Tract
brainstem and cerebellum
area postrema[50]
cerebellar flocculus[4]
locus coeruleus[29]
raphe n.[5]
forebrain
bed n. of the stria terminalis[14,60]
central n. of amygdala[15,35,49,56,60]
cerebral cortex[59,69]
hypothalamus: arcuate n.,[60] paraventricular n.,[60,64] posterolateral n.[60]

Output from Nucleus of the Solitary Tract
cord, brainstem and cerebellum
area postrema[50]
A1 catecholamine cell group[28]
ambiguus n.[28,37]
cerebellar flocculus[41,52]
intermediolateral cell column of the spinal cord[28]
Kolliker-Fuse n.[17,28]
lateral cuneate n.[28]
lateral parabrachial n.[17,28,37]
lateral periaqueductal grey matter[28]
lateral reticular formation[37]
locus coeruleus[10,42]
medial accessory olivary n.[28]
medial parabrachial n.[17,28]
paramedian reticular formation[28]
parvicellular reticular formation[58]
n. of the phrenic nerve[28]
raphe n.[1]
retrofacial n.[28]
thoracic ventral horn of the spinal cord[28]
vermis of cerebellum[41,52]
forebrain
bed n. of the stria terminalis[37]
central n. of the amygdala[37]
dorsomedial hypothalamic n.[37]
arcuate hypothalamic n.[37]
medial preoptic n.[37]
periventricular hypothalamic n.[37]
periventricular thalamic n.[37]

On the other hand, although the AP sends out direct information to many of the same central nervous system regions as does the NTS and receives direct reciprocal information from some of these, the number of brain regions so involved seems to be much fewer (Table 2). Of course, given the direct connections between AP and NTS, this difference in numbers of *direct* connections to the two nuclei may be of little functional significance.

In a recent review of the central connections of the vagus nerve, Sawchenko[46] recognized four levels of organization of the outputs from the NTS and AP. First, there is a direct projection to the autonomic motor nuclei to provide an anatomical substrate for short autonomic reflex loops. The parasympathetic preganglionic neurons involved are those in the DMX and the NA. Sympathetic preganglionic neurons in the intermediolateral cell column of the spinal cord also receive direct projections from the NTS.

The second level of organization involves vagal sensory relays to the motor components of ingestion found in the trigeminal, facial, and hypoglossal nuclei, and the special visceral efferent (accessory component) of the NA. Thirdly, gustatory and visceral information is relayed to more rostral regions of the brainstem via efferents from NTS to the parabrachial nuclei as well as to the A1 and A5 catecholaminergic cell groups of Dahlstrom and Fuxe.[12] Finally, long projections from NTS terminate in hypothalamic and limbic areas of the brain to provide integrative mechanisms for control of neuroendocrine and behavioral functions.

At every level along the vagal afferent pathways there are characteristically large numbers of neurotransmitter and neuromodulatory compounds and their receptors. This is exemplified by the large number of neuroactive substances found within the NTS.[24] In light of the extent of ramifying nervous pathways

TABLE 2
Central Connections of the Area Postrema

Input to the Area Postrema
brainstem
caudal nucleus of the solitary tract[50]
lateral parabrachial n.[50]
forebrain
hypothalamus: dorsomedial n.,[50] paraventricular n.[50,60]

Output from the Area Postrema
brainstem and cerebellum
dorsal motor n. of the vagus[50]
dorsal n. of the spinal trigeminal tract[50]
lateral parabrachial n.[50]
paratrigeminal n.[50]
n. ambiguus[50]
n. of the solitary tract[50]
ventrolateral medullary catecholamine cell group[50]
vermis of the cerebellum[50]

from the DVC, it seems likely that the neuroactive compounds distributed in different populations of these relay nuclei are somehow important in providing functional specificity for the system.

The central organization of the vagus nerve provides a good example of how spatial localization of neural pathways cannot fully account for functional differentiation. For example, it is well established that there is a large amount of anatomical overlap within the DVC in the terminal fields of afferent fibers from thoracic and abdominal viscera.[16] Is it possible that neurochemical specificity could account for functional differentiation in the vagus nerve? The simplest neurochemical code would be one neurotransmitter mediating one function and vice versa. However, just as functions fail to map simply onto spatially discrete pathways, they also fail to map onto individual neurotransmitters on a one-to-one basis. Each function involves more than one neurotransmitter, and each transmitter is involved in more than one function. For example, noradrenaline and opiates are involved in arousal, fear, nociception, ingestion, vomiting, gastrointestinal motility and secretion, heart rate, blood pressure, and endocrine and respiratory functions. Conversely, heart rate and blood pressure are influenced by opiates, noradrenaline, serotonin, somatostatin, angiotensin II, atrial natriuretic factor, substance P, vasopressin and corticotrophin-releasing factor. Clearly, there are many levels of complexity in any neuronal system at which functional specificity could be achieved. Examples of some of these include: spatially discrete neuronal wiring circuits, temporal integration of inputs due to various cable properties of neuronal membranes, the existence of several receptor subtypes for individual neuroactive substances, and the occurrence of several second and even "third messenger" systems within the postsynaptic neuron.

CENTRAL CONNECTIONS OF THE VAGAL MOTOR NUCLEI

The DMX is the principal source of preganglionic parasympathetic fibers which innervate the abdominal, and to a lesser extent the thoracic viscera. The DMX comprises a column of morphologically distinct subnuclei arranged longitudinally throughout the dorsal medulla oblongata and within which viscerotopic organization is preserved.[13] Parasympathetic efferent fibers project from medium-sized neurons in the DMX[30] and the majority of them innervate the stomach.[27] Dendritic processes from DMX neurons extend beyond the confines of the nucleus into the NTS, including its SNG.[50] Some reach the AP and the subependymal region of the fourth ventricle and even gain access through the ependymal layer to the ventricle itself.[50] These projections into areas with a poor blood-brain diffusion barrier may allow direct humoral modulation of DMX activity.

Vagal afferent fibers communicate directly with DMX neurons either within the boundary of the nucleus[33] or via the widespread dendritic arborizations of the motor neurons. These monosynaptic contacts provide an anatomical basis for vago-vagal reflex arcs.[38,50]

The NA is the other major source of preganglionic vagal efferent fibers. It fulfills a general visceral efferent function in addition to belonging to the special visceral efferent column made up of the nucleus retroambiguus, the NA itself and the nucleus retrofacialis. As with the DMX, a large degree of viscerotopic representation is present within the NA.[2,6]

The DMX and the NA have broadly similar central connections and in general, regions which receive an input from the vagal sensory nuclei project back to both the motor nuclei. As with the vagal sensory nuclei, different levels of connectivity of the motor nuclei can be defined. Not surprisingly, the largest input to the DMX and NA seems to come from the NTS and AP,[50] providing the circuitry for short visceral reflex loops.

There are outputs from the vagal motor nuclei to the cerebellum,[41,69] and electrical stimulation of the cerebellar fastigial nucleus elicits a pressor response[32] which may be mediated by a fastigio-vagal pathway.

The nucleus parabrachialis (PBN) receives inputs from vagal sensory and motor nuclei[17] and in turn relays on to the hypothalamus, amygdala and cortex.[44] In addition, there are descending pathways from the PBN to the motor nuclei of the vagus.[58] These reciprocal innervations between the PBN and the vagal motor nuclei are implicated in cardiovascular and respiratory control, and the PBN probably forms one level of complex integration of gastrointestinal, cardiovascular and respiratory activity which occurs in autonomic reflexes such as vomiting.

Other brainstem relay nuclei contribute inputs to the vagal motor nuclei although the functions performed by these connections from the raphe nuclei, periaqueductal grey, parvicellular and gigantocellular reticular formation are largely unknown. Higher brain areas also influence vagal outflow via projections from hypothalamic, limbic and cortical areas; these pathways are discussed below. For a summary of the afferent and efferent connections of the DMX and NA, see Tables 3 and 4.

Hypothalamic-vagal interactions have been recognized for many years, but good anatomical evidence for monosynaptic pathways between the hypothalamus and the DVC and NA has only recently become available. Initial experiments suggested that the paraventricular (PVH) and lateral (LH) hypothalamic nuclei had direct communications with the DMX and NA;[45] this has subsequently been confirmed by a number of investigators (see Tables 3 and 4). Using the push-pull perfusion technique, Landgraf *et al.*[20] demonstrated that both oxytocin and vasopressin are released in the DVC in response to electrical stimulation of the PVH, confirming earlier indirect evidence that these peptides are implicated in autonomic regulation.[47,53]

Many neuroactive substances, including oxytocin, vasopressin, substance P, dopamine, somatostatin, neurotensin, enkephalin and corticotrophin-releasing factor,[20,46] have been identified in the PVH-DVC pathways. As discussed

TABLE 3
Central Connections of the Dorsal Motor Nucleus of the Vagus

Input to Dorsal Motor Nucleus of the Vagus
brainstem
area postrema[50]
nucleus of the solitary tract[39]
parabrachial n.[58]
parvicellular reticular n.[39,58]
periaqueductal grey matter[58]
principal sensory trigeminal n.[39]
raphe n.[39,58]
forebrain
bed n. of the stria terminalis[14,34,48,49]
central n. of amygdala[15,34,35,48,49,56]
hypothalamus: dorsomedial n.,[58] lateral n.[58]
                paraventricular n.[39,45,54,58,60,61,64]
                ventromedial n.[58]

Output from Dorsal Motor Nucleus of the Vagus
brainstem and cerebellum
anterior and posterior cerebellar cortex[69]
Kolliker-Fuse n.[17]
parabrachial n.[17]

TABLE 4
Central Connections of the Nucleus Ambiguus

Input to the Nucleus Ambiguus
brainstem
area postrema[50]
lateral reticular n.[58]
nucleus of the solitary tract[28,37,58]
parabrachial n.[58]
periaqueductal grey[58]
forebrain
bed n. of the stria terminalis[14,15,58]
central n. of the amygdala[15]
hypothalamus: lateral n.,[45] paraventricular n.[58]

Output from the Nucleus Ambiguus
cerebellum
cerebellar cortex[41]

above, it seems unlikely that the maintenance of specificity among neurons controlling diverse functions in the vagal motor nuclei can be achieved simply by "function-specific" neurotransmitters, and the interactions between many neuroactive agents have yet to be explored.

The brain area referred to as the visceral forebrain is composed of both subcortical and cortical structures. The principal subcortical structures are the central nucleus of the amygdala (ACE), lateral bed nucleus of the stria terminalis

(BNSTL) and PVH. Cortical structures of the visceral forebrain are the insular cortex and the infralimbic-anterior cingulate cortex. The BNSTL and the ACE will be considered together since they share a number of anatomical features[14,49] and may indeed serve common functions. In the broadest terms, the amygdala is involved in the expression of somatic and autonomic components of defense, emotion and motivation. Until the mid 1970s the influence of the amygdala on autonomic components of emotional behavior was thought to be exerted indirectly via the hypothalamus, but ample evidence now exists to show that there are direct projections from the ACE and BNSTL to the DVC, and in particular to the DMX, and the NA in a variety of species (Tables 3 and 4). The demonstration of these monosynaptic connections with the vagal motor nuclei supports the notion that limbic structures may directly modulate parasympathetic outflow.

Direct pathways to the vagal sensory and motor nuclei from the visceral sensory insular cortex have been described in rodents[43,51,60] and from the orbito-insular cortex to the NTS in the cat.[63] A monosynaptic pathway from the rat medial prefrontal cortex to the NTS, DMX and NA has also been described.[59] These latter authors postulate a functional progression in the rat cortex going from medial to lateral, with the visceral motor medial frontal cortex most medially, progressing through the frontal eye fields, somatic motor cortex, somatic sensory cortex, visceral sensory cortex (insular cortex) and most laterally, the olfactory or piriform cortex.

THE PARAVENTRICULAR SYSTEM: AN HYPOTHESIS

The vagus and the DVC are remarkable for the number of functions in which they participate (Table 5). Some of these are readily predicted by a consideration of the organs that the vagus innervates; for example, 1) mediation of vagovagal reflexes relaxing the corpus of the stomach and enhancing antral motility, 2) increasing gastric and pancreatic secretion, 3) mediation of vagal chemoceptor-evoked changes in respiration, 4) decreasing cardiac output, and 5) detecting emetic stimuli in the stomach leading to the expulsion of its contents. As outlined by Andrews and Lawes in chapter 12 of this volume, however, there are many other homeostatic functions involving the vagus. Surprisingly, given the large number of functions which it subserves, the vagus is composed of a relatively small number of fibers (about 20,000). It would be of great interest to learn how so few fibers evoke so many different responses and how such complexity evolved. In particular, it is unclear how individual functions are divided among subsets of vagal fibers and/or their target neurons.

Many of the functions mediated by the vagus and its DVC are homeostatic. In mammals, they generally involve autonomic and endocrine processes, freeing somatic behavior for other purposes. In classes that evolved before mammals, however, this liberation of somatic behavior by visceral mechanisms was not always the case. In phylogenetically older classes, homeostasis is often

TABLE 5
Some Functions Involving the Vagus Nerve and its Nuclei

Arousal
Food and water intake
Taste preference
Vomiting
Gastrointestinal secretion and motility
Cardiovascular responses
Respiration
Osmoregulation
Endocrine effects

achieved by escape from, and subsequent avoidance of, suboptimal conditions. Thermoregulation in elasmobranchs is an example; sharks, lacking the heat dissipating and conserving mechanisms available to mammals, must swim between higher and lower temperatures to thermoregulate. For species living in brackish water, probably applicable to most vertebrate ancestral lines, osmoregulation is achieved by swimming between hypertonic sea water and hypotonic river water. In the lower classes of vertebrates, many homeostatic mechanisms are much less dependent upon central, integrative processes.

The hypothesis proposed here is that maintenance of homeostasis by escape and avoidance behavior in early vertebrates was governed by a set of anatomically identifiable nuclei in the brain. Such a collection of nuclei has been termed the "paraventricular system."[23] Evolution is, in one sense, a parsimonious process, part or all of a working mechanism often being adapted by slight changes to achieve a different end. Thus, as the central nervous system became more responsible for control of internal organs with the elaboration of the "autonomic" nervous system, peripheral nervous control became less autonomous. The brain nuclei governing escape from suboptimal conditions may thus have become the nuclei responsible for regulating internal homeostatic functions. Escape from, and avoidance of external threats, then, developed into more complex behaviors involving extensive autonomic, endocrine, and somatic responses.

Characteristically, the nuclei of the paraventricular system are subependymal or subpial; many of them have a blood-brain diffusion barrier of limited effectiveness. They contain a large variety of neuroactive compounds, some which seem to be almost exclusively distributed in the paraventricular system. Paraventricular nuclei participate in cardiovascular, respiratory, gastrointestinal, neuroendocrine, osmoregulatory, thermoregulatory and defensive processes. Their defining characteristics, however, are that they are all within two principal synapses of the DVC and that they are all connected to at least two other members of the set.[23]

It has been proposed[22] that the vagus is one of many routes into the set of nuclei whose ancient function was escape and avoidance behavior, but whose contemporary functions include the homeostatic processes that have replaced or supplemented escape and avoidance. The DVC is an integral part of this paraventricular system and as such, its functions are not only homeostatic but protective and defensive as well; its role in vomiting, conditioned taste aversion and behavioral defense[7] emphasize this. From this primordial defensive and protective system have evolved the four levels of central vagal connections recognized by Sawchenko:[46] autonomic efferent nuclei, ingestive branchial nuclei, centripetal gustatory and visceral afferent paths, and finally, the circuitry for neuroendocrine and behavioral functions. It is at these latter nodes of the system, such as in the forebrain and hypothalamus, that the more complex processes of the limbic system are brought to bear on the paraventricular system, resulting in the integration of autonomic, endocrine, protective and defensive functions in general behavior. The paraventricular system may also provide the neural substrate mediating the effect of threatening and noxious stimuli on psychosomatic phenomena.

In early vertebrates (as in modern "lower" vertebrates) homeostasis was achieved largely by behavioral means because these vertebrates lacked sufficient central control of an autonomous periphery. Control over the periphery was mediated in later vertebrates by the ironically named "autonomic nervous system" and by neuroendocrine mechanisms. This neural and neuroendocrine domination over the internal environment liberated behavioral processes to deal with the external environment. The central neural structures that gave rise to the behavioral mechanisms preceding homeostasis, according to this hypothesis, were transformed into the structures responsible for homeostasis itself. This is to be expected otherwise two independent systems would have governed the internal environment during the transition from escape-avoidance to homeostasis.

Such an evolutionary process has its disadvantages. The original neural system generated escape and avoidance in response to threatening situations. The same system in modern vertebrates still detects threatening situations and generates appropriate visceral and endocrine responses. The penalty for this, however, is that threat (or stress) of any kind, whether physiological or psychological, may create visceral and endocrine reactions that are not always advantageous.

Central nervous system involvement in a wide variety of disease states has been recognized for a very long time. Although the term psychosomatic illness, first developed in the 1930s, has been overused, it is clear that psychological factors may influence the development and natural history of many illnesses. Indeed, the cortical input to the DVC outlined earlier may help to explain these "psychological factors." It should be emphasized here, however, that central nervous involvement in disease states including peptic ulceration, hypertension and asthma, may occur at a number of *subcortical* levels, such as with nuclei of the paraventricular system.

Within the vagally related system of nuclei, whatever the code responsible for separation of functions, one from another, there are also mechanisms in place to coordinate these same functions in certain circumstances. For example, fear, anxiety and the perception of any kind of threat can, if sufficiently intense, result in disordered cardiovascular, respiratory and gastrointestinal functions, as every examination candidate knows. Hence, responses (in humans) such as vomiting, appropriate to the threat of noxious gastrointestinal stimuli, can be evoked seemingly inappropriately in response to the threat of extreme physical violence. However, a pelican with a stomach full of fish might view things differently. In its case, emptying its gastrointestinal tract of a heavy load in response to attack is entirely appropriate to its survival efforts.

PROSPECTS FOR FUTURE RESEARCH

It is clear from a perusal of Table 4, for example, that little information is yet available about central connections of some important vagal nuclei. Only much further painstaking research will fill these gaps in our knowledge. It is a hopeful sign that relevant work is appearing in the current literature, but this is an area of research that could be usefully expanded.

With the advent of new tracing technologies, our current understanding of the organization of the vagus nerve connections with central nervous structures has progressed a long way in the last few years. An initial flurry of research activity yielded a large amount of fresh information in a relatively short time. The limitations of the new techniques as they were applied to the very small, anatomically related brain nuclei discussed here, however, soon became apparent. Some current advances in tracing techniques and data analysis are beginning to provide more detailed anatomical information about the connectivity of these structures. For example, lectin- and cholera toxin-conjugated HRP, *Phaseolus vulgaris* leukoagglutinin (PHA-L) and biocytin may exhibit more limited spread than previously used tracers and provide better visualization of labeled subcellular elements. Also, progress in computer-aided image analysis and morphometry will help to refine these techniques and provide more detailed hodological information. Finally, double-labeling studies using axonal transport, along with immunohistochemical identification of endogenous neurochemicals at the light or electron microscopic levels are time-consuming but powerful ways of approaching the problem.

Identification of neuronal connections using lesioning techniques has been hampered by the lack of selectivity of the physical means employed to produce lesions (usually coagulation or knife cuts). Toxins such as kainic acid can be used to achieve discrete lesions which destroy neuronal cell bodies but leave fibers of passage (relatively) intact.[11] Other neurotoxins exert their cytotoxic action on populations of neurons with specific uptake sites (5,7-dihydroxytryptamine for serotonergic neurons or 6-OH-dopamine for catecholaminergic neurons, for example). The use of neurotransmitter-selective lesions may well provide more evidence to unravel the complexity of neurotransmitter interactions within the paraventricular system. Another kind of approach that may be exploited is the use of functional mapping with such brain imaging techniques as radiolabeled 2-deoxyglucose uptake (Andrews *et al.*[3] and Brizzee and Mehler[8] for example, have applied this to vagal studies), and cytochrome oxidase histochemistry.[68] The most recent development in this field involves the localization of immediate-early gene products using immunohistochemistry or *in situ* hybridization. For example, many studies have now appeared in the literature which indicate that the immediate-early gene c-fos may be selectively induced in cells of the central nervous system during neuronal activity.[40]

Electrophysiological methods have already been applied to the study of central vagal pathways; future developments along these lines will certainly provide much new and valuable information. *In vivo* brain microdialysis, although technically demanding in such small brain regions as the vagal nuclei, will probably provide new insights into the organization of neurotransmitter-specific signalling in the vagal pathways.

REFERENCES

1. **Aghajanian, G.K., and Wang, R.Y.,** Habenular and other midbrain raphe afferents demonstrated by a modified retrograde tracing technique, *Brain Res.*, 122, 229-242, 1977.
2. **Altschuler, S.M., Bao, X., Bieger, D., Hopkins, D.A., and Miselis, R.R.,** Viscerotopic representation of the upper alimentary tract in the rat: Sensory ganglia and nuclei of the solitary and spinal trigeminal tracts, *J. Comp. Neurol.*, 283, 248-269, 1989.
3. **Andrews, P.L.R., Davis, C.J., Grahame-Smith, D.G., and Leslie, R.A.,** Increase in [^{3}H]-2-deoxyglucose uptake in the ferret area postrema produced by apomorphine administration or electrical stimulation of the abdominal vagus, *J. Physiol.*, 382, 187P, 1986.
4. **Angaut, P., and Brodal, A.,** The projection of the "vestibulocerebellum" onto the vestibular nuclei in the cat, *Arch. Ital. Biol.*, 105, 441-479, 1967.
5. **Basbaum, A.J., Clanton, C.H., and Fields, H.L.,** Three bulbospinal pathways from the rostral medulla of the cat: An autoradiographic study of pain modulating systems, *J. Comp. Neurol.*, 178, 209-224, 1978.
6. **Bieger, D., and Hopkins, D.A.,** Viscerotopic representation of the upper alimentary tract in the medulla oblongata in the rat: The nucleus ambiguus, *J. Comp. Neurol.*, 262, 546-562, 1987.
7. **Bizzi, E., Libretti, A., Malliani, A., and Zanchetti, A.,** Reflex chemoceptive excitation of diencephalic sham rage behavior, *Am. J. Physiol.*, 200, 923-926, 1961.
8. **Brizzee, K.R., and Mehler, W.R.,** The central nervous connections involved in the vomiting reflex, in *Nausea and Vomiting: Mechanisms and Treatment*, Davis, C.J., Lake-Bakaar, G.V., and Grahame-Smith, D.G., Eds., Springer Verlag, Berlin, 1986, 31-55.
9. **Brodal, A.,** *Neurological Anatomy In Relation to Clinical Medicine*, Oxford University Press, Oxford, 1981.
10. **Cedarbaum, J.M., and Aghajanian, G.K.,** Afferent projections to the rat locus coeruleus as determined by a retrograde tracing technique, *J. Comp. Neurol.*, 178, 1-16, 1978.
11. **Coyle, J.T., Molliver, M.E., and Kuhar, M.J.,** *In situ* injection of kainic acid: A new method for selectively lesioning neuronal cell bodies while sparing axons of passage, *J. Comp. Neurol.*, 180, 301-324, 1978.
12. **Dahlstrom, A., and Fuxe, K.,** Evidence for the existence of monoamine-containing neurons in the central nervous system, *Acta Physiol. Scand.*, 62, Suppl. 323, 1-55, 1964.

13. Fox, E.A., and Powley, T.L., Longitudinal columnar organization within the dorsal motor nucleus represents separate branches of the abdominal vagus, *Brain Res.*, 341, 269-282, 1985.

14. Holstege, G., Meiners, L., and Tan, K., Projections of the stria terminalis to the mesencephalon, pons, and medulla oblongata in the cat, *Exp. Brain Res.*, 58, 379-391, 1985.

15. Hopkins, D.A., and Holstege, G., Amygdaloid projections to the mesencephalon, pons and medulla oblongata in the cat, *Exp. Brain Res.*, 32, 529-547, 1978.

16. Kalia, M., and Mesulam, M.-M., Brainstem projections of sensory and motor components of the vagus complex in the cat. II. Laryngeal, tracheobronchial, pulmonary, cardiac and gastrointestinal branches, *J. Comp. Neurol.*, 193, 467-508, 1980.

17. King, G.W., Topology of ascending brainstem projections to nucleus parabrachialis in the cat, *J. Comp. Neurol.*, 191, 615-638, 1980.

18. King, L.S., Cellular morphology in the area postrema, *J. Comp. Neurol.*, 66, 1-21, 1937.

19. Klara, P.M., and Brizzee, K.R., Ultrastructure of the feline area postrema, *J. Comp. Neurol.*, 171, 409-432, 1977.

20. Landgraf, R., Malkinson, T., Horn, T., Veale, W.L., Lederis, K., and Pittman, Q.J., Release of vasopressin and oxytocin by paraventricular stimulation in rats, *Am. J. Physiol.*, 258, R155-R159, 1990.

21. LaVail, J.H., and LaVail, M.M., Retrograde axonal transport in the central nervous system, *Science*, 176, 1416-1417, 1972.

22. Lawes, I.N.C., The Central Connections of Area Postrema, *Symposium on the Chemoprophylaxis of Radiation Induced Vomiting*, NATO, 1985.

23. Lawes, I.N.C., The origin of the vomiting response: A neuroanatomical hypothesis, *Can. J. Physiol. Pharmacol.*, 68, 254-259, 1990.

24. Leslie, R.A., Neuroactive substances in the dorsal vagal complex of the medulla oblongata: Nucleus of the tractus solitarius, area postrema, and dorsal motor nucleus of the vagus, *Neurochem. Internat.*, 7, 191-211, 1985.

25. Leslie, R.A., Comparative aspects of the area postrema: Fine-structural considerations help to determine its function, *Cell. Mol. Neurobiol.*, 6, 95-120, 1986.

26. Leslie, R.A., Gwyn, D.G., and Hopkins, D.A., The ultrastructure of the subnucleus gelatinosus of the nucleus of the tractus solitarius in the cat, *J. Comp. Neurol.*, 206, 109-118, 1982.

27. Leslie, R.A., Gwyn, D.G., and Hopkins, D.A., The central distribution of the cervical vagus nerve and gastric afferent and efferent projections in the rat, *Brain Res. Bull.*, 8, 37-43, 1982.

28. Loewy, A.D., and Burton, H., Nuclei of the solitary tract: Efferent projections to the lower brain stem and spinal cord of the cat, *J. Comp. Neurol.*, 181, 421-450, 1978.

29. Loizu, L.A., Projections of the nucleus locus coeruleus in the albino rat, *Brain Res.*, 15, 563-566, 1969.

30. McLean, J.H., and Hopkins, D.A., Ultrastructural identification of labelled neurons in the dorsal motor nucleus of the vagus nerve following injections of horseradish peroxidase into the vagus nerve and brainstem, *J. Comp. Neurol.*, 206, 243-252, 1982.

31. Mesulam, M.-M., Tetramethylbenzidine for horseradish peroxidase neurohistochemistry: A non-carcinogenic blue reaction product with superior sensitivity for visualizing neural afferents and efferents, *J. Histochem. Cytochem.*, 26, 106-117, 1978.

32. Miura, M., and Reis, D.J., Cerebellum: A pressor response elicited from the fastigial nucleus and its efferent pathway in brainstem, *Brain Res.*, 13, 595-599, 1969.

33. Neuheuber, W.L., and Sandoz, P.A., Vagal primary afferent terminals in the dorsal motor nucleus of the rat: Are they making monosynaptic contacts on preganglionic efferent neurons?, *Neurosci. Lett.*, 69, 126-130, 1986.

34. Onai, T., Takayama, K., and Miura, M., Projections to areas of the nucleus tractus solitarii related to circulatory and respiratory responses in cats, *J. Auton. Nerv. Syst.*, 18, 163-175, 1987.

35. Price, J.L., and Amaral, D.G., An autoradiographic study of the projections of the central nucleus of the monkey amygdala, *J. Neurosci.*, 1, 1242-1259, 1981.

36. **Retzius, G.,** *Das Menschenhirn. Studien in der makroskopischen morphologie*, Norstedt, Stockholm, 1896.
37. **Ricardo, J.A., and Koh, E.T.,** Anatomical evidence of direct projections from the nucleus of the solitary tract to the hypothalamus, amygdala, and other forebrain structures in the rat, *Brain Res.*, 153, 1-26, 1978.
38. **Rinaman, L., Card, J.P., Schwaber, J.S., and Miselis, R.R.,** Ultrastructural demonstration of a gastric monosynaptic vagal circuit in the nucleus of the solitary tract in rat, *J. Neurosci.*, 9, 1985-1996, 1989.
39. **Rogers, R.C., Kita, H., Butcher, L.L., and Novin, D.,** Afferent projections to the dorsal motor nucleus of the vagus, *Brain Res. Bull.*, 5, 365-373, 1980.
40. **Sagar, S.M., Sharp, F.R., and Curran, T.,** Expression of c-fos protein in brain: Metabolic mapping at the cellular level, *Science*, 240, 1328-1331, 1988.
41. **Saigal, R.P., Karamanlidis, A.N., Voogd, J., Micheloudi, H., and Mangana, O.,** Cerebellar afferents from motor nuclei of cranial nerves, the nucleus of the solitary tract, and nuclei coeruleus and parabrachialis in sheep, demonstrated with retrograde transport of horseradish peroxidase, *Brain Res.*, 197, 200-206, 1980.
42. **Sakai, K., Touret, M., Salvert, D., Leger, L., and Jouvet, M.,** Afferent projections to the cat locus coeruleus as visualized by the horseradish peroxidase technique, *Brain Res.*, 119, 21-41, 1977.
43. **Saper, C.B.,** Convergence of autonomic and limbic connections in the insular cortex of the rat, *J. Comp. Neurol.*, 210, 163-173, 1982.
44. **Saper, C.B., and Loewy, A.D.,** Efferent connections of the parabrachial nucleus in the rat, *Brain Res.*, 197, 291-317, 1980.
45. **Saper, C.B., Loewy, A.D., Swanson, L.W., and Cowan, W.M.,** Direct hypothalamo-autonomic connections, *Brain Res.*, 117, 305-312, 1976.
46. **Sawchenko, P.E.,** Central connections of the sensory and motor nuclei of the vagus nerve, *J. Auton. Nerv. Sys.*, 9, 13-26, 1983.
47. **Sawchenko, P.E., and Swanson, L.W.,** The organization of noradrenergic pathways from the brainstem to the paraventricular and supraoptic nuclei in the rat, *Brain Res. Rev.*, 4, 275-325, 1982.
48. **Schwaber, J.S., Kapp, B.S., and Higgins, G.,** The origin and extent of direct amygdala projections to the region of the dorsal motor nucleus of the vagus and the nucleus of the solitary tract, *Neurosci. Lett.*, 20, 15-20, 1980.
49. **Schwaber, J.S., Kapp, B.S., Higgins, G.A., and Rapp, P.R.,** Amygdaloid and basal forebrain direct connections with the nucleus of the solitary tract and the dorsal motor nucleus, *J. Neurosci.*, 2, 1424-1438, 1982.
50. **Shapiro, R.E., and Miselis, R.R.,** The central neural connections of the area postrema of the rat, *J. Comp. Neurol.*, 234, 344-364, 1985.
51. **Shipley, M.T.,** Insular cortex projection to the nucleus of the solitary tract and brainstem visceromotor regions in the mouse, *Brain Res. Bull.*, 8, 139-148, 1982.
52. **Somana, R., and Walberg, F.,** Cerebellar afferents from the nucleus of the solitary tract, *Neurosci. Lett.*, 11, 41-47, 1979.
53. **Swanson, L.W.,** Immunohistochemical evidence for a neurophysin-containing autonomic pathway arising in the paraventricular nucleus of the hypothalamus, *Brain Res.*, 128, 346-353, 1977.
54. **Swanson, L.W., and Kuypers, H.G.J.M.,** The paraventricular nucleus of the hypothalamus: Cytoarchitectonic subdivisions and the organization of projections to the pituitary, dorsal vagal complex and spinal cord as demonstrated by retrograde fluorescence double labeling methods, *J. Comp. Neurol.*, 194, 555-570, 1980.
55. **Taber, E.,** The cytoarchitecture of the brainstem of the cat. 1. Brainstem nuclei of the cat, *J. Comp. Neurol.*, 116, 27-69, 1961.
56. **Takeuchi, Y., Matsushima, S., Matsushima, R., and Hopkins, D.A.,** Direct amygdaloid projections to the dorsal motor nucleus of the vagus nerve: A light and electron microscopic study in the rat, *Brain Res.*, 280, 143-147, 1983.

57. **Taylor, A.C., and Weiss, P.,** Demonstration of axonal flow by the movement of tritium-labeled protein in mature optic nerve fibers, *Proc. Natl. Acad. Sci.* (USA), 54, 1521-1527, 1965.

58. **ter Horst, G.J., Luiten, P.G.M., and Kuipers, F.,** Descending pathways from hypothalamus to dorsal motor vagus and ambiguus nuclei in the rat, *J. Auton. Nerv. Syst.*, 11, 59-75, 1984.

59. **Terreberry, R.R., and Neafsey, E.J.,** Rat medial frontal cortex: A visceral motor region with a direct projection to the solitary nucleus, *Brain Res.*, 278, 245-249, 1983.

60. **Van der Kooy, D., Koda, L.Y., McGinty, J.F., Gerfen, C.R., and Bloom, F.E.,** The organization of projections from the cortex, amygdala, and hypothalamus to the nucleus of the solitary tract in rat, *J. Comp. Neurol.*, 224, 1-24, 1984.

61. **Veening, J.G., Swanson, L.W., and Sawchenko, P.E.,** The organization of projections from the central nucleus of the amygdala to brainstem sites involved in central autonomic regulation: A combined retrograde transport-immunohistochemical study, *Brain Res.*, 303, 337-357, 1984.

62. **Wan, X.S.T., Trojanowski, J.Q., and Gonatas, J.O.,** Cholera toxin and wheat germ agglutinin conjugates as neuroanatomical probes: Their uptake and clearance, transganglionic, and retrograde transport and sensitivity, *Brain Res.*, 243, 215-224, 1982.

63. **Willett, C.J., Gwyn, D.G., Rutherford, J.G., and Leslie, R.A.,** Cortical projections to the nucleus of the tractus solitarius: An HRP study in the cat, *Brain Res. Bull.*, 16, 497-505, 1986.

64. **Willett, C.J., Rutherford, J.G., Gwyn, D.G., and Leslie, R.A.,** Projections between the hypothalamus and the dorsal vagal complex in the cat: An HRP and autoradiographic study, *Brain Res. Bull.*, 18, 63-71, 1987.

65. **Wilson, J.T.,** On the anatomy of the calamus region in the human bulb with an account of the hitherto undescribed nucleus postremus, *J. Anat. Physiol.*, 40, 210-241, 1906.

66. **Wislocki, G.B., and LeDuc, E.H.,** Vital staining of the hematoencephalic barrier by silver nitrate and trypan blue, and cytological comparisons of neurohypophysis, pineal body, area postrema, intercolumnar tubercle and supraoptic crest, *J. Comp. Neurol.*, 96, 371-413, 1952.

67. **Wislocki, G.B., and Putnam, T.J.,** Note on the anatomy of the areae postremae, *Anat. Rec.*, 19, 281-287, 1920.

68. **Wong-Riley, M.T.,** Cytochrome oxidase: An endogenous marker for neuronal activity, *Trends Neurosci.*, 12, 94-101, 1989.

69. **Zheng, Z.H., Dietrichs, E., and Walberg, F.,** Cerebellar afferent fibres from the dorsal motor vagal nucleus in the cat, *Neurosci. Lett.*, 32, 113-118, 1982.

Chapter 5

CENTRAL REGULATION OF BRAINSTEM GASTRIC VAGO-VAGAL CONTROL CIRCUITS

R.C. Rogers and G.E. Hermann

TABLE OF CONTENTS

LIST OF ABBREVIATIONS

5HT = serotonin
BST, BNST = bed nucleus of the stria terminalis
CNA = central nucleus of the amygdala
DMN = dorsal motor nucleus of the vagus
DVC = dorsal vagal complex
NA = nucleus ambiguus
nRO = nucleus raphe obscurus
NST = nucleus of the solitary tract
PVH, PVN = paraventricular nucleus of the hypothalamus
SST = somatostatin
TRH = thyrotropin releasing hormone

EXTERNAL SENSORY EVENTS AND THE CONTROL OF THE GASTROINTESTINAL TRACT: AN INTRODUCTION

Physicians and natural scientists have probably always suspected that events external to the organism have a profound influence on the efficiency of digestive processes.[10] Indeed, it is a rare individual who does not associate the effects of different emotional states with the elicitation of diarrhea, gastric acid reflux, or gastrointestinal pain. These suspicions were validated during the nineteenth and early twentieth centuries by pioneering investigators such as Beaumont,[7] Pavlov,[68] Cannon,[12,13,14] Cannon and Leib.[15] Their work provided the basis for the earliest empirical understanding of the adaptive value of central neural modulation of gastrointestinal performance.

Cannon, in particular, provided support for the notion that rapid and effective control of the digestive apparatus by the brain is important to the survival of organisms. Most hunting animals, including man in the wild, must pursue, capture, kill, consume and assimilate nutrients quickly in order to avoid predation themselves.[12-15] In hunting animals, sustained aggression is a necessary part of the act of pursuing a meal. It follows that the efficiency of digestion could be maximized if the external stimuli which provoke the aggressive behaviors necessary for prey capture could also be used by the brain to initiate the process of digestion.[2] Cannon's experiments on the effects of aggression-provoking stimuli on autonomic functions provided evidence that events which produce sustained hostility are associated with an increase in gastric motility and secretion.[12-15] Such a neurological sharing of exteroceptive information produces a system which anticipates the arrival of nutrients in the gastrointestinal tract by incrementing digestive processes.[102]

Pavlov[68] and Cannon and Lieb,[15] also have demonstrated clearly that the central nervous system exerts considerable anticipatory control over digestive processes. In the classical conditioning paradigm, exterosensory events related to the imminent initiation of ingestion and digestion (i.e., sight, smell, auditory signals, taste) are powerful initiators of salivation, fundic (receptive) relaxation, antral contractions, gastric secretion, pancreatic endocrine and exocrine secretion as well as changes in the overall motility patterns of the intestine. On the other hand, foraging and hunting animals often (and quite suddenly) become the object of predation or attack while ingesting a meal. When faced with such a threat, the organism must prepare either to fight or flee and to suppress the digestive process at once. The termination of gastrointestinal function is essential if skeletal muscle blood flow is to be maximized to meet the threat.

Beaumont,[7] Cannon,[12,13,15] and Wolf and Wolf[112] provide conclusive evidence that if the brain's interpretation of external sensory events elicits fear, gastrointestinal motility and secretion will show suppression proportional to the degree of the fear response. These observers also noted that stimuli which provoke hostility, resentment or attack were associated with increased motility and secretion. On the basis of these observations, Cannon concluded that the autonomic changes induced in gastrointestinal function were essential parallels to the cognitive appreciation of external stimuli as threatening or rewarding. Thus, even in modern human society, the appreciation of an environment as threatening or fear producing may be expected to evoke a suppression of digestive function. Likewise, stimuli evoking hostility, attack or the desire to feed may provoke an increase in digestive efficiency in anticipation of tearing into either an "enemy" or the paper of a scientific rival; one's prey or a meal in a five-star restaurant.

This adaptation of gastrointestinal function by the central nervous system results from the modulation of "lower-level" circuits in the caudal medulla whose main function is the reflexive control of the digestive process.

NERVOUS CONTROL OF THE STOMACH: INTRINSIC INNERVATION AND VAGO-VAGAL INFLUENCES

The stomach, indeed the entire digestive system, is endowed with its own division of the autonomic nervous system, the enteric plexus.[113,114] This extensive neuronal network is located between the mucosa and the circular and longitudinal muscle layers of the abdominal viscera. It is capable of regulating a limited array of functions independent of any connection with the central nervous system. For example, the enteric plexal neuronal network is fully capable of generating periodic increases and decreases in digestive tract motility and secretion in absence of any connections with the brain or spinal cord.[113,114] It is now clear that the enteric plexus is not a simple post-ganglionic relay between the central nervous system and effector tissues in the gut. Rather, it is an independent, sensorimotor programmer of local gastrointestinal events. Although this plexus is capable of limited independent regulatory function, it is equally clear that vagal efferent preganglionic input to the plexus provides the overall coordination and control over the proximal gastrointestinal tract. This overall controlling input from the central nervous system is essential to the rapid changes induced in digestive function by feeding, or by the appreciation of provocative environmental stimuli[21,111] (Figures 1 and 2).

Much of the basic central neural circuitry coordinating gastrointestinal function involves the vago-vagal interconnections of the nucleus of the solitary tract (NST) with the dorsal motor nucleus of the vagus (DMN)[31] and the nucleus ambiguus (NA) in the caudal medulla.[18,49,66,117] The NST receives first-order sensory input from the special and general visceral divisions of the cranial nerves VII, IX and X.[19] Of interest to this review is the fact that vagal chemosensory and mechanosensory afferent axons terminate in a region of the NST which lies directly above the gastric division of the dorsal motor nucleus.[5,31,49,74,75] This area of the NST projects, in turn, to the subjacent gastric-DMN.[31,65,80] The final common pathway to the stomach emanates primarily from the medial part of the DMN.[27] This vagal-NST-DMN connection probably carries viscero-gastric vago-vagal reflexes.[5,31] A similar reflexive

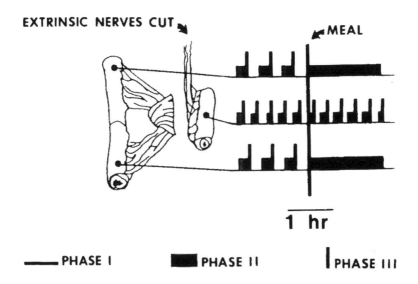

FIGURE 1. The migrating myoelectric complex is an example of a periodic gastrointestinal motility function that is entirely mediated by the enteric plexus of the bowel. This schematic diagram shows that the extrinsically denervated bowel segment on the right maintains an orderly resting motility pattern (phase I = a non-motile state, phase II = a segmenting state, phase III = propulsive contractions). Note, however, that the rapid conversion of the contractile state of the bowel to a pattern of continuous segmentation seen following a meal is entirely dependent on intact extrinsic autonomic innervation (segment on the left). (Redrawn from Sarr, MG, and Kelly, KA, *Gastroenterology*, 81, 303-310, 1981, and AGA Undergraduate Teaching Project Unit 20.)

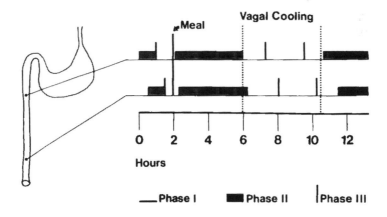

FIGURE 2. Illustration of the primary importance of the vagus in coordinating the overall motility state of the gut in response to abrupt changes in behavior (feeding). Reversible conduction block (cooling) of the vagus nerves results in the complete disruption of overall central control over gastrointestinal motility. The motility pattern that remains after vagal block is the resting periodic migrating myoelectric complex activity, elaborated by the enteric plexus. (Redrawn from Hall, KE, *et al.*, *Am. J. Physiol.*, 243, G276-284, 1982, and AGA Undergraduate Teaching Project Unit 20.)

connection between the NST and NA has been demonstrated anatomically [8,65] and may be involved with the control of the esophagus and proximal stomach.[31]

Having two types of efferent vagal input to the stomach, excitatory and inhibitory, allows for a considerable range of control over gastric function by visceral (vagal) reflex inputs. The excitatory vagal-enteric input to smooth muscle and secretory epithelial effector cells is principally cholinergic. Inhibitory vagal input to the stomach is neither adrenergic or cholinergic; it is likely that either adenosine or peptide-containing neurons in the enteric plexus mediate this powerful inhibitory vagal input to the stomach[30] (Figure 3). No clearly defined histological segregation of excitatory or inhibitory "clusters" of preganglionic vagal neurons has been made to date. In fact, electrical stimulation of subpopulations of gastric vagal efferents in the DMN evokes a mixed pattern of excitatory and inhibitory vagal influences over the stomach.[89] However, a number of physiological studies have clearly shown that this mixed excitatory/inhibitory vagal input to the stomach is not functionally random. Specific, identifiable visceral sensory inputs evoke the appropriate activation of the

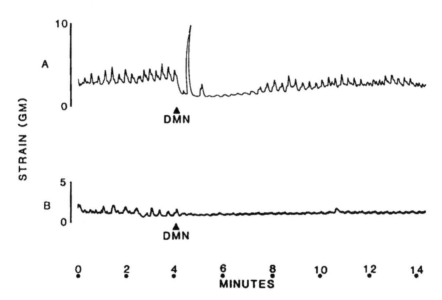

FIGURE 3. Demonstration of the existence of non-cholinergic vagal efferent innervation of the stomach. A miniature extraluminal strain gauge is placed on the corpus of the stomach to measure the contractile state of gastric circular smooth muscle. *A:* control stimulation of the DMN (10 μA, 10 Hz, 0.3 msec. for 2 sec) before atropine methyl nitrate treatment. Note sharp phasic contraction superimposed on marked reduction in gastric tone and motility. *B:* Effects of the same DMN stimulation as A above after peripheral atropinization (400 μg/kg atropine methyl nitrate i.p.). Note complete absence of augmented phasic contractions which depend on the function of a muscarinic synapse and the reduction of background motility which persists. This persistent reduction in motility following DMN stimulation is evidence for a non-cholinergic gastric-vagal inhibitory pathway. (From *Peptides*, 8, 505-513, 1987. With permission.)

excitatory or the inhibitory efferent vagal population. For example, Martinson,[61] Abrahamsson,[1] and Grundy *et al.*,[34] have clearly identified esophageal, corpus, antral and intestinal mechanoreceptive afferent projections to the medulla which evoke gastric relaxation via vagal inhibitory efferents. Likewise, the coordinated and sustained high levels of gastrointestinal motility observed after feeding requires intact vagal excitatory efferent innervation of the gut.[21] Although the full nature and extent of vago-vagal reflex control of gastric function is reviewed in detail elsewhere,[31,83] the reader should appreciate that basic medullary vagal control circuits are fully capable of "bidirectional" (i.e., excitatory and inhibitory) control over the stomach and that vagal efferent projections from the DMN and NA represent the final common motor pathway between the brain and the enteric nervous system. One would predict that any descending central nervous system inputs to these basic gastric control circuits might also produce increments or reductions in gastric function.

NERVOUS CONTROL OF THE STOMACH: CENTRAL NERVOUS SYSTEM MECHANISMS

The hypothalamus and limbic system have long been associated with the overall coordination of the *milieu interieur* in response to ongoing or anticipated changes in behavior. However, until about 10 years ago, the literature describing central nervous system modulation of autonomic function consisted largely of a morass of conflicting reports (see Grijalva *et al.*,[32] for review). The almost rampant confusion about central nervous system control of autonomic functions lay in the general lack of knowledge regarding the efferent connections of the hypothalamus and limbic system on the one hand, and the afferent connections of vago-vagal reflex circuits on the other. As a consequence, a mechanistic understanding of central nervous system control over gastric function based on forebrain lesion and electrical stimulation studies alone was not possible. The situation improved dramatically in the late 1970s when a number of investigators began to apply advanced neurohistochemical and immunocytochemical tracing techniques to limbic and hypothalamic nuclei and to the autonomic preganglionic nuclei of the brainstem and spinal cord.[31,41,51,54,59,73,80,85-87,91,95,98-101,104,106,117] These neuroanatomical tracing studies revealed that the sensory and motor components of the gastric vago-vagal reflexes, (i.e., the NST and DMN) receive significant and discrete inputs from several sources (Figure 4). As a result, the notion has developed that, although basic gastric functions can be maintained by vago-vagal reflexes localized within the brainstem, these reflexes may be modulated by extrinsic central nervous system inputs to these basic control circuits. These extrinsic inputs to basic vago-vagal control circuitry are implicated in the coordination of gastric function with behavior.

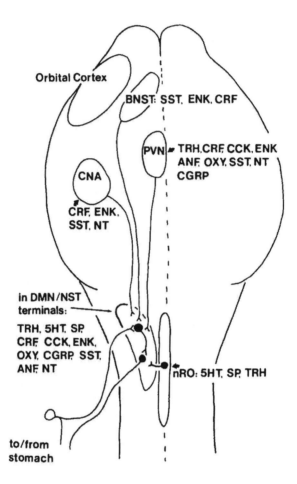

FIGURE 4. At least four major forebrain inputs to gastrointestinal/autonomic control centers in the brainstem have been identified: The bed nucleus of the stria terminalis (BNST), paraventricular nucleus of the hypothalamus, (PVN), central nucleus of the amygdala (CNA) and the orbital frontal cortex region. These four forebrain structures receive vast amounts of input from limbic and cortical regions involved in interpreting the significance of, and establishing the emotional responses to, sensory inputs from the external environment. All four areas also receive inputs from autonomic sensory "relay" nuclei such as the nucleus of the solitary tract (NST) and the parabrachial nuclei. In general then, it is believed that the BNST, CNA, PVN and certain cortical regions are critically-involved in adapting the organisms' internal state to match the current or anticipated behavioral state. A large number of putative peptide neurotransmitters may be found in at least some of these forebrain projections to the dorsal vagal complex (DVC). The peptides listed for these descending pathways have all been shown to provoke changes in gastrointestinal function when injected into the brain. This is far from an exhaustive list and one should not infer that the structures listed are the only sources of terminations in the DVC for the listed peptide or transmitter. It is very likely that peptide effects on gastrointestinal function are mediated by receptors on the sensory (NST) and motor (DMN) components of vago-vagal reflexes. Abbreviations, Anatomical structures: BNST, bed nucleus of the stria terminalis; CNA, central nucleus of the amygdala; DMN, dorsal motor nucleus of the vagus; nRO, nucleus raphe obscurus; NST, nucleus of the solitary tract.

VENTRAL FOREBRAIN INPUTS
TO VAGO-VAGAL REFLEX CIRCUITS

Three structures in the ventral forebrain, i.e., the paraventricular nucleus of the hypothalamus (PVH), the central nucleus of the amygdala (CNA), and the bed nucleus of the stria terminalis (BST), all send a considerable number of axons directly to the vagal medullary region which contains the NST as well as the DMN and NA.[45,59,85,86,95,104] Detailed anatomical studies have revealed that the PVH, CNA, and BST together form a continuous interconnected band of "pre-vagal" neurons that extends laterally from the PVH through the dorsal part of the lateral hypothalamus.[86,98] This lateral extension of the PVH is continuous with the CNA which, in turn, merges medially with the BST.[86,98] These recent anatomical observations indicate that the entire dorsal half of the lateral hypothalamus may belong to this band of forebrain, pre-vagal neurons.[86,98] Note that this hypothalamic area has long been associated with the regulation of gastric function.[48,92] By virtue of these anatomical connections, this interconnected band of three limbic-hypothalamic structures has been implicated in the control of gastric function via synaptic projections directly to the DMN, or it may change the gain of viscero-gastric vago-vagal reflexes by its direct synaptic connections with the NST.[31]

A number of investigators have recently demonstrated that injection of endogenous neuropeptides into specific cerebral nuclei or the ventricular system can greatly affect gastric function (for review, see Gillis *et al.*,[31] Morley *et al.*,[63] and Tache[102]). As a result of these studies, it is now thought that the central neural regulation of gastric function involves a delicate balance of interacting neuropeptides within the synaptic circuitry of the dorsal vagal complex (DVC).[63,77] Immunocytochemical methods indicate that the limbic and hypothalamic areas involved in the regulation of gastrointestinal function are replete with brain-gut peptides.[41,100] Numerous peptide-specific pathways from the PVH, CNA and BST are now known to terminate in the neuropil of the neurons within brainstem nuclei that represent the final common path for central control of gastric events (Figure 4). Thus, the possibility exists that specific gastrointestinal responses may be "encoded" by peptidergic projections to the DVC from PVH, CNA, BST and cortical neurons.

INFLUENCE OF PARAVENTRICULAR NUCLEUS OF THE
HYPOTHALAMUS (PVH) ON GASTRIC FUNCTIONS

Electrophysiological studies have shown that neurons of the NST which receive sensory input from the stomach via the vagus may also receive direct input from the PVH.[75,76,82] Similar electrophysiological evidence indicates an interaction between descending PVH neurons and vagal motor neurons of the DMN.[55] Microstimulation of the PVH enhances neuronal responses of NST neurons to gastric inflation (Figures 5, 6), while destruction of the PVH sharply

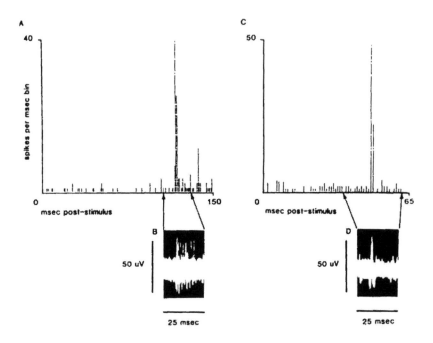

FIGURE 5. Convergence of input from the PVH and gastric vagal afferents onto single NST neurons. *A:* Post-stimulus histogram response profile of single NST neuron following stimulation of ventral gastric branch of vagus nerve (0.5 Hz, 1 ms, 200 μA, 100 trials) *B:* Oscilloscope record of same NST unit as in A, responding to stimulation of vagal branch; 10 superimposed sweeps. Record correlates with the histogram in time indicated by the arrows. *C:* Post-stimulus histogram response profile of same NST unit illustrated in A and B following microstimulation of PVH (0.5 Hz, 0.1 ms, 20 μA, 100 trials) *D:* Parallel oscilloscope traces of same NST unit responding to stimulation of PVH; 10 superimposed sweeps. Although the constancy of the NST response to PVH stimulation is suggestive of antidromic invasion of the NST, this neuron failed to follow PVH stimulation greater than a few Hz, indicating orthodromic activation of this NST unit by the PVH. (From *J. Auton. Nerv. Sys.*, 14, 351-362, 1985. With permission.)

reduces the sensitivity of the vago-vagal reflex which controls acid secretion (Figure 7). Thus, the PVH is in position to control gastric function by controlling basic vago-vagal reflex sensitivity as well as the activity of vagal efferent projections to the stomach.

Immunohistochemical tracing studies have revealed that this PVH-DVC pathway contains several peptides, including oxytocin.[23,44,95,100,117] Our studies[77-79] indicate that oxytocin is a very likely neuroeffector candidate in the regulation of gastric function by the PVH. Specifically, microstimulation of the PVH evokes increased gastric acid secretion and enhanced phasic gastric contractions, superimposed on a reduction of circular smooth muscle activity (Figures 8, 9). Picomolar injections of oxytocin into the DVC mimics the increased acid secretion and decreased tone seen following PVH stimulation (Figures 10, 11). These particular PVH-stimulation effects (i.e., enhanced gastric secretion and reduced gastric motility) are blocked by picomolar injections

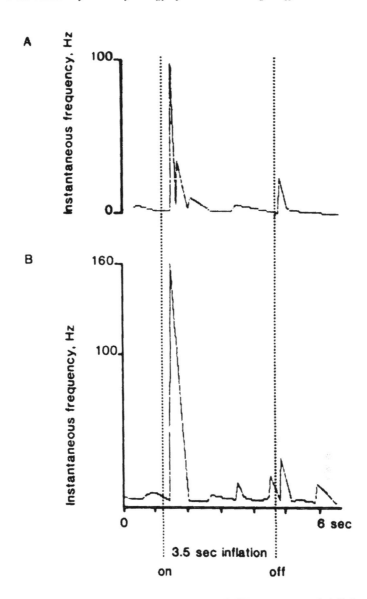

FIGURE 6. Microstimulation of PVH enhances responses of NST neurons to gastric inflation. *A:* Instantaneous frequency plot of the activity of a single medial NST neuron responding to rapid gastric inflation and deflation. Gastric inflation (3 ml air injected rapidly, held for 3.5 sec and withdrawn via indwelling catheter; max. inflation pressure of 10 cm H_2O) was delivered by digital linear actuator-based pump. Note phasic activation pattern of NST neuron activity. *B:* Instantaneous frequency plot of same NST cell as in (A) now responding to gastric inflation (as above) during simultaneous PVH microstimulation background. Half-threshold PVH stimulation (2 Hz, 0.1 ms, 10 μA) was initiated 1 min prior to the onset of gastric inflation. Note the approximate 60% increase in instantaneous firing rate compared to the control condition in A. (From *J. Auton. Nerv. Sys.*, 14, 351-362, 1985. With permission.)

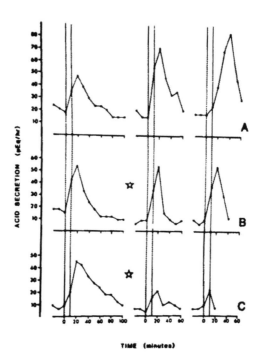

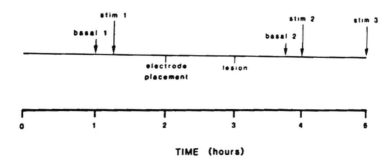

FIGURE 7. Destruction of PVH sharply reduces sensitivity of vago-vagal reflex involved in gastric acid secretion. *Upper:* Gastric acid secretion evoked by vagal afferent stimulation. Secretion results presented left to right occurred following vagal stimulation delivered at points 1, 2, and 3 as depicted in time line. Panel A—no lesion control: acid secretion following vagal afferent stimulation; Panel B—extra-PVH lesion control: acid secretion in response to vagal afferent stimulation before and after control lesion; Panel C—PVH lesion: acid secretion in response to vagal afferent stimulation before and after PVH lesion (* denotes time of lesion). *Lower:* Time-line representation of experimental stimulation sequence. Two lesion groups (PVH and extra-PVH control) were prepared for electrode placement and lesion during hours 2-3. All animals were exposed to three vagal afferent stimulation periods at the times indicated. Vagal stimulation parameters: 5V, 2 ms, 10 sec ON, 10 sec OFF. (From *J. Auton. Nerv. Sys.*, 13, 191-199, 1985. With permission.)

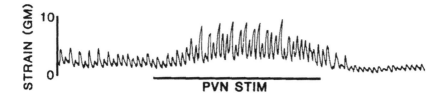

FIGURE 8. Microstimulation of PVN (20 Hz, 50 µA, 0.3 msec for 5 min; stimulation on at "PVN STIM" bar) evokes enhanced phasic gastric contractions. Note modest reduction in post-stimulus motility. (From *Peptides*, 8, 505-513, 1987. With permission.)

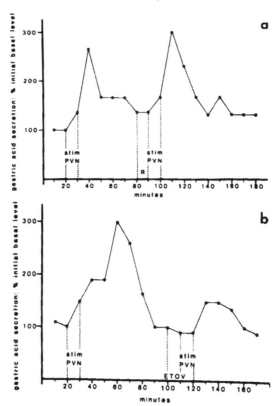

FIGURE 9. Oxytocin antagonist (ETOV) blocks effects of PVN microstimulation on gastric acid secretion. *A:* Typical control case illustrating the effect of PVN microstimulation on gastric acid output. The first PVN stimulation, at 20-30 minutes (10 Hz, 50 µA, 0.3 msec for 10 min at "stim PVN"), evokes a substantial rise in acid production. An injection of artificial CSF (5 nanoliters; at "R") into the ipsilateral DMN has no effect on the acid output evoked by a second, identical PVN stimulation ("stim PVN" at 90-100 min). *B:* Typical case illustrating the effect of the oxytocin antagonist, ETOV, on PVN stimulation-evoked gastric acid production. Although the initial PVN stimulation (same parameters as above; "stim PVN") evokes a large increase in gastric acid output, injection of ETOV (25 picomoles in 5 nanoliters artificial CSF) into the DMN greatly reduces the response to the second PVN stimulation. (From *Peptides*, 7, 695-700, 1985. With permission.)

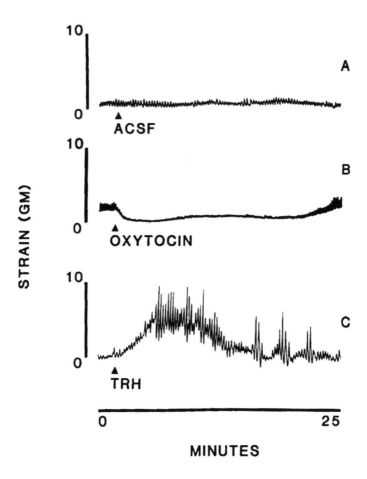

FIGURE 10. Effects on gastric motility following injections of ACSF, oxytocin, or TRH into the DMN. *A:* ACSF (2 nanoliters) *B:* oxytocin (4 picomoles in 2 nanoliters) *C:* TRH (4 picomoles in 2 nanoliters). (From *Peptides,* 8, 505-513, 1987. With permission.)

of an oxytocin antagonist into this same brainstem site (Figures 9, 12). *In vitro* studies by Dreifuss and colleagues have revealed that oxytocin has direct excitatory effects on neurons in the DMN.[17,22] Our own preliminary electro-physiological studies indicate that DVC neurons receiving input from gastric vagal mechanoreceptors are also excited by oxytocin (Figure 13). Other studies from our laboratory indicate that oxytocin inhibits gastric motility by activating non-cholinergic vagal efferent projections.[62] This notion of inhibitory PVH-oxytocin control over gastric motility is strongly supported by the work of Ricardo and Koh[71] and Verbalis *et al.,*[107] who found evidence that oxytocin release by hypothalamic neurons is a central feature in the inhibition of gastric motility observed following systemic lithium chloride and cholecystokinin administration. It is interesting to note that the pattern of gastric function

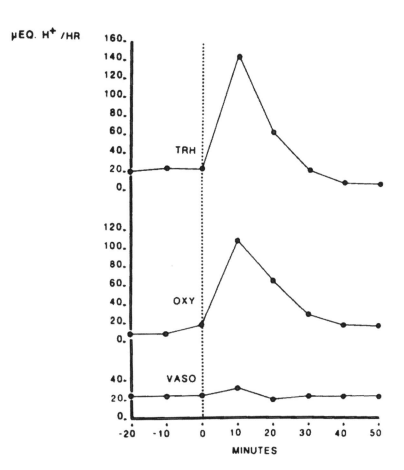

FIGURE 11. Typical time course of the gastric secretory responses following central application of TRH (11 picomoles), oxytocin (11 picomoles), or vasopressin (a structural control for oxytocin; 11 picomoles) injected into the DMN area at time "0." (From *Peptides*, 6, 1143-1148, 1985. With permission.)

changes elicited by oxytocin injections into the DVC mimic those seen immediately following the initiation of feeding. It has been recognized since Pavlov's time that the initial portion of the cephalic phase of digestion is characterized by a reduction in fundus/corpus motility and tone (receptive relaxation) and an increase in gastric secretion.[83] Perhaps those regions of the central nervous system involved in interpretating external sensory events linked to the arrival of food are using the PVH-DVC oxytocinergic pathway as a conduit to evoke the appropriate changes in gastrointestinal function.

This PVH-dorsal medullary connection has recently been implicated in the production of stress-related pathology. Thus, PVH microstimulation produces increases in gastric acid secretion and gastroduodenal erosions similar to those observed during cold and restraint.[26] Whether this PVH stimulation effect on

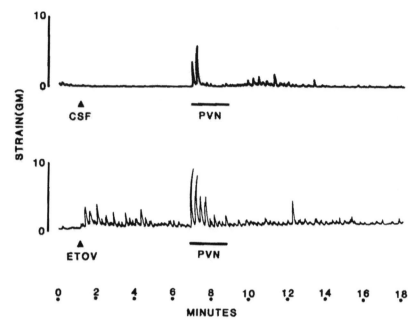

FIGURE 12. Underlying inhibitory PVN-stimulation effects on motility are blocked by picomolar injections of oxytocin antagonist (ETOV) into the DMN. *Upper* (control): effect of PVN stimulation (20 Hz, 50 μA, 0.3 msec for 2 min) on gastric motility following a control injection of artificial CSF (2 nanoliters) into the DMN. *Lower*: effect of PVN stimulation (as above) on gastric motility following an ETOV (2 nanoliter × 2 mM) injection into the DMN. Note the immediate increase in motility following the central injection of the oxytocin antagonist, as well as the augmented effect PVN stimulation has on motility. (From *Peptides*, 7, 695-700, 1985. With permission.)

gastric pathophysiology is due to the release of oxytocin into the neuropil of the DVC remains to be established.

CENTRAL NUCLEUS OF THE AMYGDALA (CNA)

Amygdalar involvement in the control of autonomic function has been appreciated for some time.[20,29,33,36,50,57,93] In particular, the CNA has been associated with augmentation of gastric acid secretion and gastric motility.[31,35,36,92] Until recently, the control of the stomach by the CNA had been explained in terms of complex interactions involving limbic, hypothalamic, reticular, and autonomic preganglionic nuclei.[35] However, anatomical data have since indicated that direct reciprocal connections exist between the CNA and regions of the DVC.[16,71,86,104,106] Recent data support the view that the CNA evaluates the "stressfulness" of aversive stimulation and coordinates visceral responses accordingly.[38]

Electrophysiological studies confirmed that the CNA does maintain direct connections with the medullary DVC.[20,73] In our experiments, NST neurons

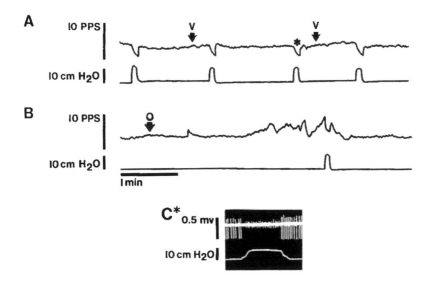

FIGURE 13. Oxytocin activates NST neurons which respond to gastric inflation. *Panel A:* rate meter record of the activity of a single NST unit's activity in response to gastric distension (see corresponding pressure record below ratemeter record) and vehicle control (artificial cerebrospinal fluid) injections (167 picoliters at "V"). Note that the applications of vehicle had no effect on the activity of the recorded cell. Asterisk (*) indicates the portion of the record from which the oscillograph record (lower panel) was taken. *Panel B:* response of the recorded unit to oxytocin (O) and gastric distension. Delayed activation of DVC neurons by this peptide (as seen here) has also been reported in *in vitro* preparations.[22] Note that oxytocin elevates the firing rate for the recorded NST unit but does not alter the basic response to inflation.

were identified by their response to cervical vagal stimulation. In turn, CNA neurons were antidromically identified following stimulation of the identified NST population, demonstrating that a monosynaptic CNA-NST projection exists. Conversely, approximately 15% of identified NST cells were orthodromically activated by CNA stimulation. Thus, these NST neurons were receiving convergent input from the vagus and CNA. Such reciprocal connections between these nuclei could put this limbic structure in position to process internal visceral sensory cues and then alter a variety of autonomic functions by changing the setpoint or gain of autonomic reflexes. The CNA could accomplish this by altering the excitability of NST or DMN neurons in a manner similar to that described for the PVH-DVC pathway.[75,76]

A substantial number of somatostatin (SST)-containing neurons exist in the CNA, and these cells appear to maintain a long, descending connection with neurons in the DVC.[16,51,73,85,104,106] Therefore, it seems reasonable to suspect that the CNA may directly influence gastric function by activating a descending somatostatinergic pathway to the DVC region. This hypothesis is generally supported by the observation that intracerebroventricular injections of SST evoke increases in duodenal motility.[9]

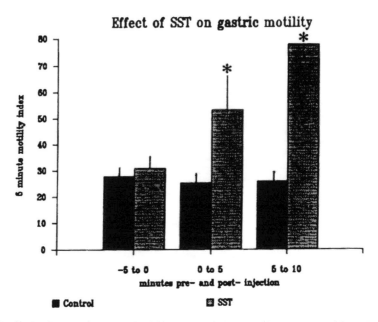

FIGURE 14. Injection of somatostatin (SST; 5 picomoles in 5 nanoliters) into the DMN evokes a significant increase in gastric motility relative to the motility seen following injection of artificial CSF (5 nanoliters) (* = $p < 0.05$, Sign test). (From *Neurosci. Abs.*, 13, 204.16, 1987. With permission.)

If a somatostatinergic path between the CNA and dorsal medulla is responsible for increases in gastric motility, then the injection of small amounts of SST into the DMN area should markedly increment gastric motility. Also, if a CNA-dorsal medullary somatostatinergic path controls gastric motility, then increases in motility induced by microstimulation of the CNA should be blocked by an antagonist of SST action (i.e., cyclo[7-aminoheptanoyl-Phe-d-Trp-Lys-Thr-(oBzl)] or CPP1, from Bachem Labs).[28]

Microinjection of SST (5 picomoles) into the DMN region does evoke phasic gastric contractions (Figure 14). This increase in gastric motility can be mimicked by microstimulation of the CNA and can be completely abolished by systemic pretreatment with atropine methyl nitrate, which suggests that a muscarinic synapse is required for the elaboration of this effect.[40] Similar injections of SST into the DVC also evoke significant elevations in gastric acid secretion (Figure 15). Additionally, when the SST antagonist (i.e., CPP1) is injected into the DMN prior to CNA microstimulation, subsequent CNA-induced changes in gastric motility are reduced (Figure 16). Thus, these data suggest that a somatostatinergic projection between the limbic forebrain and the dorsal vagal nuclei may play a role in regulating parasympathetic input to the stomach.[40]

The precise mechanism of SST effects on the dorsal medullary neurons which control gastric function are unknown. The issue is confused by a number of reports which demonstrate seemingly contradictory roles for SST as a central

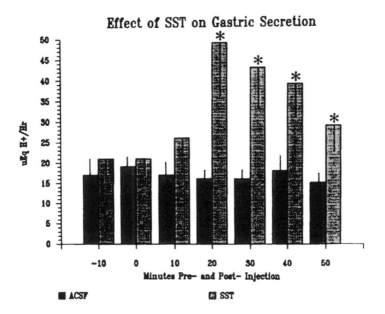

FIGURE 15. Injection of SST (5 picomoles in 5 nanoliters) into the DMN evokes a marked increase in gastric acid secretion relative to secretion levels seen after injection of artificial CSF (5 nanoliters) (* = $p < 0.05$, Sign test). (From *Neurosci Abs.*, 13, 204.16, 1987. With permission.)

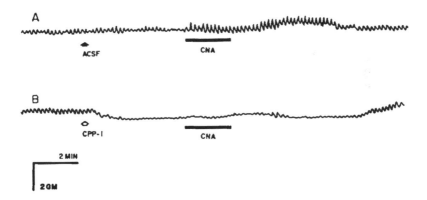

FIGURE 16. Effects on gastric motility following microstimulation of CNA. *A*: Changes in gastric motility and circular muscle tone evoked by injection of artificial CSF (ACSF; 5 nanoliter) into the DMN, followed 5 minutes later by electrical stimulation of the CNA (25 Hz, 50 μA, 0.3 msec for 2 min). *B*: Reduction in gastric tone and motility evoked by injection of SST antagonist (CPP-1; 5 picomoles in 5 nanoliters) into the DMN also suppresses motility increases normally elicited by microstimulation of CNA. (From *Neurosci. Abs.*, 13, 204.16, 1987. With permission.)

effector substance. For example, SST has been observed to both increase[60,64] and decrease[68,110] the excitability of central neurons through a variety of mechanisms. Thus, an apparent increase in parasympathetic outflow to the stomach may be the result of (a) direct, excitatory action on the efferent vagal neurons, (b) indirect presynaptic facilitation, or, (c) disinhibition. Intracellular recordings from known gastric efferent neurons will be required to determine which mechanism is responsible for this change in parasympathetic efferent activity.

BED NUCLEUS OF THE STRIA TERMINALIS (BST)

As mentioned above, anatomical studies have revealed that the PVH, CNA and the BST together form a continuous interconnected band of "pre-vagal" neurons.[45,71,86,98] Like the PVH and CNA, the BST makes direct projections to nuclei of the DVC.[45] Thus, it is reasonable to suspect that this nucleus may also be involved in the potential modulation of vagally mediated gastric function.

Preliminary work from our laboratory indicates that microstimulation of the BST elicits an increase in contractility and/or tone of the gastric musculature. This increase in gastric activity can be mimicked by micropressure injections of glutamate into the BST and can be abolished following systemic administration of atropine methyl nitrate[39] (Figure 17).

Immunohistochemical studies on the distribution of neuropeptides reveals that cell bodies and fibers in the BST contain SST, enkephalin and corticotropin-releasing factor as well as fibers which contain thyrotropin releasing hormone (TRH) and bombesin[3,23,87,101,108,115] oxytocin and vasopressin.[11,105] These neurochemicals have also been localized to terminal endings within the NST and DMN.[3,11,23,44,87,101,105,108,115] It remains to be seen, however, which of these neurochemical candidates from the BST may be responsible for modulating gastric functions.

CEREBRAL CORTEX

Cortical influence on autonomic systems has been known for some time.[47,58,94,109] It has long been recognized that emotions and stress have a powerful influence on gastrointestinal motility, and cortical involvement in the process is very likely. For example, gastrointestinal activity is normally dramatically reduced in response to fear-inducing stimulation.[13,112] Data from electrical stimulation and lesion studies suggest that the cortex exerts an inhibitory influence on ongoing gastrointestinal activity[4,24,43,90,96,97] in a manner similar to that observed following fear-inducing stimulation.

Anatomical studies have recently indicated the existence of direct projections from the infralimbic and insular cortex (also referred to as the "visceral sensory and motor" cortex) to the medullary DVC.[46,84,91,103,104] Given that this area of the medial frontal cortex is considered to be part of the limbic system,[103] its direct connections with the medullary DVC may provide a conduit through

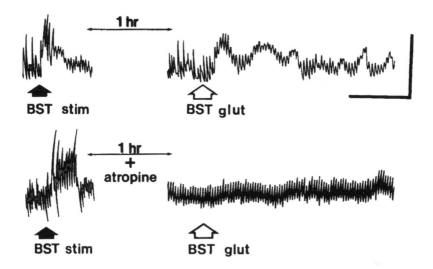

FIGURE 17. Bed nucleus of the stria terminalis (BST) and gastric contractility. *Upper Panel:* Electrical microstimulation of the BST (100 μA, 20 Hz, 0.5 msec, 20 sec at dark arrow) produces an abrupt increase in gastric contractility measured by extraluminal miniature strain gauges. One hour later, an injection of glutamate (2 nanomole in 2 nanoliters) via a micropipette in parallel with the metal stimulation electrode also elicits an increase in gastric contractility. This result shows that the activation of cell bodies in the BST produces an increase in gastric contractility. *Lower Panel:* peripheral atropinization with atropine methyl nitrate (400 μg/kg, i.p.) eliminates the effect of glutamate in the BST on gastric motility. This result implicates vagal efferent connections with muscarinic neurons in the enteric plexus as the final pathway between the BST and gastric circular smooth muscle. (From *Neurosci. Abs.*, 14, 217.8, 1988. With permission.)

which various emotions may attenuate ongoing gastrointestinal function and, ultimately, may also be responsible for the development of stress-induced gastric ulcers.[38]

RECAPITULATION: PERCEPTION OF EXTERNAL EVENTS AND FOREBRAIN CONTROL OVER GASTROINTESTINAL FUNCTION

We have seen that a distinct cortical region and three interrelated ventral forebrain structures provide a substantial amount of input to gastric vago-vagal control circuits of the dorsal medulla. Peptide-containing neural pathways from these forebrain structures may modulate vagal control of the stomach by directly influencing the excitability of vagal efferent neurons in the DMN. These same pathways may also affect the gain and/or setpoint of the reflex control of gastric function by altering the excitability of second order visceral relay neurons in the NST. These findings provide insight into the means by which forebrain structures alter vagal control of the stomach. However, the mechanism by which the brain converts perceptions of the outside world into appro-

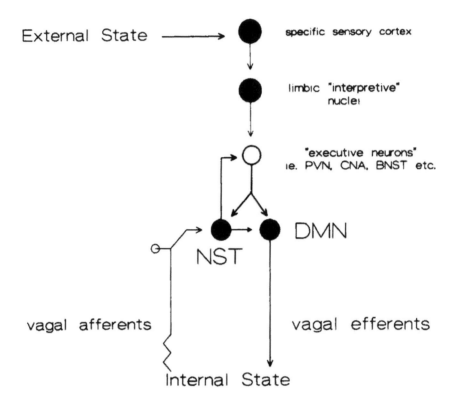

FIGURE 18. Schematic diagram of the proposed relationship between exterosensory systems, limbic "interpretive" circuits, forebrain autonomic "executive" areas and the central components of vago-vagal reflexes. Forebrain "executive" areas, such as the BST, central amygdala and paraventricular hypothalamus, are in a unique position to evaluate the state of the *"milieu interieur"* (by virtue of inputs from brainstem visceral afferent pathways) as well as the current or anticipated behavioral state (via input from limbic nuclei whose function is to evaluate the significance of exteroceptive signals). These executive nuclei are capable of altering the internal state, including gastrointestinal functions, to accommodate the behavioral state of the organism.

priate autonomic function has not been addressed, largely because the process is, at best, poorly understood. Fortunately, the hodology of these forebrain structures which control gastric vago-vagal circuits has been studied with advanced tracing methods. Based on these anatomical data, one can now construct at least a rough outline of how the brain may maintain the *milieu interieur* by making appropriate autonomic responses to changes in the environment.

Extensive anatomical studies provide convincing evidence that the orbital cortical region, the PVH, CNA and BST all receive a substantial amount of information from complex cortical sensory processing regions as well as from limbic structures thought to be involved in assigning significance to sensory inputs.[70] Additionally, the PVH, CNA, BST and orbital cortex receive a large amount of afferent input from visceral sensory "relays," the NST and parabrachial nuclei.[70,99] As stated before, these forebrain structures also send neural projections to the NST and the preganglionic autonomic neurons in the DMN. Given this arrangement, the orbital cortex, PVH, CNA and BST emerge as autonomic "executive" nuclei. It is possible that these structures are kept informed of the current state of the *milieu interieur* as well as the perceived status of the organism in the environment (i.e., threatened, presented with an opportunity to feed, etc.). Should an "error signal" result from the comparison between current (or expected) external events and the current status of the autonomic nervous system, these forebrain "executive" nuclei are in a position to alter the internal state accordingly (Figure 18). Obviously, a substantial amount of behavioral and physiological work will be necessary to convert this speculative model into a framework for the understanding of central autonomic control.

BRAINSTEM INPUTS TO VAGO-VAGAL REFLEX CIRCUITS: NUCLEUS RAPHE OBSCURUS (nRO) AND THE DIURNAL REGULATION OF GASTRIC FUNCTION

Peroxidase histochemical and immunocytochemical tracing studies have revealed that the medullary raphe nuclei and neurons in the adjacent reticular formation are sources of a significant amount of afferent input for the NST and DMN. Although little is known about the nature of reticular formation control over gastric function, the nucleus raphe obscurus (nRO) in the caudal medulla is emerging as an important modulator of vagal gastrointestinal control circuits. Activation of the nRO by either electrical microstimulation or microinjections of glutamate evokes a significant increase in gastric motility and tone[62] (Figure 19). This nRO-induced effect is probably due to the activation of cholinergic DMN efferent projections to the stomach because peripheral muscarinic blockade eliminates nRO stimulation-evoked changes in gastric contractility. Preliminary electrophysiological data indicate that, like the PVH, the nRO may alter gastric functions by changing the excitability of NST neurons which form the afferent limb of vago-vagal reflexes. As Figure 20 shows, NST neurons activated by gastric inflation are strongly inhibited after stimulation of the nRO.

The triamino peptide TRH and the indolamine serotonin (5HT) are contained within the nRO-DVC projection. Indeed, 5HT and TRH have been reported to be co-localized within cell bodies of the nRO.[25,53,67] Recent data implicate both TRH and 5HT as potential neuroeffector substances involved in communication between the nRO and DVC regarding the regulation of gastric function.

TRH appears to be a potent activator of gastric motility and secretion. When amounts of TRH as small as 4 picomole are pressure injected into the DMN region, a significant increase in motility and acid secretion is evoked[60,62] (Figures 10, 11). Our electrophysiological studies on the effects of TRH on NST and DMN neuron activity reveal an interesting pattern of responses. Approximately 50% of DMN neurons tested were activated by TRH; none were inhibited.[64,81] Of NST neurons tested, approximately 50% were inhibited by TRH;

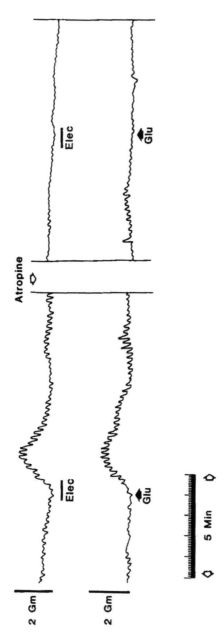

FIGURE 19. Gastric corpus strain gauge records of circular smooth muscle contractions. Electrical microstimulation (10 μA, 20 Hz, 0.5 msec for 60 sec) of the nRO or glutamate microinjections (1.7 nanomole in 17 nanoliters of vehicle) into the nRO both elicit a significant increase in contractions. The same stimuli were repeated 10 minutes after an i.p. injection of the peripheral muscarinic blocker atropine methyl nitrate. The results indicate that nRO stimulation effects on gastric motility require intact muscarinic synapses between vagal post-ganglionic neurons in the enteric plexus and gastric circular smooth muscle. (From *Brain Res.*, 486, 181-184, 1989. With permission.)

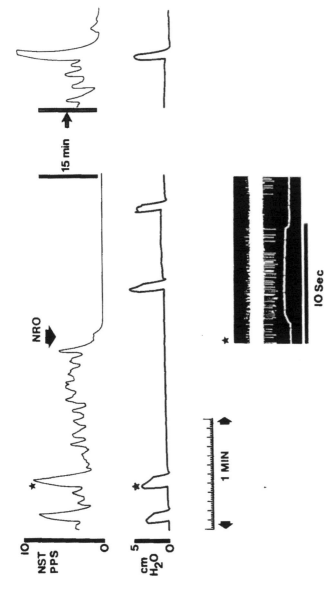

FIGURE 20. Effect of nRO microstimulation on the activity of gastric inflation-related NST neurons. Upper trace shows plot of action potential frequency vs. time illustrating the excitation of an NST neuron in response to gastric distention produced by inflating a balloon in the corpus/antrum region. Inflation pressures are shown in the middle trace. Lower trace shows the raw unit activity (top) in response to inflation (bottom) for the trial marked by the star. Note that a brief train of nRO stimulation (3 pulses, 25 µA, 0.3 msec duration at 0.5 Hz; at NRO) reduce background activity as well as activity in response to inflation. The NST unitary response to inflation returns 15 min later.

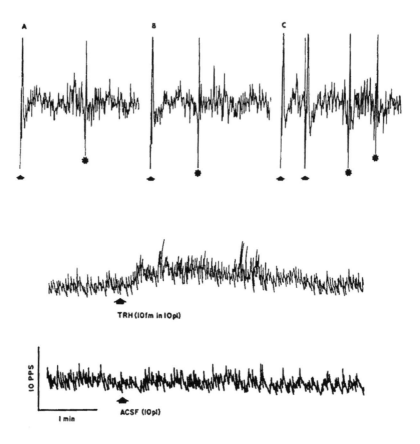

FIGURE 21. Excitatory effects of TRH on DMN neurons. *Upper:* Antidromic identification of a DMN neuron. A—antidromic response at 32 msec. B—"collision" with a spontaneously occurring spike; C—response following at high frequency (100 Hz) vagal stimulations; antidromic spike at *. (Scale bars = 100 uV/32 msec.) *Middle:* Rate-meter plot of the activity of the DMN cell identified above. Cell firing rate doubled following the micropressure injection of TRH (10 femtomoles in 10 picoliters) into the DMN region. *Lower:* Rate-meter plot of the activity of the same DMN cell following control microinjection of artificial CSF (10 picoliters) into the DMN region. (From *J. Auton. Nerv. Sys.*, 26, 107–112, 1989. With permission.)

none were excited (Figures 21–23). This differential pattern of effects on NST and DMN neurons may be important to a general understanding of central nervous system control over gastric functions. For example, the control of gastric corpus tone and motility involves an inhibitory vago-vagal reflex loop whereby antral inflation yields a reduction in corpus contractility.[1,88] Thus, we propose that when TRH is microinjected into the DVC, it activates the gastric vagal efferents in the DMN to enhance motility while, at the same time, it reduces the inhibitory component of the vagal reflex in the NST. This combination of effects on gastric vagal efferents on the one hand, and on compensatory reflexes on the other, may contribute to the large increases in gastric

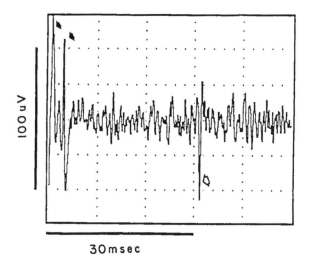

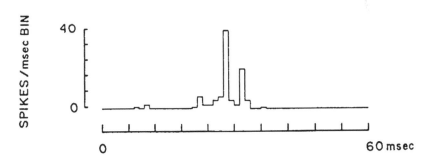

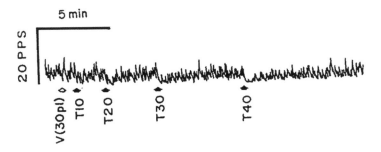

FIGURE 22. Inhibitory effects of TRH on NST neurons. *Upper:* Orthodromically identified NST neuron's response to vagal stimulation. Note failure to follow high frequency vagal stimulation pulses (arrows). *Middle:* Peristimulus histogram of the same NST neuron responding to 100 vagal stimulations. Note typical orthodromic (i.e., irregular latency) pattern of activation of the unit following vagal stimulation. *Lower:* Effects of TRH on activity pattern of the NST neuron identified above. T10-T40 = 10-40 femtomoles of TRH applied by micropressure injection represents volumes from 10-40 picoliters, respectively. Artificial CSF (V30 pl = 30 picoliters) injection had no effect on unit activity.

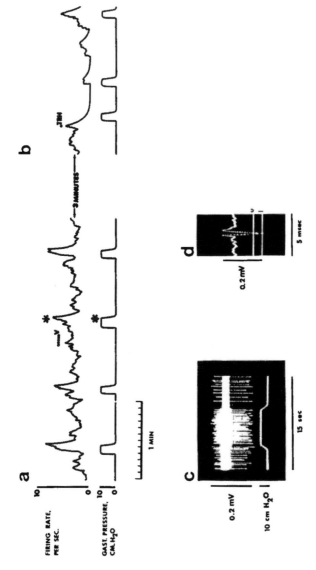

FIGURE 23. The effects of TRH on a gastric inflation-activated neuron in the NST. *a*: Rate meter and gastric distension pressure record showing the cumulative unit firing rate vs. time in response to gastric inflation. Five micropressure applications (at dots) of vehicle (V) solution (20 picoliters/dot) had no effect on the unit response to gastric inflation. *b*: Rate meter and gastric pressure record taken from the same unit three minutes later. Note that a single injection of the TRH solution (TRH at dot; 20 femtomole in 20 picoliters) produced an immediate suppression of both spontaneous activity and the activation produced by gastric inflation. *c*: Storage oscillograph tracing of the same unit's response to gastric inflation. This tracing corresponds to the firing rate/gastric pressure record marked by an asterisk (*) in panel a. *d*: Oscillograph illustrating the isolation of the single unit used to produce the tracings in panel a. u = upper window discriminator level, l = lower discriminator level. (From *J. Auton. Nerv. Sys.*, 26, 107–112, 1989. With permission.)

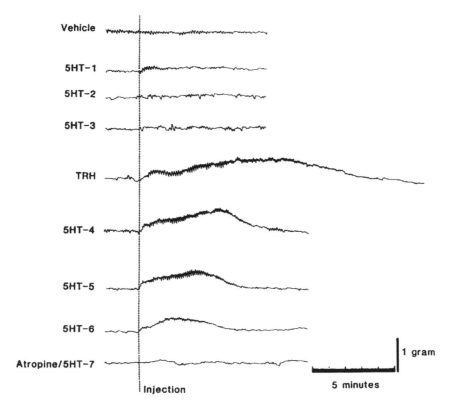

FIGURE 24. Interaction between serotonin (5HT) and TRH in the control of gastric motility by the dorsal medulla. TRH appears to augment the effectiveness of 5HT-evoked changes in gastric motility. *Vehicle*: effects on gastric motility following injection of artificial CSF (4 nanoliters) into the DMN. *5HT-1 through 3*: injection of 5HT (8 picomoles in 4 nanoliters) into the DMN at intervals of 20 min between the end of the record and the beginning of the next injection. *TRH*: application of TRH (1 nanomole in 1 microliter) onto the dorsal medulla. *5HT-4 through 6*: injection of 5HT (8 picomoles in 4 nanoliters) beginning 20 min after the end of the TRH record. *Atropine/5HT-7*: atropine methyl nitrate (1 mg/kg, s.c.) completely suppresses the gastric response to subsequent injections of 5HT into the DMN.

motility and secretion seen following application of TRH to the dorsal medulla[102] (Figure 24).

Recent studies from our laboratory[62] have demonstrated that when 5HT alone is microinjected into the DMN, a modest increase in gastric motility and circular muscle tone can be elicited (Figure 11). As shown earlier, application of TRH to the DMN evokes a massive increase in both gastric motility and tone which lasts approximately 20 minutes. If 5HT is applied to the DMN well after the primary effects of TRH on these motility indices have subsided, this subsequent exposure to 5HT results in greatly amplified effects on gastric function. This amplification of 5HT's effect by TRH is quite long-lasting, on the order of several hours. Although the mechanism by which TRH enhances the effects of 5HT is not known, long-lasting intracellular changes in a second messenger cascade have been observed after TRH administration to cultured pituitary cells.[6] Thus, it is tempting to speculate that the excitability level of neurons within the vagal nuclei can be adjusted by one neurochemical (e.g., TRH) such that the efficacy of another neurochemical (e.g., 5HT) can be regulated.

The physiological significance of the nRO input to the DVC is not known at this time. It is interesting to note, however, that the raphe nuclei, in general, appear to be involved in the transition between sleep and wakefulness.[42] Such changes in arousal are highly correlated with gross changes in gastrointestinal motility.[52,54] Thus, it is possible that the raphe nuclei control the transitions from sleep and waking as well as the associated changes in gastrointestinal function appropriate to the arousal state. The understanding of this mechanism may be significant to elucidating the causes of the arousal related onset of irritable bowel syndrome.[52,54]

SUMMARY

Nuclei of the DVC (i.e., the NST and DMN) are primary components responsible for the direct autonomic control of gastrointestinal functions. These brainstem nuclei receive direct input from the cortex, PVH, BST, CNA, and nRO of the medullary reticular area. This anatomical arrangement allows the basic vago-vagal reflex circuits in the DVC to be influenced by these extrinsic sources of neuronal input which contain a bewildering array of mediator substances. This diversity of central nervous system input may provide a variety of options to elicit different responses within the DVC and, ultimately, in gastrointestinal functions. This review gives a few examples of how different putative neurochemical agents contained in the central projections to the DVC can modify or attenuate the basic vago-vagal reflexes involved in controlling gastric function. Given that these DVC neurons are also involved in the control of other visceral autonomic functions, it is tempting to speculate that the delicate balancing of various interacting neurochemicals within the synaptic microenvironment of the DVC may be responsible for orchestrating the full array of parasympathetically controlled autonomic functions.

ACKNOWLEDGMENTS

This work was supported by NINCDS grant NS 24530 to RCR.

REFERENCES

1. **Abrahamsson, H.,** Studies on the inhibitory nervous control of gastric motility, *Acta. Physiol. Scand. (Suppl.)*, 390, 5-33, 1973.

2. **Almy, T.P.,** The gastrointestinal tract in man under stress, in *Gastrointestinal Disease*, Slesenger, M.H., and Fordtran, J.S., Eds., Saunders, New York, 1972, 3-12.

3. **Atweh, S.F., Murrin, L.C., and Kuhar, M.J.,** Presynaptic localization of opiate receptors in vagal and accessory optic systems; an autoradiographic study, *Neuropharmacology*, 17, 65-71, 1978.

4. **Babkin, B.P., and Speakman, T.J.,** Cortical inhibition of gastric motility, *J. Neurophysiol.*, 13, 55-63, 1950.

5. **Barber, W.D., and Burks, T.F.,** Brainstem response to phasic gastric distension, *Am. J. Physiol.*, 245, G242-248, 1983.

6. **Barker, J.L., Duffy, B., Harrison, N.L., Owen, D.G., and MacDonald, J.F.,** Signal transduction mechanisms in cultured CNS neurons and clonal pituitary cells, *Neuropharmacology*, 26, 941-955, 1987.

7. **Beaumont, W.,** *Experiments and Observations on Gastric Juice and the Physiology of Digestion*, Allen, Plattsburg, NY, 1833.

8. **Beckstead, R.M., Morse, J.R., and Norgren, R.,** The nucleus tractus solitarius in the monkey: Projections to the thalamus and brainstem, *J. Comp. Neurol.*, 190, 259-282, 1980.

9. **Bueno, L., and Ferre, J.P.,** Central regulation of intestinal motility by somatostatin and cholecystokinin octapeptide, *Science*, 216, 1427-1429, 1982.

10. **Cabanis, P.J.G.,** "Introduction" on the relations between the physical and moral aspects of man, 1802; translated by Saidi, M.P., and edited by Mora, G., for Johns Hopkins Univ. Press, Baltimore, MD, 1981.

11. **Caffe, A.R., and Van Leeuwen, F.W.,** Vasopressin-immunoreactive cells in the dorsomedial hypothalamic region, medial amygdaloid nucleus and locus coeruleus of the rat, *Cell Tissue Res.*, 233, 23-33, 1983.

12. **Cannon, W.B.,** The movements of the intestines studied by means of Roentgen rays, *Am. J. Physiol.*, 6, 251, 1902.

13. **Cannon, W.B.,** The influence of emotional states on the functions of the alimentary canal, *Amer. J. Med. Sci.*, 137, 480-487, 1909.

14. **Cannon, W.B.,** *Bodily Changes in Pain, Hunger, Fear and Rage*, Appleton, New York, 1929.

15. **Cannon, W.B., and Leib, C.W.,** The receptive relaxation of the stomach, *Am. J. Physiol.*, 29, 267-273, 1911.

16. **Cassell, M.D., Gray, T.S., and Kiss, J.Z.,** Neuronal architecture in the rat central nucleus of the amygdala: A cytological, hodological and immunocytochemical study, *J. Comp. Neurol.*, 246, 478-499, 1986.

17. **Charpak, S., Armstrong, W.E., Muhlethaler, M., and Dreifuss, J.J.,** Stimulatory action of oxytocin on neurones of the dorsal motor nucleus of the vagus nerve, *Brain Res.*, 300, 83-89, 1984.

18. **Coil, J., and Norgren, R.,** Cells of origin of motor axons in the subdiaphragmatic vagus of the rat, *J. Auton. Nerv. Syst.*, 1, 203-210, 1979.

19. **Contreras, R.J., Beckstead, R.M., Norgren, R.,** Central projections of trigeminal, facial glossopharyngeal, and the vagus nerves: An autoradiographic study in the rat, *J. Auton. Nerv. Syst.*, 6, 303-322, 1982.

20. **Cox, G.E., Jordan, D., Moruzzi, P., Schwaber, J.S., Spyer, K.M., and Turner, S.A.,** Amygdaloid influences on brainstem neurons in the rabbit, *J. Physiol.*, 381, 135-148, 1986.

21. **Diamont, N.E., Hall, K.E., Mui, H., and El Sharkway, T.Y.,** Vagal control of feeding motor pattern in the lower esophageal sphincter, stomach and small intestine of dog, in *Gastrointestinal Motility*, Christenson, J., Ed., Raven Press, New York, 1980, 365-390.

22. **Dreifuss, J.J., Raggenbass, M., Charpak, S., Dubois-Dauphin, M., and Tribollet, E.,** A role of central oxytocin in autonomic functions: Its action in the motor nucleus of the vagus nerve, *Brain Res. Bull.*, 20, 765-770, 1988.

23. **Elde, R., and Hokfelt, T.,** Localization of hypophysiotrophic peptides and other biologically active peptides within the brain, *Annu. Rev. Neurosci.,* 41, 587-602, 1979.

24. **Eliasson, S.,** Cerebral influence on gastric motility in cat, *Acta Physiol. Scand.,* 26 (Suppl. 95), 1-70, 1952.

25. **Eskay, R.L., Long, R.T., and Palkovits, M.,** Localization of immunoreactive thyrotropin-releasing hormone in the lower brainstem of the rat, *Brain Res.,* 277, 159-162, 1983.

26. **Ferguson, A.V., Marcus, P., Spencer, J., and Wallace, J.L.,** Paraventricular nucleus stimulation causes gastroduodenal mucosal necrosis in the rat, *Am. J. Physiol.,* 255, R861-865, 1988.

27. **Fox, E.A., and Powley, T.L.,** Longitudinal columnar organization within the dorsal motor nucleus represents separate branches of abdominal vagus, *Brain Res.,* 341, 269-282, 1985.

28. **Fries, J.L., Murphy, W.A., Sueiras-Diaz, J., and Coy, D.H.,** Somatostatin antagonist analog increases GH, insulin and glucagon release in the rat, *Peptides,* 3, 811-814, 1982.

29. **Gebber, G.L., and Klevans, L.R.,** Central nervous system control of cardiovascular reflexes, *Fed. Proc.,* 31, 1245-1252, 1972.

30. **Gillespie, J.S.,** Non-adrenergic, non-cholinergic inhibitory control of gastrointestinal motility, in *Motility of the gastrointestinal tract,* Weinbeck, M., Ed., Raven Press, New York, 1982, 51-66.

31. **Gillis, R.A., Quest, J.A., Pagani, F.D., and Norman, W.P.,** Control centers in the central nervous system for regulating gastrointestinal motility, in *Handbook of Physiology,* Wood, J.D., Ed., American Physiological Society, Bethesda, MD, 1988.

32. **Grijalva, C.V., Lindholm, E., and Novin, D.,** Physiological and morphological changes in the gastrointestinal tract induced by hypothalamic intervention: An overview, *Brain Res. Bull.,* 5 (Suppl. 1), 19-31, 1980.

33. **Grijalva, C.V., Tache, Y., Gunion, M.W., Walsh, J.H., and Geiselman, P.J.,** Amygdaloid lesions attenuate neurogenic gastric mucosal erosions but do not alter gastric secretory changes induced by intercisternal bombesin, *Brain Res. Bull.,* 16, 55-61, 1986.

34. **Grundy, D., Salih, A.A., and Scratcherd, T.,** Modulation of vagal efferent fiber discharge by mechanoreceptors in the stomach, duodenum and colon of the ferret, *J. Physiol.,* 319, 43-52, 1981.

35. **Henke, P.G.,** The hypothalamus-amygdala axis and experimental gastric ulcers, *Neurosci. Biobehav. Rev.,* 3, 75-82, 1979.

36. **Henke, P.G.,** The telencephalic limbic system and experimental gastric pathology: A review, *Neurosci. Biobehav. Rev.,* 6, 381-390, 1982.

37. **Henke, P.G.,** Recent studies of the central nucleus of the amygdala and stress ulcers, *Neurosci. Biobehav. Rev.,* 12, 143-150, 1988.

38. **Henke, P.G., and Savoie, R.J.,** The cingulate cortex and gastric pathology, *Brain Res. Bull.,* 8, 489-492, 1982.

39. **Hermann, G.E., McCann, M.J., and Rogers, R.C.,** Bed nucleus of stria terminalis influence over gastric function, *Auton. Nerv. Sys.,* 30,123-128, 1990.

40. **Hermann, G.E., and Rogers, R.C.,** Dorsal medullary somatostatin causes an increase in gastric acid secretion, *Neurosci. Abs.,* 17, 737, 1987.

41. **Hermann, G., and Rogers, R.C.,** Extrinsic neural control of brainstem gastric vago-vagal reflex circuits, in *Nerves and the Gastrointestinal Tract,* Singer, M.V., and Goebell, H., Eds., MTP Press, 1989, 345-346.

42. **Hobson, J.A., and Scheibel, A.B.,** The brainstem core: Sensorimotor integration and behavioral state control, *Neurosci. Res. Prog. Bull.,* 18, 173, 1980.

43. **Hoffman, B.L., and Rasmussen, T.,** Stimulation studies of insular cortex of macaca mulatta, *J. Neurophysiol.,* 16, 343-351, 1953.

44. **Hokfelt, T., Fuxe, K., Johansson, O., Jeffcoate, S., and White, N.,** Thyrotropin-releasing hormone (TRH) containing nerve terminals in certain brainstem nuclei and in the spinal cord, *Neurosci. Lett.,* 1, 133-139, 1975.

45. **Holstege, G., Meiners, L., and Tan, K.,** Projections of the bed nucleus of the stria terminalis to the mesencephalon, pons, and medulla oblongata in the cat, *Exp. Brain Res.*, 58, 379-391, 1985.

46. **Hurley-Guis, K.M., and Neafsay, E.J.,** The medial frontal cortex and gastric motility: Microstimulation results and their possible significance for the overall pattern of organization of rat frontal and parietal cortex, *Brain Res.*, 365, 241-248, 1986.

47. **Kaada, B.R., Pribram, K.H., and Epstein, J.A.,** Respiratory and vascular responses in monkeys from temporal pole, insula, orbital surface, and cingulate gyrus, *J. Neurophysiol.*, 12, 347-356, 1949.

48. **Kadekaro, M., Timo-Iaria, C., and Vincenti, M. de L.M.,** Control of gastric secretion by the central nervous system, in *Nerves and the Gut*, Brooks, F.P., Evers, P.W., and Slack, C.B., Eds., Thorofare, NJ, 1977, 377-429.

49. **Kalia, M., and Mesulam, M.M.,** Brainstem projections of sensory and motor components of the vagus complex in the cat. II. Laryngeal, tracheobronchial, pulmonary, cardiac and gastrointestinal branches, *J. Comp. Neurol.*, 193, 467-508, 1980.

50. **Kapp, B.S., Gallagher, M., Underwood, M.D., McNall, C.L., and Whitehorn, D.,** Cardiovascular responses elicited by electrical stimulation of the amygdala central nucleus in the rabbit, *Brain Res.*, 234, 251-262, 1982.

51. **Kawai, Y., Inagaki, S., Shiosaka, S., Senba, E., Hara, Y., Sakanaka, M., Takatsuki, K., and Tohyama, M.,** Long descending projections from amygdaloid somatostatin containing cells to the lower brain stem, *Brain Res.*, 239, 603-607, 1982.

52. **Kellow, J.E., Gill, R.C., and Wingate, D.L.,** Proximal gut motor activity in irritable bowel syndrome: Patients at home and at work, *Gastroenterology*, 92 (part 2), 1463, 1987.

53. **Kubek, M.J., Rea, M.A., Hodes, Z.I., and Aprison, M.H.,** Quantitation and characterization of thyrotropin releasing hormone in vagal nuclei and other regions of the medulla oblongata of the rat, *J. Neurochem.*, 40, 1307-1313, 1983.

54. **Kumar, D., and Wingate, D.L.,** The irritable bowel syndrome: A paroxysmal motor disorder, *Lancet*, 2, 973-977, 1985.

55. **Lawrence, D., and Pittman, Q.J.,** Interaction between descending paraventricular neurons and vagal motor neurons, *Brain Res.*, 332, 158-160, 1985.

56. **Lechan, R.M., Snapper, S.B., and Jackson, I.M.D.,** Evidence that spinal cord TRH is independent of the paraventricular nucleus of the hypothalamus, *Neurosci. Lett.*, 43, 61-65, 1983.

57. **Loewy, A.D., and McKellar, S.,** The neuroanatomical basis of central cardiovascular control, *Fed. Proc.*, 39, 2495-2503, 1980.

58. **Lofving, B.,** Cardiovascular adjustments induced from the rostral cingulate gyrus, *Acta Physiol. Scand.*, (Suppl. 53), 1841-1884, 1961.

59. **Luiten, P.G.M., ter Horst, G.J., Karst, H., and Steffens, A.B.,** The course of paraventricular hypothalamic efferents to autonomic structures in medulla and spinal cord, *Brain Res.*, 329, 374-378, 1985.

60. **Mancillas, J.R., Siggins, G.R., and Bloom, F.E.,** Somatostatin selectively enhances acetlycholine-induced excitations in the rat hippocampus and cortex, *Proc. Natl. Acad. Sci. USA*, 83, 7518-7521, 1986.

61. **Martinson, J.,** Studies on the efferent vagal control of the stomach, *Acta Physiol. Scand.*, 65 (Suppl. 255), 1-24, 1973.

62. **McCann, M.J., Hermann, G.E., and Rogers, R.C.,** Thyrotropin-releasing hormone (TRH) potentiates the gastric responses evoked by dorsal medullary serotonin (5HT), *J. Auton. Nerv. Sys.*, 25, 35-40, 1988.

63. **Morley, J.E., Levine, A.S., and Silvis, S.E.,** Minireview: Central regulation of gastric acid secretion: The role of neuropeptides, *Life Sci.*, 31, 399-410, 1982.

64. **Mueller, A.L., Kunkel, D.D., and Schwartzkroin, P.A.,** Electrophysiological actions of somatostatin in hippocampus: An *in vitro* study, *Cell Mol. Neurobiol.*, 6, 363-379, 1986.

65. **Norgren, R.,** Projections from the nucleus tractus solitarius in the rat, *Neuroscience*, 3, 207-218, 1978.

66. **Pagani, F.D., Norman, W.P., Kasbekar, D.K., and Gillis, R.A.,** Localization of sites within the dorsal motor nucleus of the vagus that affect gastric motility, *Am. J. Physiol.*, 249, G73-84, 1985.

67. **Palkovits, M., Mezey, E., Eskay, R.L., and Brownstein, M.J.,** Innervation of the nucleus of the solitary tract and dorsal vagal nucleus by thyrotropin-releasing hormone containing raphe neurons, *Brain Res.*, 373, 246-251, 1986.

68. **Pavlov, I.P.,** *The work of the digestive glands,* transl. by Thompson, W.H., C. Griffith, London, 1910.

69. **Pittman, Q.J., and Siggins, G.R.,** Somatostatin hyperpolarizes hippocampal pyramidal cells in vitro, *Brain Res.*, 221, 402-408, 1981.

70. **Price, J.L.,** Integrated systems of the CNS: I, hypothalamus, hippocampus amygdala and retina, in *Handbook of Chemical Neuroanatomy*, Price, J.L., Ed., Elsevier Scientific, Amsterdam, 1987, 1-79.

71. **Ricardo, J.A., and Koh, E.T.,** Anatomical evidence of direct projections from the nucleus of the solitary tract to the hypothalamus, amygdala and other forebrain structures in the rat, *Brain Res.*, 153, 1-26, 1978.

72. **Renaud, L.P., Tang, M., McCann, M.J., Striker, E.M., and Verbalis, J.G.,** Cholecystokinin and gastric distension activate oxytocinergic cells in the rat hypothalamus, *Am. J. Physiol.*, 253, R661-665, 1987.

73. **Rogers, R.C., and Fryman, D.L.,** Direct connections between the central nucleus of the amygdala and the nucleus of the solitary tract: An electrophysiological study in the rat, *J. Auton. Nerv. Syst.*, 22, 83-87, 1988.

74. **Rogers, R.C., and Hermann, G.E.,** Central connections of the hepatic branch of the vagus nerve: A horseradish peroxidase study, *J. Auton. Nerv. Syst.*, 7, 165, 1983.

75. **Rogers, R.C., and Hermann, G.E.,** Gastric vagal solitary neurons excited by paraventricular nucleus microstimulation, *J. Auton. Nerv. Syst.*, 14, 351-362, 1985.

76. **Rogers, R.C., and Hermann, G.E.,** Vagal afferent stimulation-evoked gastric secretion suppressed by paraventricular nucleus lesion, *J. Auton. Nerv Syst.*, 13, 191-199, 1985.

77. **Rogers, R.C., and Hermann, G.E.,** Dorsal medullary oxytocin, vasopressin and TRH effects on gastric secretion and heart rate, *Peptides*, 6, 1143-1148, 1985.

78. **Rogers, R.C., and Hermann, G.E.,** Hypothalamic paraventricular nucleus stimulation-induced gastric acid secretion and bradycardia suppressed by oxytocin antagonist, *Peptides*, 7, 695-700, 1986.

79. **Rogers, R.C., and Hermann, G.E.,** Oxytocin, oxytocin antagonist, TRH and hypothalamic paraventricular nucleus stimulation effects on gastric motility, *Peptides*, 8, 505-513, 1987.

80. **Rogers, R.C., Kita, H., Butcher, L.L., and Novin, D.,** Afferent projections to the dorsal motor nucleus of the vagus, *Brain Res. Bull.*, 5, 365-373, 1980.

81. **Rogers, R.C., McCann, M.J., and Hermann, G.E.,** TRH effects on physiologically-identified neurons in the dorsal vagal complex: *In vivo* and *in vitro* studies, *Neuroscience Abs.*, 14, 538, 1988.

82. **Rogers, R.C., and Nelson, D.O.,** Neurons of the vagal division of the solitary nucleus activated by the paraventricular nucleus of the hypothalamus, *J. Auton. Nerv. Syst.*, 10, 193-197, 1984.

83. **Roman, C., and Gonella, J.,** Extrinsic control of digestive tract motility, in *Physiology of the Gastrointestinal Tract*, Johnson, L.R., Ed., Raven Press, New York, 1987, 507-553.

84. **Saper, C.B.,** Convergence of autonomic and limbic connections in the insular cortex of the rat, *J. Comp. Neurol.*, 210, 163-173, 1982.

85. **Schwaber, J.S., Kapp, B.S., and Higgins, G.,** The origin and extent of direct amygdala projections to the region of the dorsal motor nucleus of the vagus and the nucleus of the solitary tract, *Neurosci. Lett.*, 20, 15-20, 1980.

86. **Schwaber, J.S., Kapp, B.S., Higgins, G.A., and Rapp, P.R.,** Amygdaloid and basal forebrain connections with the nucleus of the solitary tract and the dorsal motor nucleus, *J. Neurosci.*, 2, 1424-1438, 1982.

87. **Schwaber, J.S., Wray, S., Higgins, G.A., and Hoffman, G.,** The central nucleus of the amygdala: Descending autonomic connections and neuropeptide systems in the rat, *Anat. Res.,* 199, 228A, 1981.

88. **Scratcherd, T., and Grundy, D.,** Reflex control of gastric motility by stimuli acting from within the stomach, in *Nerves and the Gastrointestinal Tract,* Singer, M.V., and Goebell, H., Eds., MTP Press, 1989, 373-382.

89. **Semba, T., Kimura, H., and Fugii, K.,** Bulbar influence on gastric motility, *Jpn. J. Physiol.,* 19, 521-533, 1969.

90. **Sheehan, D.,** The effect of cortical stimulation on gastric movements in the monkey, *J. Physiol.,* 83, 177-184, 1957.

91. **Shipley, M.T.,** Insular cortex projection to the nucleus of the solitary tract and brainstem visceromotor regions in the mouse, *Brain Res. Bull.,* 8, 138-148, 1982.

92. **Smith, G.P., and McHugh, P.R.,** Gastric secretory response to amygdaloid or hypothalamic stimulation in monkeys, *Am. J. Physiol.,* 213, 640-644, 1967.

93. **Smith, O.A., and deVito, J.L.,** Central neural integration for the control of autonomic responses associated with emotion, *Annu. Rev. Neurosci.,*7, 43-65, 1984.

94. **Smith, W.K.,** The functional significance of the rostral cingular cortex as revealed by its response to electrical stimulation, *J. Neurophysiol.,* 8, 241-255, 1945.

95. **Sofroniew, M.V., and Schrell, U.,** Evidence for a direct projection from oxytocin and vasopressin neurons in hypothalamic paraventricular nucleus to the medulla oblongata: Immunohistochemical visualization of both the horseradish peroxidase transported and the peptide produced by the same neurons, *Neurosci. Lett.,* 22, 211-217, 1981.

96. **Spiegel, E.A., Weston, K., and Oppenheimer, M.J.,** Postmotor foci influencing the gastrointestinal tract and their descending pathways, *J. Neuropathol. Exp. Neurol.,* 2, 45-53, 1943.

97. **Strom, G., and Uvnas, B.,** Motor responses of gastrointestinal tract and bladder to topical stimulation of frontal lobe, basal ganglia, and hypothalamus in cat, *Acta Physiol. Scand.,* 21, 90-104, 1950.

98. **Swanson, L.W., and Kuypers, H.G.J.M.,** The paraventricular nucleus of the hypothalamus: Cytoarchitectonic subdivisions and the organization of projections to the pituitary, the dorsal vagal complex and spinal cord as demonstrated by retrograde fluorescence double-labeling methods, *J. Comp. Neurol.,* 194, 555-570, 1980.

99. **Swanson, L.W., and Mogenson, G.,** Neural mechanisms for functional coupling of autonomic, endocrine and skeletomotor responses in adaptive behavior, *Brain Res. Rev.,* 3, 1-24, 1981.

100. **Swanson, L.W., and Sawchenko, P.E.,** Hypothalamic integration: Organization of the paraventricular and supraoptic nuclei, *Annu. Rev. Neurosci.,* 6, 269-325, 1983.

101. **Swanson, L.W., Sawchenko, P.E., Rivier, J., and Vale, W.W.,** Organization of ovine corticotropin-releasing factor immunoreactive cells and fibers in the rat brain: An immunohistochemical study, *Neuroendocrinology,* 36, 165-186, 1985.

102. **Tache, Y.,** Central nervous system regulation of gastric acid secretion, in *Physiology of the Gastrointestinal Tract,* Johnson, L.R., Ed., Raven Press, New York, 1987, 911-930.

103. **Terreberry, R.R., and Neafsay, E.J.,** Rat medial frontal cortex: A visceral motor region with a direct projection to the solitary nucleus, *Brain Res.,* 278, 245-249, 1983.

104. **van der Kooy, D., Koda, L., McGinty, J.F., Gerfen, C.R., and Bloom, F.,** The organization of projections from the cortex, amygdala and hypothalamus to the nucleus of the solitary tract in rat, *J. Comp. Neurol.,* 224, 1-24, 1984.

105. **Van Leeuwen, F., and Caffe, R.,** Vasopressin-immunoreactive cell bodies in the bed nucleus of the stria terminalis of the cat, *Cell Tissue Res.,* 228, 525-534, 1983.

106. **Veening, J.G., Swanson, L.W., and Sawchenko, P.E.,** The organization of projections from the central nucleus of the amygdala to brainstem sites in central autonomic regulation: A combined retrograde transport-immunohistochemical study, *Brain Res.,* 303, 337-357, 1982.

107. **Verbalis, J.G., McCann, M.J., McHale, C.M., and Striker, E.M.,** Oxytocin secretion in response to CCK and food; differentiation of nausea from satiety, *Science,* 232, 1417-1419, 1983.

108. **Villarreal, J.A., and Brown, M.R.,** Bombesin-like peptide in hypothalamus: Chemical and immunological characterization, *Life Sci.,* 23, 2729-2733, 1978.
109. **Ward, A.A., Jr.,** The cingulate gyrus: Area 24, *J. Neurophysiol.,* 11, 13-23, 1948.
110. **Watson, T.W., and Pittman, Q.J.,** Mechanism of action of somatostatin in the hippocampal slice, *Proc. West. Pharmacol. Soc.,* 30, 361-363, 1987.
111. **Witty, R.T., and Long, J.F.,** Effects of ambient temperature on gastric secretion and food intake in the rat, *Am. J. Physiol.,* 219, 1359-1362, 1970.
112. **Wolf, S., and Wolf, H.G.,** *Human Gastric Function: An Experimental Study of Man and His Stomach,* Oxford University Press, New York, 1943.
113. **Wood, J.D.,** Physiology of the enteric nervous system, in *Physiology of the Gastrointestinal Tract,* Johnson, L.R., Ed., Raven Press, New York, 1986, 67-110.
114. **Wood, J.D.,** Signal transduction in intestinal neurons, in *Proceedings of Xth International Symposium on Gastrointestinal Motility,* Szurszewski, Ed., Elsevier Science Publications, Amsterdam, 1987, 55-69.
115. **Wray, S., Schwaber, J.S., and Hoffman, G.,** Neuropeptide localization in the rat central nucleus of the amygdala, *Anat. Rec.,* 199, 282A, 1981.
116. **Wyrwicka, W., and Garcia, R.,** Effect of electrical stimulation of the dorsal nucleus of the vagus nerve on gastric acid secretion in cats, *Exp. Neurol.,* 65, 315-325, 1979.
117. **Zimmerman, E.A., Nilaver, G., Hou-Yu, A., and Silverman, A.J.,** Vasopressinergic and oxytocinergic pathways in the central nervous system, *Fed. Proc.,* 43, 91-96, 1984.

Chapter 6

VAGAL AFFERENT INNERVATION OF THE ENTERIC NERVOUS SYSTEM

C. Sternini

TABLE OF CONTENTS

LIST OF ABBREVIATIONS

CGRP = calcitonin gene-related peptide
ENS = enteric nervous system
HRP = horseradish peroxidase
NKA = neurokinin A
NKB = neurokinin B
PPT = preprotachykinins
SP = substance P
TK = tachykinins

THE ENTERIC NERVOUS SYSTEM: ANATOMICAL ORGANIZATION

The digestive tract is innervated by a complex neural network, referred to as the enteric nervous system (ENS), which consists of numerous intrinsic neurons that are organized into two major ganglionated plexuses.[18,21,23,69] The myenteric or Auerbach's plexus lies between the longitudinal and circular muscle layers, and the submucosal or Meissner's plexus is located within the submucosa. Intramural neurons give rise to nerve fibers that connect the ganglia within the plexus and the ganglionated plexuses to each other; fibers emerging from the ganglionated plexuses innervate the different layers of the gut and blood vessels. The majority of enteric axons originates from intrinsic neurons, which represent the chief component of the nervous apparatus controlling digestive functions. This is supported by the observation that decentralization causes little effect on most of the spontaneous and reflex activities, which in turn provides strong evidence for the existence of sensory receptors, intrinsic primary afferent neurons, interneurons and motor neurons within the ENS (see Furness and Costa[19] for review).

The ENS also comprises efferent (parasympathetic and sympathetic) and afferent inputs, which contribute to the fiber network and which integrate with the intrinsic neurons in regulating digestive functions. Extrinsic afferent fibers originate from the nodose and dorsal root ganglia. There is also indirect evidence that at least a portion of the sensory nerves supplying the gut originates from intramural neurons; however, these neurons have not yet been unequivocally identified.[21] Visceral afferents are likely to play a considerably more complex role than pain transmission and are likely to be involved in visceral regulation and coordination via different neuronal pathways.[2,36,37,52] Therefore, the definition of the morphological and neurochemical organization of the sensory innervation of the digestive system has become a fundamental issue for understanding the functional role of visceral afferents in the neural coordination and integration of digestive functions.

This chapter will focus on an analysis of the extrinsic afferent innervation of the upper gastrointestinal tract and pancreas and will include a description of the origin, peripheral distribution and neurochemistry of afferent fibers as visualized by combining retrograde tracing approaches and immunohistochemistry, with a particular emphasis on vagal afferents.

AFFERENT INNERVATION OF THE GASTROINTESTINAL TRACT AND PANCREAS

Retrograde Tracing Studies

The digestive system, like other viscera, receives a double sensory innervation, which is made up of sensory fibers running through the vagi and the sympathetic nerves, where they generally are intermingled with efferent fibers.[2,37,52] Within visceral nerves, the proportion of afferents exceeds that of efferents; the vagus, which is the largest autonomic nerve, contains mainly afferent fibers. Afferent fibers are unmyelinated (the majority) or thinly myelinated and are characterized by slow conduction; the proportion of unmyelinated versus thinly myelinated fibers increases from oral to aboral areas, and at the intestinal level afferents are almost entirely unmyelinated.[52]

An important achievement in understanding the anatomical substrates of visceral reflexes, including intestinal reflex activities, has been obtained with the application of neurochemical approaches. These approaches rely on peripheral injections of substances that are taken up from terminals and axonally transported, leading to the elucidation of the origin and termination sites of afferent fibers. A multiplicity of substances, including horseradish peroxidase (HRP), wheat germ agglutinin-HRP, cholera toxin-HRP and fluorescent dyes, have proven to be good markers for axonal tracing of neuronal pathways and have been utilized by numerous investigators.[13,42,53,59,63,68,79] Retrograde tracing studies have shown that extrinsic afferent fibers innervating the abdominal viscera arise bilaterally from neurons located in the nodose and dorsal root ganglia.[13,30,31,51,64,65,70,76] Vagal afferent neurons are preferentially concentrated within the body and caudal pole of the nodose ganglia.[13,30,31] A certain degree of viscerotopic segregation has been found in the nodose ganglia. Vagal afferents supplying the ventral surface of the stomach and the duodenal lobe of the pancreas preferentially arise from the left nodose ganglion.[13,64,65] Conversely, the pyloric antrum,[30] the proximal duodenum (see below) and the splenic lobe of the pancreas[64,65] receive more vagal afferents from the right nodose ganglion. Spinal afferents supplying digestive viscera arise from neurons distributed throughout the ganglia, which are located at different spinal levels according to the region of the alimentary tract, even though there is an extensive overlap. In fact, the cervical esophagus receives afferents from C_1-T_1, the stomach and pancreas from T_5-L_1/L_2, the gallbladder from T_5-T_{11}, the proximal duodenum from T_9-L_3 and the distal colon from two sets of ganglia, T_{13}-L_1 and L_6-S_1.[30,31,51,65,70,76]

Axonal tracing approaches have mapped the sensory and motor connections between the viscera and the central nervous system and have unraveled visceral afferent pathways. The possibility of combining fluorescent retrograde tracers with immunohistochemistry, which allows for the simultaneous visualization of retrogradely labeled and immunohistochemically labeled neurons, has enabled the identification of neurochemically characterized sensory neurons giving rise to afferents innervating a given viscus. Sensory neurons and terminals can be visualized by immunohistochemical labeling for several peptides. Using immunocytochemistry, which relies on the availability of specific antibodies raised against given substances, together with other tools, such as capsaicin, a selective sensory neurotoxin that primarily affects small-diameter sensory neurons,[55] and retrogradely transported fluorescent tracers (e.g., True Blue, Fast Blue and Fluoro-Gold), it has been possible to begin to characterize neuronal pathways and their chemical coding.[13,30,31,71,76]

Peptide Sensory Markers

Visceral afferent neurons are characterized by a diversity of biochemical properties which enable specific and selective histochemical and immunohistochemical staining. A substantial proportion of afferents contains a multiplicity of peptides,[13,24,33,40,61] but there are also non-peptidergic afferent neurons and terminals that express special biochemical properties, including a variety of species-specific membrane surface glycoconjugates and acid phosphatase isoenzymes.[14,15,61,66,67,75] Even though afferent systems can be characterized by different neurochemical properties, it is the visualization of visceral afferents by immunohistochemical labeling for bioactive peptides that has significantly contributed to our knowledge on the peripheral distribution, origin and neurochemistry of different visceral systems.

Among the many peptides, which have been found to be suitable markers for sensory neurons and terminals and which are also present in the ENS, substance P (SP) has been regarded for a long time as the most generalized peptide sensory marker.[38,39,58] SP belongs to a family of structurally related peptides, the tachykinins (TK), which in mammals also include neurokinin A (NKA; also known as substance K), neurokinin B (NKB; also known as neuromedin K) and the N-terminally extended peptides, neuropeptide K and neuropeptide-γ.[41,50] It is noteworthy to point out that nearly all the antisera used so far to study the distribution of SP immunoreactivity have been directed to the C-terminal portion of this peptide, which is common to all TK peptides and which therefore cannot discern which TK is expressed in a particular population of neurons. Therefore it is more appropriate to refer to the immunoreactive staining obtained with these antibodies as TK immunoreactivity, a term that will be used throughout this chapter for simplicity and brevity. TK is expressed in a population of small- to medium-size sensory neurons and in a variety of sites known to contain nociceptive endings, such as the skin and vascular system.[38,39,58] In addition to SP or related TKs, other peptides are present in sensory neurons, including somatostatin, galanin, dynorphin, cholecystokinin, vasoactive intestinal polypeptide, bombesin (or its related peptide, gastrin releasing peptide) and the more recently discovered peptide, calcitonin gene-related peptide (CGRP).[6,24,33,34,40,46,60,61] CGRP, a peptide generated by alternative RNA processing of the primary transcript of the calcitonin gene,[60] is now generally accepted as the most ubiquitous bioactive peptide sensory marker. CGRP immunoreactivity is present in the largest number of small- to medium-size sensory neurons than any other peptide described to date and in some large-size sensory neurons.[29,40,46] In the periphery, CGRP immunoreactivity is localized in a great number of unmyelinated and thinly myelinated axons widely distributed to a variety of tissues and viscera.[29,46,60]

Some peptides label distinct populations (e.g., TK and somatostatin, even though there has been some recent controversy concerning this concept);[22,34,40,47] whereas others colocalize in subpopulations of neurons and processes [e.g., CGRP and TK colocalize extensively (Figure 1); other examples include cho-

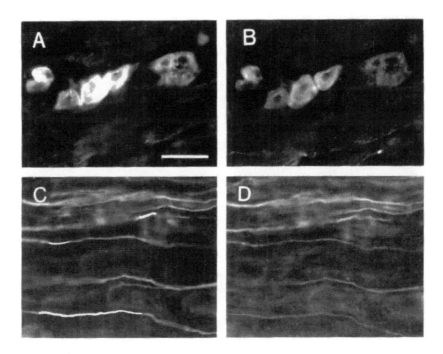

FIGURE 1. Cryostat sections of the left nodose ganglion (A and B; rostral pole) and vagus nerve (C and D) of the rat double-labeled for CGRP (A and C) and TK (B and D) immunoreactivities, using a mixture of guinea pig CGRP and rabbit NKA antisera. (Immunofluorescence technique; calibration bar: 50 μm.)

lecystokinin and TKs or CGRP, galanin and CGRP or TK].[24,40] A multiplicity of peptides can be expressed in the same neuron[24,40] and different classes of neurons can be distinguished by their chemistry and projection patterns. The same peptide may also colocalize with different combinations of peptides in different neuronal populations. For example, four major populations of capsaicin-sensitive neurons have been identified; they are immunoreactive for both CGRP and TK, but differ on the basis of their immunoreactivity to either cholecystokinin and/or dynorphin.[24] Moreover, the CGRP and TK combination appears to be the only one present in capsaicin-sensitive afferents innervating most of the abdominal viscera and their vasculature.

In the nodose ganglion, neurons containing peptide immunoreactivity are preferentially concentrated at the rostral region (Figures 1A, B), where they can be clustered together, whereas the percentage of peptide-containing neurons in the caudal part is usually much lower, with the exception of those neurons positive for vasoactive intestinal polypeptide immunoreactivity, which are slightly more numerous in the caudal than rostral pole.[33]

Peptides synthesized in sensory neurons are axonally transported both peripherad and centrad, and the axonal transport velocities for some of these peptides have been determined in the vagus and splanchnic nerves of several species. The amount of peptide transported to the periphery is usually higher than that transported toward the central terminations.[13] Moreover, the axonal transport rates estimated for TK and CGRP in the vagus nerve are quite similar, as anticipated by their extensive co-occurrence in sensory neurons.[26,80] This observation, together with the ultrastructural evidence that TK and CGRP immunoreactivities are stored in the same large vesicles in peripheral nerves,[32] suggests that after stimulation these peptides might be released simultaneously at the peripheral endings.

The identification of peptide-containing afferents innervating the ENS is problematic because the same peptides that are expressed in sensory neurons and terminals are also found in intrinsic neurons and terminals. Among the numerous peptides that can be used for labeling sensory structures, CGRP and SP or related TKs appear to be the best markers for the visualization of a subpopulation of digestive afferents, as indicated by immunoassay studies in association with chemical and surgical denervation procedures and axonal tracing approaches. These studies have clearly demonstrated that these peptides are expressed in both enteric and extrinsic afferent fibers innervating the digestive system and that particularly CGRP is a valuable marker for the visualization of a major subset of extrinsic afferent fibers supplying the alimentary canal.

CGRP AND TK INNERVATION OF THE
DIGESTIVE SYSTEM

CGRP and TKs are widely distributed throughout the ENS where they are present in nerve fibers innervating all the layers of the gut, the pancreas and hepatobiliary tract in several species.[8,9,11,12,28,73,74,76] Interestingly, unlike TK immunoreactivity, which is found in intrinsic ganglion cells in all the regions of the gut,[9,11,12] including the ganglionated plexus of the gallbladder,[28,51] CGRP immunoreactivity has a differential distribution in different regions of the alimentary canal. It is restricted to nerve fibers in the esophagus, stomach, pancreas and biliary tract, but it is present in both nerve fibers and enteric ganglion cells in both the small and large intestines[8,27,28,51,73,74,76] (Figure 2).

Neonatal treatment with the sensory neurotoxin capsaicin depletes the CGRP fibers innervating the esophagus, stomach (Figure 3) and pancreas, and causes a dramatic reduction of those supplying the biliary tract and the vasculature as well as a marked decrease of non-vascular fibers distributed to the gut wall.[27,73,74] Quantitative analysis by radioimmunoassay has shown > 95% decrease in CGRP immunoreactive concentrations in extracts from the esophagus and stomach, a 60% reduction in pancreatic extracts (the presence of CGRP-containing endocrine cells in the islets accounts for the remaining 40%) and < 50% decrease in intestinal extracts of capsaicin-treated rats, when compared to their littermate controls.[74] On the other hand, the absence of CGRP immunoreactivity within the celiac ganglia[76] and the lack of sensitivity of CGRP-containing fibers in the digestive tract to the sympathetic neurotoxin, 6-

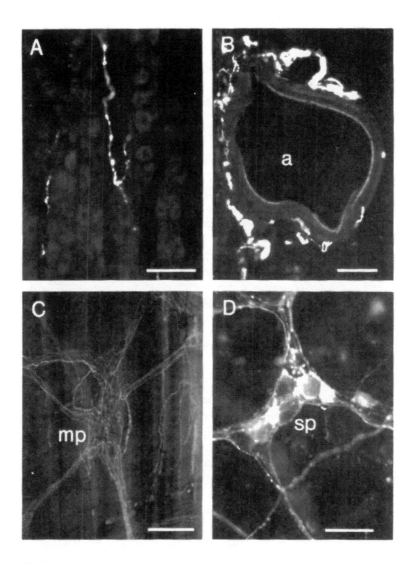

FIGURE 2. Photomicrographs showing the distribution of CGRP immunoreactivity in the rat gastrointestinal tract, using a rabbit CGRP antiserum. A and B: cryostat sections of the gastric mucosa (A) and submucosa (B) showing varicose fibers immunoreactive for CGRP, running parallel to the parietal cells (A) and bundles of fibers associated with a blood vessel (B), which has the anatomical appearance of a small artery (a). C and D: whole mount preparations of the muscle layer of rat stomach (C) and of the submucosal layer of rat ileum (D), illustrating the network of CGRP immunoreactive fibers in the myenteric (mp) and submucosal (sp) plexuses and the presence of CGRP-containing enteric neurons in the intestinal submucosal plexus (D). (Immunofluorescence method; calibration bars: 50 μm in A, B and D; 150 μm in C.)

A

B

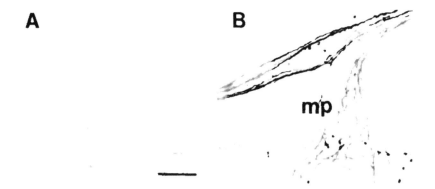

mp

FIGURE 3. Comparable regions from muscle layer preparations (containing the myenteric plexus) of the stomach from a rat treated at birth with capsaicin (A) and from its littermate control (B) processed for CGRP immunohistochemistry. Capsaicin treatment causes a depletion of CGRP innervation (A), whereas the CGRP immunoreactive pattern in the littermate control (B) is comparable to that in normal animals (Figure 2 C). Antiserum as in Figure 2. (Avidin-biotin peroxidase anti-peroxidase method; calibration bar: 50 μm. Used with permission by *Gastroenterology*, from Sternini *et al.*[74])

hydroxydopamine,[73,74,76] rule out a possible sympathetic origin of the CGRP extrinsic innervation. These findings clearly indicate that the extrinsic CGRP fibers form a major component of the sensory innervation of the gut. The bulk of the extrinsic CGRP fibers likely originates from the CGRP-containing neurons located in dorsal root sensory ganglia, since bilateral vagotomy does not cause detectable reduction of the CGRP innervation of the gut, unlike celiac and superior mesenteric ganglionectomy, which dramatically reduces the CGRP innervation of the upper gut, pancreas and biliary tract.[27,76,80] (Sternini, unpublished data).

CGRP and TK immunoreactivities colocalize in a subpopulation of fibers, namely those innervating the blood vessels (Figure 4) and the submucosa, in some fibers in the mucosa (Figure 4) and in a few fibers in the muscle layer, but not in intrinsic ganglion cells, clearly indicating that only the extrinsic component of the CGRP gastrointestinal innervation contains TK immunoreactivity. The colocalization of CGRP and TK immunoreactivities in capsaicin-sensitive sensory axons has been demonstrated in several tissues.[25] Unlike the CGRP afferents, however, the extrinsic sensory TK-containing nerves form only a minor population in the digestive system, being mainly confined to a perivascular location and only in a lesser degree to the gut wall.[11,25]

CGRP AND TK AFFERENTS: VAGAL VERSUS SPINAL ORIGIN

The proportion of CGRP- and TK-containing sensory neurons supplying different structures and viscera has been determined in several species by

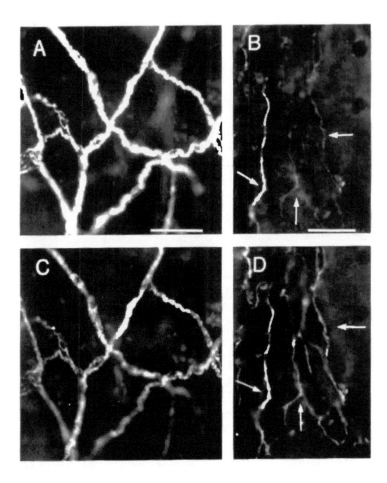

FIGURE 4. Simultaneous visualization of CGRP (A and B) and TK (C and D) immunoreactivities in fibers innervating the guinea pig vena porta (A and C, whole mount preparation) and a villus of the rat duodenum (B and D, cryostat section). CGRP and TK immunostainings were obtained with a mixture of rabbit CGRP antiserum and rat monoclonal SP antibody (Pel-Freeze) in A and C (used with permission by *Cell Tissue Res.*, from Goehler *et al.*[28]), and with a mixture of guinea pig CGRP and rabbit NKA antisera in B and D. Arrows in B and D indicate processes expressing both CGRP and NKA/TK immunoreactivities. (Immunofluorescence technique; calibration bars: 50 μm.)

combining retrograde transport of fluorescent dyes and CGRP or TK immuno-histochemistry. Most studies have been carried out in rats. The stomach and pancreas have been analyzed most extensively, even though there are some data concerning other areas of the alimentary tract and other species.[30,31,65,76,80]

Green and Dockray[30,31] have reported that CGRP or TK immunoreactivity is present in < 10% or < 5%, respectively, of True Blue retrogradely labeled neurons visualized in the nodose ganglion after injection of the tracer into the gastric wall or the pyloric antrum of the rat. In other studies, which also have relied on the injection of True Blue as a retrograde tracer into the stomach and pancreas, no TK immunoreactivity has been visualized in either gastric or pancreatic vagal afferents.[65,76] On the other hand, the proportion of CGRP- or TK-containing vagal afferents innervating the cervical esophagus is higher than that observed for other regions of the gut (about 26% and 14%, respectively[30]).

In contrast, the percentages of neurons containing the retrogradely transported True Blue and CGRP immunoreactivity, following injection into the rat esophagus (cervical), stomach (ventral surface), pancreas and descending colon, were much higher than those observed within the nodose ganglia, ranging from 70% for the esophagus to 80-95% for the other regions examined. The proportions of True Blue retrogradely labeled and TK immunoreactive neurons were also higher in the spinal than in the nodose ganglia, with the highest percentages observed when the tracer was injected into the stomach wall (up to 55%) and the lowest proportion identified following injection into the pancreas (11-20%).[30,31,65,76]

In our studies, combining retrograde tracing techniques with immunohistochemistry for either CGRP or for the simultaneous visualization of CGRP and TK immunoreactivities, we have used as fluorescent tracers either Fast Blue or Fluoro-Gold, both previously shown to be suitable for unraveling neuronal pathways.[51,62,79] Fast Blue or Fluoro-Gold were used at concentrations of 5% and 3-4%, respectively, and injected in a volume of 10 µl into the wall (both anterior and posterior surfaces) of the abdominal esophagus, stomach (from the cardias to the pylorus) and proximal duodenum, and into the pancreatic parenchyma (both splenic and duodenal lobes) of the rat. For each experiment, 5-10 injections were made in each viscus, using a fine gauge needle held in place for 15-30 seconds after each injection to prevent possible leakage of the dye from the injection site. The injection sites were then carefully swabbed and a physical barrier (e.g., plastic wound spray) was applied[17] to prevent diffusion of the dye to adjacent organs. Following a survival time of 5-10 days, animals were sacrificed and tissues (nodose ganglia and dorsal root ganglia T_5-L_3) were fixed in paraformaldehyde solutions, sectioned and processed for immunohistochemistry using immunofluorescence procedures.[73] For the visualization of CGRP immunoreactive neurons, a rabbit CGRP antiserum (dilutions 1:3000-1:5000) was used.[73,74] For the simultaneous visualization of CGRP and TK immunoreactivities, a mixture of guinea pig CGRP antiserum (1:200-1:500 dilutions) and either rabbit SP (1:500; provided by Drs. R. Murphy and J.B. Furness) or rabbit NKA (1:500; provided by H. Wong and Dr. J.H. Walsh) was used, and the antibody-antigen complexes were visualized using secondary antibodies conjugated with different fluorophores (e.g., fluorescein and rhodamine).[10,28] The guinea pig CGRP antiserum was raised against synthetic [Tyr] rat α-$CGRP_{23-37}$ conjugated to keyhole lympet hemocyanin via glutaraldehyde. This antiserum does not cross react with different TK peptides and gives an immunoreactive pattern comparable to that obtained with the rabbit CGRP antiserum.[71] Immunoreactive staining obtained with the guinea pig CGRP antiserum was totally abolished after preabsorption with either [Tyr] rat α-CGRP$_{23-37}$ or rat α-CGRP$_{1-37}$. The immunoreactive patterns obtained using SP or NKA antisera were comparable, and they were completely abolished after preabsorption with synthetic SP and NKA peptides, respectively. In addition, the SP immunoreaction was eliminated with an excess of either NKA or NKB, and the NKA immunoreaction was completely blocked by NKB and almost totally blocked by an excess of SP, indicating that both SP and NKA antisera are good generalized markers for the mammalian TKs.

When Fast Blue or Fluoro-Gold were injected into the esophageal or gastric wall or into the pancreas, similar proportions of retrogradely labeled neurons were observed in both nodose ganglia. When the upper duodenal wall was injected, retrogradely labeled neurons were usually more abundant in the right than in the left nodose ganglion. In our experiments, the fluorescent tracer was injected into both the ventral and posterior surfaces of the stomach, from the cardias to the pylorus, and into the whole pancreatic gland, unlike in previous studies where the tracer injections were confined to the ventral surface of the gastric body or to either the splenic or duodenal lobes of the pancreas.[30,64,65] This could account for the apparent discrepancies between our and previous results, which have shown differences between the proportions of left and right vagal neurons supplying the stomach and pancreas.[30,64,65] The number of retrogradely labeled neurons visualized in the nodose ganglia varied depending on the viscus injected. Thus, Fast Blue or Fluoro-Gold labeled neurons were more numerous following injection of the tracer into the esophagus than when it was injected into the stomach or the pancreas; even fewer neurons were visualized following the injection into the proximal duodenum. Figure 5 is a typical example of fluorescent tracer localization in the nodose ganglion following injection into the esophageal wall. Within the dorsal root ganglia, Fast Blue or Fluoro-Gold was retrogradely transported to neurons located at levels T_5-L_2, when injected into the stomach or pancreas (mainly at levels T_8-T_{13} and T_8-T_{12}, respectively), and at levels T_9-L_3 (mainly T_{10}-L_1) when injected into the proximal duodenal wall. Detailed analysis of the spinal origin of esophageal afferents was not carried out.

In agreement with other studies, the proportions of vagal neurons retrogradely labeled with either Fast Blue or Fluoro-Gold and immunoreactive for CGRP were usually quite low, ranging between 2% and 8%. Similarly, low proportions of retrogradely labeled neurons containing CGRP immunoreactivity were found in the nodose ganglia when the fluorescent tracer was injected into the abdominal esophagus (Figure 6), indicating that the vagal afferent contribution to the esophageal innervation varies depending on the portion of the esophagus. The percentages of CGRP/TK-containing vagal neurons supplying the upper gastrointestinal tract and pancreas were even lower, ranging from 1% to 7%. On the other hand, the majority of either Fast Blue or Fluoro-Gold retrogradely labeled cells visualized in the dorsal root ganglia was immunoreactive for CGRP, with the highest percentages observed when the fluorescent

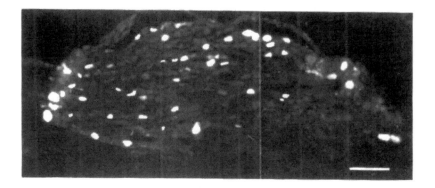

FIGURE 5. Localization of the fluorescent dye Fluoro-Gold in neurons of the left nodose ganglion (caudal region is on the left) of rat following injection of tracer (10 μl of a 4% solution) into the wall (both surfaces) of the abdominal esophagus. Survival time 8 days. (Calibration bar: 150 μm.)

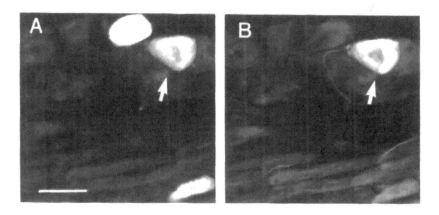

FIGURE 6. Localization of Fluoro-Gold retrogradely labeled cells in the left nodose ganglion (A: rostral pole) of rat as visualized after injection of the tracer into the abdominal esophageal wall. B: the same section showing CGRP immunoreactivity. Arrow indicates the same cell retrogradely labeled with Fluoro-Gold and immunoreactive for CGRP. (Calibration bar: 50 μm; CGRP antiserum as in Figure 4B.)

tracer was injected into the stomach or the proximal duodenal wall (up to 89%). About 50% of spinal neurons innervating the digestive tract contained both CGRP and TK immunoreactivities (Figure 7).

TK AND CGRP mRNA EXPRESSION IN SENSORY GANGLIA

The identification of neuropeptides in visceral afferent neurons has depended on immunohistochemical and radioimmunoassay approaches that rely

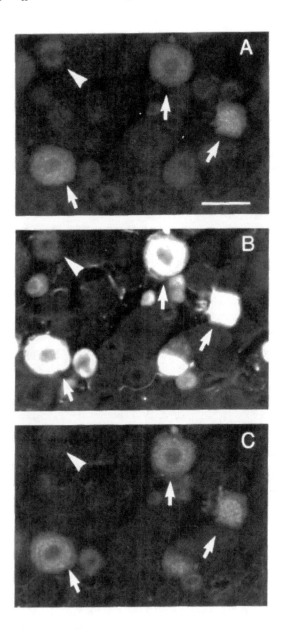

FIGURE 7. Simultaneous visualization of Fluoro-Gold retrogradely labeled (A), CGRP (B) and TK (C) immunolabeled cells in the dorsal root ganglion T_8 of rat. The fluorescent tracer was injected into both the anterior and posterior surfaces of the gastric wall, from the cardias to the pylorus. Arrows indicate neurons containing the retrogradely transported fluorescent dye, CGRP and TK immunoreactivities; arrowheads indicate neurons retrogradely labeled with Fluoro-Gold and immunoreactive for CGRP, but lacking TK immunoreactivity. (CGRP and TK antisera as in Figures 4B and D; calibration bar: 50 μm; CGRP and TK immunostaining were obtained with a mixture of guinea pig CGRP and rabbit NKA antisera.)

upon the availability of antibodies generated against the known amino acid sequences of peptides. Progress in molecular biology has resulted in defining the nucleotide sequences of mRNAs encoding different peptides, thus enabling an unambiguous identification of their sites of biosynthesis. This approach has been particularly valuable for the TK peptides, which share the COOH-terminal region against which most of the TK antibodies are raised. The TKs are generated from precursors, the preprotachykinins (PPT) that are encoded by two related but separate genes: one encoding SP and NKA (known as PPT I or PPT A gene), and the other only encoding NKB (known as PPT II or PPT B gene).[4,43,44,56] Similarly, CGRP immunohistochemistry does not allow discernment between the products of two distinct genes, the calcitonin/α-CGRP and the β-CGRP genes, which generate two highly homologous peptides, the α- and β-CGRP.[1,60] The availability of probes complementary to the TK or CGRP precursor mRNAs and the development of techniques such as the *in situ* hybridization histochemistry now allow the study of the cellular localization of these mRNAs, thus providing information about which TK or CGRP peptide is expressed in a particular population of neurons.

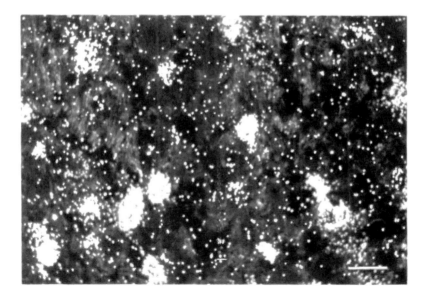

FIGURE 8. Dark field photomicrograph of a dorsal root ganglion of rat showing selected ganglion cells expressing SP/NKA-encoding transcripts. Clusters of grains over cell bodies indicate specific hybridization. Tissue was hybridized with ^{35}S-labeled RNA probe (1 ng/slide; specific activity 3-5 x 10[8] cpm/µg RNA) complementary to the nucleotide sequence of PPT I mRNAs encoding the tachykinin peptides SP and NKA and processed for autoradiography (7-day exposure time). (Calibration bar: 50 µm.)

In situ hybridization histochemistry was performed in aldehyde fixed sections of rat sensory ganglia with ^{35}S-labeled single-stranded RNA probes complementary to the SP/NKA-encoding PPT mRNAs, the NKB-encoding PPT mRNA,[4,44] or to specific sequences of the α- and β-CGRP mRNAs.[1] These studies demonstrated that: 1) SP/NKA-encoding transcripts (Figure 8) and α- and β-CGRP mRNAs are present in selected neurons within the sensory ganglia, characterized by a small to medium size;[71,72] 2) α-CGRP mRNA is more abundant than β-CGRP mRNA in small- and medium-sized neurons, and it is the predominant form expressed in large-size neurons;[57,71] and 3) NKB-encoding mRNA does not appear to be expressed in sensory ganglia, since specific hybridization signals could not be detected in sensory ganglia hybridized with the NKB RNA probe (Sternini, unpublished data). Neurons expressing the SP/NKA- or the CGRP-encoding mRNAs have a regional distribution similar to neurons containing TK or CGRP immunoreactivity, suggesting that specific mRNAs and the posttranslationally processed peptides are expressed in the same populations of neurons.

CONCLUDING REMARKS

Visceral afferents are characterized by a diversity of biochemical properties and can be distinguished on the basis of a variety of specific cytochemical markers. A large proportion of visceral afferents, either originating from vagal or spinal sensory ganglia, express an array of bioactive peptides, the most useful for the identification of afferents supplying the ENS being CGRP (the most ubiquitous peptide sensory marker) and the TK peptides (even though at a lesser degree than CGRP). The contribution of vagal or spinal peptidergic neurons, as visualized by immunohistochemical labeling for CGRP and TKs in combination with retrograde tracing axonal techniques, to the total afferent innervation of different viscera varies depending on the viscus. The major source for the peptidergic afferent innervation of abdominal viscera, including the alimentary tract, is the dorsal root ganglia. Peptide-containing vagal neurons mainly supply thoracic structures, including the cervical esophagus.[30,49] Only a small proportion of peptidergic afferents projecting to the gut arises from vagal sensory neurons. This finding is not surprising, in view of the observation that peptide-containing neurons in the nodose ganglion are preferentially concentrated in the rostral pole;[33] whereas the majority of neurons giving rise to afferents supplying the abdominal viscera, as visualized by retrograde tracing techniques, is preferentially located in the body and caudal pole of the ganglion.[30,31]

The occurrence of CGRP immunoreactivity in a high proportion of spinal gastro-enteric and pancreatic afferents, together with results reported on other organs,[7,77] provides evidence that CGRP is a useful, generalized marker for a major subset of visceral afferent neurons. CGRP immunoreactivity in afferent neurons reflects the expression of the two CGRP genes, the calcitonin/α-CGRP and the β-CGRP genes,[1,60] even though the α-CGRP mRNA is the most prominent form.[54,57,71] Furthermore, the presence of SP/NKA-encoding transcripts in sensory neurons[72] and the lack of specific hybridization with RNA probes complementary to the NKB-encoding mRNA (Sternini, unpublished data), strongly support the hypothesis that sensory neurons only synthesize the TK peptides, SP and NKA (and perhaps also the N-terminally extended forms of NKA, neuropeptide K and neuropeptide-γ, which are posttranslational processing products of the same precursor mRNAs from which SP and NKA are generated), but not the TK peptide, NKB. Sensory neurons containing CGRP and SP/NKA mRNAs have the same appearance and distribution as those identified with immunohistochemical techniques and have been shown to give rise to a subpopulation of afferents supplying the digestive system. These findings, together with the axonal transport and immunohistochemistry results, indicate that a substantial population of abdominal visceral afferents express α-CGRP, β-CGRP and PPT I genes.

The significance and functional implications of the co-existence of bioactive peptides in the same neuronal population is not well understood. The multiplicity of chemical messengers in individual sensory neurons supports the possibility of co-release and interactions. It might also indicate that neurons with selected biochemical properties have different targets and are likely to have different functions. The principles of plurichemical coding and plurichemical transmission,[20,35] which have been introduced in the last decade and which may apply to all neuronal systems, might also imply that individual neurons are capable of exerting multiple functions.

In view of the relative abundance of TK- and CGRP/TK-containing afferents and particularly of the exceptionally vast supply of CGRP immunoreactive afferents innervating the digestive system, together with the variety of targets supplied by these peptidergic afferents, it is difficult to explain their functional roles only as "sensory." The concept of local effector roles for sensory endings in regulating multiple functions, including blood flow, neurogenic inflammatory processes and "axon reflexes," trophic effects and autonomic and visceral activities, has been gaining increasing acceptance (for reviews see Holzer[36]; Kruger [45]). Afferent neurons might therefore subserve double functions, both afferent and efferent. It is possible that their major role is to maintain effector control of target tissues.[45,46] The observation that most visceral afferents, including those supplying the digestive system, are unmyelinated or thinly myelinated and are derived from small- to medium-size sensory neurons, together with the possible local effector role of sensory endings, has led to the introduction of the concept of "noceffector," which indicates the capability of a neuron to combine afferent and efferent roles, obtained by nerve impulses and peptide release, respectively.[45,46]

The biological effects of putative neurotransmitters and/or neuromodulators such as TKs and CGRP in sensory afferents supplying the alimentary tract is still largely unknown. The differentiation between the activities of afferents and enteric, intrinsic neurons is complicated by the fact that these neuron populations may express the same bioactive peptides. CGRP and TKs exert a variety of biological activities in the digestive system, which include inhibition of gastric acid secretion, coordination of gastrointestinal motility, excitation of myenteric neurons and vasodilatation.[3,29,36,58,78] CGRP is a particularly powerful vasodilator, being far more potent than SP.[5] The extensive distribution of CGRP immunoreactive axons to blood vessels along with CGRP profound vasodilator effect are consistent with an effector functional role of this peptide. Moreover, TKs and CGRP have been suggested as putative mediators of sensory neurons implicated in gastric mucosal protection, in view of their inhibitory effects on gastric acid secretion and vasodilator effect.[29,36] However, despite the great abundance of CGRP fibers innervating blood vessels, the CGRP inhibition of gastric acid secretion does not appear to be associated with modifications of gastric mucosal blood flow.[48] On the other hand, it has been recently demonstrated that CGRP is a potent stimulator of gastrointestinal somatostatin release, leading to the speculation that CGRP effects on gastric acid secretion might be mediated by somatostatin.[16] CGRP and TK release from visceral afferents may be responsible for the regulation of different functions, including vasomotor tone, motility and secretion, by influencing a variety of target tissues, either by direct or indirect effects. Afferent axons may therefore contribute to many effector roles in addition to being involved with sensory transmission, even though their mechanisms of action still need to be fully elucidated.

ACKNOWLEDGMENTS

Original work presented here was supported by NIH grants DK38752 and DK40469. The author wishes to express her deep appreciation to K. Anderson for his important contributions, to M. Lai and P. Svensson for expert technical assistance and to Dr. N. Brecha for his helpful comments on the manuscript. The author also wishes to thank H. Wong and Dr. J.H. Walsh for providing the NKA antiserum, Drs. R. Murphy and J.B. Furness for the SP antiserum, Drs. T.I. Bonner and J.E. Krause for SP/NKA and NKB cDNAs, respectively, and Dr. S.G. Amara for CGRP cDNAs.

REFERENCES

1.   Amara, S.G., Arriza, J.L., Leff, S.E., Swanson, L.W., Evans, R.M., and Rosenfeld, M.G., Expression in brain of a messenger RNA encoding a novel neuropeptide homologous to calcitonin gene-related peptide, *Science*, 229, 1094-1097, 1985.
2.   Andrews, P.L.R., Vagal afferent innervation of the gastrointestinal tract, in *Progress in Brain Research*, Vol. 67, *Visceral Sensation*, Cervero, F., and Morrison, J.F.B., Eds., Elsevier, New York, 1986, 65-86.
3.   Barthó, L., and Holzer, P., Search for a physiological role of substance P in gastrointestinal motility, *Neuroscience*, 16, 1-32, 1985.
4.   Bonner, T.I., Affolter, H.-U., Young, A.C., and Young, W.S., III, A cDNA encoding the precursor of the rat neuropeptide, neurokinin B, *Mol. Brain Res.*, 2, 243-249, 1987.

5. **Brain, S.D., Williams, T.J., Tippins, J.R., Morris, H.R., and MacIntyre, I.,** Calcitonin gene-related peptide is a potent vasodilator, *Nature*, 313, 54-56, 1985.

6. **Buck, S.H., Walsh, J.H., Yamamura, H.I., and Burks, T.F.,** Minireview: Neuropeptides in sensory neurons, *Life Sci.*, 30, 1857-1866, 1982.

7. **Cadieux, A., Springall, D.R., Mulderry, P.K., Rodrigo, J., Ghatei, M.A., Terenghi, G., Bloom, S.R., and Polak, J.M.,** Occurrence, distribution and ontogeny of CGRP immunoreactivity in the rat lower respiratory tract: Effect of capsaicin treatment and surgical denervations, *Neuroscience*, 19, 605-627, 1986.

8. **Clague, J.R., Sternini, C., and Brecha, N.,** Localization of calcitonin gene-related peptide-like immunoreactivity in neurones of the rat gastrointestinal tract, *Neurosci. Lett.*, 56, 63-68, 1985.

9. **Costa, M., Cuello, A.C., Furness, J.B., and Franco, R.,** Distribution of enteric neurons showing immunoreactivity for substance P in the guinea pig ileum, *Neuroscience*, 5, 323-331, 1980.

10. **Costa, M., Furness, J.B., and Gibbins, I.L.,** Chemical coding of enteric neurons, in *Progress in Brain Research, Vol. 68, Coexistence of neuronal messengers: A new principle in chemical transmission*, Hökfelt, T., Fuxe, K., and Pernow, B., Eds., Elsevier, New York, 1986, 217-239.

11. **Costa, M., Furness, J.B., and Llewellyn-Smith, I.J.,** Histochemistry of the enteric nervous system, in *Physiology of the Gastrointestinal Tract*, Johnson, L.R., Ed., Raven Press, New York, 1987, 1-40.

12. **Costa, M., Furness, J.B., Llewellyn-Smith, I.J., and Cuello, A.C.,** Projections of substance P neurons within the guinea pig small intestine, *Neuroscience*, 6, 411-424, 1981.

13. **Dockray, G.J., and Sharkey, K.A.,** Neurochemistry of visceral afferent neurones, in *Progress in Brain Research, Visceral Sensation, Vol. 67*, Cervero, F., and Morrison, J.F.B., Eds., Elsevier, New York, 1986, 133-148.

14. **Dodd, J., Jahr, C.E., Hamilton, P.N., Heath, M.J.S., Matthew, W.D., and Jessell, T.E.,** Cytochemical and physiological properties of sensory and dorsal horn neurons that transmit cutaneous sensation, *Cold Spring Harbor Symp. Quant. Biol.*, 48, 685-695, 1983.

15. **Dodd, J., and Jessell, T.E.,** Lactoseries carbohydrates specify subsets of dorsal root ganglion neurons projecting to the superficial dorsal horn of rat spinal cord, *J. Neurosci.*, 5, 3278-3294, 1985.

16. **Dunning, B.E., and Taborsky, G.J.,** Calcitonin gene-related peptide: A potent and selective stimulator of gastrointestinal somatostatin secretion, *Endocrinology*, 120, 1774-1781, 1987.

17. **Fox, E.A., and Powley, T.L.,** Tracer diffusion has exaggerated CNS maps of direct preganglionic innervation of the pancreas, *J. Auton. Nerv. Syst.*, 15, 55-59, 1986.

18. **Furness, J.B., and Costa, M.,** Types of nerves in the enteric nervous system, *Neuroscience*, 5, 1-20, 1980.

19. **Furness, J.B., and Costa, M.,** *The Enteric Nervous System*, Churchill Livingtsone, London, 1987.

20. **Furness, J.B., Morris, J.L., Gibbins, I.L., and Costa, M.,** Chemical coding of neurons and plurichemical transmission, *Annu. Rev. Pharmacol. Toxicol.*, 29, 289-306, 1989.

21. **Gabella, G.,** Innervation of the gastrointestinal tract, *Int. Rev. Cytol.*, 59, 129-193, 1979.

22. **Garry, M.G., Miller, K.E., and Seybold, V.S.,** Lumbar dorsal root ganglia of the cat: A quantitative study of peptide immunoreactivity and cell size, *J. Comp. Neurol.*, 284, 36-47, 1989.

23. **Gershon, M.D.,** The enteric nervous system, *Annu. Rev. Neurosci.*, 4, 227-272, 1981.

24. **Gibbins, I.L., Furness, J.B., and Costa, M.,** Pathway-specific patterns of the co-existence of substance P, calcitonin gene-related peptide, cholecystokinin and dynorphin in neurons of the dorsal root ganglia of the guinea-pig, *Cell Tissue Res.*, 248, 417-437, 1987.

25. **Gibbins, I.L., Furness, J.B., Costa, M., MacIntyre, I., Hillyard, C.J., and Girgis, S.,** Co-localization of calcitonin gene-related peptide-like immunoreactivity with substance P in cutaneous, vascular and visceral sensory neurons of the guinea pig, *Neurosci. Lett.*, 57, 125-130, 1985.

26. Gilbert, R.F.T., Emson, P.C., Fahrenkrug, J., Lee, C.M., Penman, A., and Wass, J., Axonal transport of neuropeptides in the cervical vagus nerve of the rat, *J. Neurochem.*, 34, 105-113, 1980.

27. Goehler, L.E., and Sternini, C., Effect of extrinsic denervation on calcitonin gene-related peptide immunoreactivity (CGRP-IR) in the rat hepatobiliary system, *Soc. Neurosci. Abs.*, 14, 984, 1988.

28. Goehler, L.E., Sternini, C., and Brecha, N., Calcitonin gene-related peptide immunoreactivity in the hepatobiliary system of the guinea-pig: Distribution and co-localization with substance P, *Cell Tissue Res.*, 253, 145-150, 1988.

29. Goodman, E.C., and Iversen, L.L., Calcitonin gene-related peptide: Novel neuropeptide, *Life Sci.*, 38, 2169-2178, 1986.

30. Green, T., and Dockray, G.J., Calcitonin gene-related peptide and substance P in afferents to the upper gastrointestinal tract in the rat, *Neurosci. Lett.*, 76, 151-156, 1987.

31. Green, T., and Dockray, G.J., Characterization of the peptidergic afferent innervation of the stomach in the rat, mouse and guinea-pig, *Neuroscience*, 25, 181-193, 1988.

32. Gulbenkian, S., Merighi, A., Wharton, J., Varndell, I.M., and Polak, J.M., Ultrastructural evidence for the coexistence of calcitonin gene-related peptide and substance P in secretory vesicles of peripheral nerves in the guinea pig, *J. Neurocytol.*, 15, 535-542, 1986.

33. Helke, C.J., and Hill, K.M., Immunohistochemical study of neuropeptides in vagal and glossopharyngeal afferent neurons in the rat, *Neuroscience*, 26, 539-551, 1988.

34. Hökfelt, T., Elde, R., Johansson, O., Luft, R., Nilsson, G., and Arimura, A., Immunohistochemical evidence for separate populations of somatostatin-containing and substance P-containing primary afferent neurons in the rat, *Neuroscience*, 1, 131-136, 1976.

35. Hökfelt, T., Fuxe, K., and Pernow, B., *Progress in Brain Research., Vol. 68, Coexistence of neuronal messengers: a new principle in chemical transmission*, Elsevier, New York, 1986.

36. Holzer, P., Local effector functions of capsaicin-sensitive sensory nerve endings: Involvement of tachykinins, calcitonin gene-related peptide and other neuropeptides, *Neuroscience*, 24, 739-768, 1988.

37. Jänig, W., and Morrison, J.F.B., Functional properties of spinal visceral afferents supplying abdominal and pelvic organs, with special emphasis on visceral nociception, in *Progress in Brain Research, Vol. 67, Visceral Sensation*, Cervero, F., and Morrison, J.F.B., Eds., Elsevier, New York, 1986, 87-114.

38. Jessell, T.M., Substance P in nociceptive sensory neurons, in *Substance P in the nervous system*, Ciba Foundation Symposium 91, Pitman, London, 1982, 225-248.

39. Jessell, T.M., Substance P in the nervous system, in *Handbook of Psychopharmacology, Vol. 16*, Iversen, L.L., Iversen, S.D., and Snyder, S.H., Eds., Plenum, New York, 1983, 1-105.

40. Ju, G., Hökfelt, T., Brodin, E., Fahrenkrug, J., Fisher, J.A., Frey, P., Elde, R.P., and Brown, J.C., Primary sensory neurons of the rat showing calcitonin gene-related peptide immunoreactivity and their relation to substance P-, somatostatin-, vasoactive intestinal polypeptide- and cholecystokinin-immunoreactive ganglion cells, *Cell Tissue Res.*, 247, 417-431, 1987.

41. Kage, R., McGregor, G.P., Thim, L., and Conlon, J.L., Neuropeptide-γ: a peptide isolated from rabbit intestine that is derived from γ-preprotachykinin, *J. Neurochem.*, 50, 1412-1417, 1988.

42. Kalia, M., and Sullivan, J.M., Brainstem projections of sensory and motor components of the vagus nerve in the rat, *J. Comp. Neurol.*, 211, 248-264, 1982.

43. Kotani, H., Hoshimaru, M., Nawa, H., and Nakanishi, S., Structure and gene organization of bovine neuromedin K, *Proc. Natl. Acad. Sci USA*, 83, 7074-7078, 1986.

44. Krause, J.E., Chirgwin, J.M., Carter, M.S., Xu, Z.S., and Hershey, A.D., Three rat preprotachykinin mRNAs encode the neuropeptide substance P and neurokinin A, *Proc. Natl. Acad. Sci. USA*, 84, 881-885, 1987.

45. **Kruger, L.,** Morphological correlates of "free" nerve endings- A reappraisal of thin sensory axon classification, in *Fine Afferent Nerve Fibers and Pain,* Schmidt, R.F., Schaible, H.-G., and Vahle-Hinz, C., Eds, VCH Verlagsgesellschaft mbH, Federal Republic of Germany, 1987, 3-13.
46. **Kruger, L., Silverman, J.D., Mantyh, P.W., Sternini, C., and Brecha, N.,** Peripheral patterns of calcitonin gene-related peptide general somatic sensory innervation: cutaneous and deep terminations, *J. Comp. Neurol.,* 280, 291-302, 1989.
47. **Leah, J.D., Cameron, A.A., Kelly, W.L., and Snow, P.J.,** Coexistence of peptide immunoreactivity in sensory neurons of the cat, *Neuroscience,* 16, 683-690, 1985.
48. **Leung, F.W., Tallos, E.G., Taché, Y.F., and Guth, P.H.,** Calcitonin gene-related peptide inhibits acid secretion without modifying blood flow, *Am. J. Physiol.,* 252, G215-G218, 1987.
49. **Lundberg, J.M., Hökfelt, T., Martling, C.-R., Saria, A., and Cuello, C.,** Substance P immunoreactive sensory nerves in the lower respiratory tract of various mammals including man, *Cell Tissue Res.,* 235, 251-261, 1984.
50. **Maggio, J.E.,** Tachykinins, *Annu. Rev. Neurosci.,* 11, 13-28, 1988.
51. **Mawe, G.M., and Gershon, M.D.,** Structure, afferent innervation, and transmitter content of ganglia of the guinea pig gallbladder: relationship to the enteric nervous system, *J. Comp. Neurol.,* 283, 374-390, 1989.
52. **Mei, N.,** Sensory structures in the viscera, in *Progress in Sensory Physiology 4,* Autrum, H., Ottoson, D., Perl, E.R., Schmidt, R.F., Shimazu, H., and Willis, W.D., Eds., Springer-Verlag, New York, 1983, 2-42.
53. **Mesulam, M.-M.,** Principles of horseradish peroxidase neurochemistry and their applications for tracing neural pathways-axonal transport, enzyme histochemistry, and light microscopical analysis, in *Tracing Neural Connections with Horseradish Peroxidase,* Mesulam, M.-M., Ed., Wiley, Chichester, United Kingdom, 1982, 1-151.
54. **Mulderry, P.K., Ghatei, M.A., Spokes, R.A., Jones, P.M., Pierson, A.M., Hamid, Q.A., Kanse, S., Amara, S.G., Burrin, J.M., Legon, S., Polak, J.M., and Bloom, S.R.,** Differential expression of α-CGRP and β-CGRP by primary sensory neurons and enteric autonomic neurons of the rat, *Neuroscience,* 25, 195-205, 1988.
55. **Nagy, J.I.,** Capsaicin: A chemical probe for sensory neuron mechanisms, in *Handbook of Psychopharmacology, Vol. 6,* Iversen, L.L., and Snyder, S.M., Eds., Plenum Press, New York, 1982, 185-235.
56. **Nawa, H., Kotani, H., and Nakanishi, S.,** Tissue-specific generation of two preprotachykinin mRNAs from one gene by alternative RNA splicing, *Nature,* 312, 729-734, 1984.
57. **Noguchi, K., Senba, E., Morita, Y., Sato, M., and Tohyama, M.,** Co-expression of α-CGRP and β-CGRP mRNAs in the rat dorsal root ganglion cells, *Neurosci. Lett.,* 108, 1-5, 1990.
58. **Pernow, B.,** Substance P, *Pharmacol. Rev.,* 35, 85-141, 1983.
59. **Rinaman, L., and Miselis, R.R.,** The organization of the vagal innervation of rat pancreas using cholera toxin-horseradish peroxidase conjugate, *J. Auton. Nerv. Syst.,* 21, 109-125, 1987.
60. **Rosenfeld, M.G., Mermod, J.-J., Amara, S.G., Swanson, L.W., Sawchenko, P.E., Rivier, J., Vale, W.V., and Evans, R.M.,** Production of a novel neuropeptide encoded by the calcitonin gene with tissue-specific RNA processing, *Nature,* 304, 129-135, 1983.
61. **Salt, T.E., and Hill, R.G.,** Neurotransmitter candidates of somatosensory primary afferent fibers, *Neuroscience,* 10, 1083-1103, 1983.
62. **Schmued, L.C., and Fallon, J.H.,** Fluoro-Gold: a new fluorescent retrograde axonal tracer with numerous unique properties, *Brain Res.,* 377, 147-154, 1986.
63. **Shapiro, R.E., and Miselis, R.R.,** The central organization of the vagus nerve innervating the stomach of the rat, *J. Comp. Neurol.,* 238, 473-488, 1985.
64. **Sharkey, K.A., and Williams, R.G.,** Extrinsic innervation of the rat pancreas: demonstration of vagal sensory neurones in the rat by retrograde tracing, *Neurosci. Lett.,* 42, 131-135, 1983.
65. **Sharkey, K.A., Williams, R.G., and Dockray, G.J.,** Sensory substance P innervation of the stomach and pancreas, *Gastroenterology,* 87, 914-921, 1984.

66. Silverman, J.D., and Kruger, L., Acid phosphatase as a selective marker for a class of small sensory ganglion cells in several mammals: spinal cord distribution, histochemical properties, and relation to fluoride-resistant acid phosphatase (FRAP) of rodents, *Somatosens. Res.*, 5, 219-246, 1988.

67. Silverman, J.D., and Kruger, L., Lectin and neuropeptide labeling of separate populations of dorsal root ganglion neurons and associated "nociceptor" thin axons in rat testis and cornea whole-mount preparations, *Somatosens. Res.*, 5, 259-267, 1988.

68. Skirboll, L., Hökfelt, T., Norell, G., Phillipson, O., Kuypers, H.G.M., Bentivoglio, M., Catsman-Berrevoets, C.E., Visser, T.J., Steinbusch, H., Verhofstad, A., Cuello, A.C., Goldstein, M., and Brownstein, M., A method for specific transmitter identification of retrogradely labelled neurons: immunofluorescence combined with fluorescence tracing, *Brain Res. Rev.*, 8, 99-127, 1984.

69. Sternini, C., Structural and chemical organization of the enteric nervous system, *Annu. Rev. Physiol.*, 50, 81-93, 1988.

70. Sternini, C., Neurochemistry of spinal afferents supplying the gastrointestinal tract and pancreas, in *Brain and Gut Interactions*, Taché, Y., and Wingate, D., Eds., CRC Press, 1991, 45-55.

71. Sternini, C., and Anderson, K., Calcitonin gene-related peptide-containing neurons supplying the rat digestive system: differential distribution and expression pattern, Somatosens. *Mot. Res.*, 9, 45-59, 1992.

72. Sternini, C., Anderson, K., Frantz, G., Krause, J.E., and Brecha, N., Expression of substance P/neurokinin A-encoding preprotachykinin messenger ribonucleic acids in the rat enteric nervous system, *Gastroenterology*, 97, 348-356, 1989.

73. Sternini, C., and Brecha, N., Immunocytochemical identification of islet cells and nerve fibers containing calcitonin gene-related peptide-like immunoreactivity in the rat pancreas, *Gastroenterology*, 90, 1155-1163, 1986.

74. Sternini, C., Reeve, J.R., Jr., and Brecha, N., Distribution and characterization of calcitonin gene-related peptide immunoreactivity in the digestive system of normal and capsaicin-treated rats, *Gastroenterology*, 93, 852-862, 1987.

75. Streit, W.J., Schulte, B.A., Balentine, J.D., and Spicer, S.S., Evidence for glycoconjugate in nociceptive primary sensory neurons and its origin from the Golgi complex, *Brain Res.*, 377, 1-17, 1986.

76. Su, H.C., Bishop, A.E., Power, R.F., Hamada, Y., and Polak, J.M., Dual intrinsic and extrinsic origins of CGRP- and NPY-immunoreactive nerves of the rat gut and pancreas, *J. Neurosci.*, 7, 2674-2687, 1987.

77. Su, H.C., Wharton, J., Polak, J.M., Mulderry, P.K., Ghatei, M.A., Gibson, S.J., Terenghi, G., Morrison, J.F.B., Ballesta, J., and Bloom, S.R., Calcitonin gene-related peptide immunoreactivity in afferent neurons supplying the urinary tract: combined retrograde tracing and immunohistochemistry, *Neuroscience*, 18, 727-747, 1986.

78. Takaki, M., Jin, J.-G., and Nakayama, S., Possible involvement of calcitonin gene-related peptide (CGRP) in non-cholinergic non-adrenergic relaxation induced by mesenteric nerve stimulation in guinea pig ileum, *Brain Res.*, 478, 199-203, 1989.

79. Taylor, D.C.M., Pierau, Fr.-K., and Schmid, H., The use of fluorescent tracers in the peripheral sensory nervous system, *J. Neurosci. Methods*, 8, 211-224, 1983.

80. Varro, A., Green, T., Homes, S., and Dockray, G.J., Calcitonin gene-related peptide in visceral afferent nerve fibres: quantification by radioimmunoassay and determination of axonal transport rates, *Neuroscience*, 26, 927-932, 1988.

Chapter 7

VAGAL RECEPTOR TRANSPORT

T.H. Moran and P.R. McHugh

TABLE OF CONTENTS

LIST OF ABBREVIATIONS

ANG II-angiotensin II
CCK = cholecystokinin
DMX = dorsal motor nucleus
^{3}(H-NMS) = ^{3}H-N-methyl scopolamine
NTS = nucleus tractus solitarius

INTRODUCTION

The vagus nerve contains both efferent and afferent limbs. The efferent vagus has cell bodies in the dorsal motor nucleus (DMX) of the caudal brain stem, while the afferent vagal cell bodies are contained within the nodose ganglion. Axons from the afferent cell bodies project both peripherally to the various target organs and centrally to the nucleus tractus solitarius (NTS). The efferent and afferent limbs of the vagus play a variety of roles in regulating the function of the target organs they innervate. Efferent signals can modulate cardiovascular, pulmonary and gastrointestinal functions. Afferent neurons receive information from these target organs and relay it to the brain through the NTS. There are also clear examples of vago-vagal reflexes involving vagal processing of sensory information and a vagal motor response to that afferent information.

A variety of neurotransmitters or neuromodulators are released from vagal fibers and the vagus has been demonstrated to contain neurotransmitter and peptide receptors. Since there is no synthesis of proteins in nerve terminals, some neurotransmitter molecules or receptor proteins must be synthesized at the cell body and transported to the locations where they will exert some physiological function. There are axoplasmic transport mechanisms responsible for the delivery of large and small molecules to and from nerve endings. This chapter will focus on the transport of receptors within the vagus, identify the mechanisms by which this transport is carried out, and review the available information on which receptor populations are contained and transported in both the efferent and afferent limbs of the vagus nerve.

AXONAL TRANSPORT

One of the defining characteristics of nerve cells is long axons. The cell bodies of neurons are the main sites of protein synthesis and, consequently, there is often a long distance between the site of synthesis and the nerve terminal where these proteins will be utilized. Figure 1 presents a cartoon of the three portions of the nerve cell involved in this synthesis-transport-utilization process. At the site of the cell body, protein and lipid macromolecules are synthesized through transcriptional processes and incorporated into membranes within the Golgi apparatus and the endoplasmic reticulum. These transmitters, enzymes, receptors or their precursor molecules are carried along the length of the axon through the mechanisms of axonal transport to their site of use, which may be either along the axon itself or at the nerve terminal. This use may involve the release of neurotransmitters or the incorporation of receptor molecules into the membrane. Axonal transport occurs at a variety of rates with fast and slow axonal transport occurring by different mechanisms.

The original demonstration of axonal transport was made by observing an accumulation of axoplasm proximal to an axonal constriction. The amount of

NERVE CELL

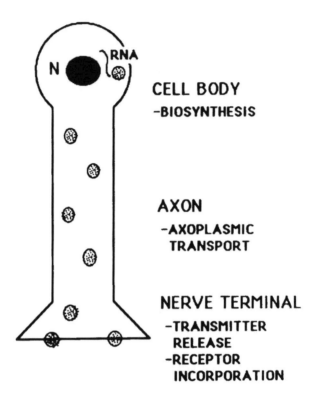

CELL BODY
-BIOSYNTHESIS

AXON
-AXOPLASMIC
TRANSPORT

NERVE TERMINAL
-TRANSMITTER
RELEASE
-RECEPTOR
INCORPORATION

FIGURE 1. Schematic of nerve cell demonstrating synthesis, axonal transport and utilization of neurotransmitters and receptors.

axoplasm accumulated increased with time, and when the constriction was removed, the accumulated material moved down the nerve fiber at the rate of 1 mm per day. This transport was termed axoplasmic flow.[24] In the early 1960s, several groups described the presence of material in nerves moving at a much more rapid rate (up to 400 mm per day). This fast axonal transport also occurs from the nerve endings back to the cell bodies, presumably to return materials for recycling. The rate of fast retrograde transport is only one-half to two-thirds that of anterograde transport. The reason for this difference in transport rate is not clear. The potential functions of this retrograde transport will be discussed.

The movement of materials involved in synaptic transmission from the perikaryon to the nerve terminal occurs by fast axonal transport. While the mechanisms underlying this transport are not completely understood, it has been demonstrated that microtubules play an essential role. Antimitotic alkyloids, or colchicine which are known to disrupt microtubules, interfere with fast transport. In contrast, the mechanism for slow axonal transport differs. It is unidirectional, dependent upon the cell body and appears to occur by bulk flow.

DISCOVERY OF AXONAL TRANSPORT OF RECEPTOR PROTEINS

In 1980, two independent reports provided evidence for the axonal transport of receptors. In the first, Young *et al.*,[26] proceeding from the standpoint that biochemical investigations had demonstrated the presence of opiate presynaptic receptors in axon nerve terminals in rat vagal nerves, utilized *in vitro* autoradiography to demonstrate both the presence of opiate receptors in the nodose ganglion and the receptor buildup on the proximal side of a ligature around the vagus nerve. Examination of the receptor distribution in the nodose ganglion revealed receptors in association with fiber bundles between the cell bodies and a marked association of receptors with the majority of the neuronal cell bodies. At the ligation site there was a 6 to 1 proximal to distal binding ratio around the ligation in nerves that had been ligated for 20 hours. The ratio was less in nerves ligated for 7 hours and not significantly different from control in the nerves ligated for only 1 to 2 minutes before processing. The original estimate suggested that the opiate receptors were moving at a range of 3 to 4 mm per hour, suggesting that transport was taking place by a mechanism of fast axonal transport.

In concluding this initial report, the authors stated that it was not surprising that receptors would undergo axonal or dendritic flow. Synthesis of receptor proteins must take place in the perikaryon and must be moved in some fashion to distal areas where they can become membrane bound. Thus, the authors suggested that axonal flow would turn out to be a common property of most or all receptors. Much future evidence would show that their speculation was correct, although, as will be demonstrated, the specifics of the transport phenomena depend upon the receptor population under study.

While this initial article on opiate receptors was in press, Laduron[11] reported the presence and axonal flow of muscarinic receptors in the dog splenic nerve. Muscarinic receptors were labeled *in vitro* with ^{3}H-dexetimide and found to accumulate on both sides of a ligature, indicating the existence and axoplasmic transport of presynaptic muscarinic cholinergic receptors. In contrast to the Young *et al.* study on opiate receptors, however, this transport appeared to be both anterograde and retrograde. This distinction, that the transport of some receptors can only be demonstrated in a proximal-distal manner while the transport of other receptors or binding sites can be shown to occur in both directions along the axon is one of the issues to be discussed in greater detail.

Proceeding from these initial demonstrations, the presence and axonal transport of binding sites has been studied in both central and peripheral neurons. Table 1 demonstrates the receptor populations for which axonal transport has been observed in peripheral nerves. In all cases, binding sites are identified as

TABLE 1
Axonal Transport of Receptors in Peripheral Nerves

RECEPTOR	NERVE	SPECIES
Non-Peptide Receptors:		
Muscarinic	Splenic	Dog
	Hypogastric	Cat
	Sciatic	Rat
	Vagus	Rat
Nicotinic	Sciatic	Rat
		Cat
		Human
	Optic	Rat
B-Adrenergic	Sciatic	Rat
Peptide Receptors:		
Opiate	Vagus	Rat
CCK	Vagus	Rat
ANG II	Vagus	Dog
Neurotensin	Vagus	Rat
Peptide YY	Vagus	Rat

they accumulate around a ligature site. Estimation of binding site distribution around a ligataure can either be done using *in vitro* autoradiography (Figure 2) or by directly counting nerve segments. The remainder of this chapter will focus on vagal receptor transport.

VAGAL TRANSPORT OF NON-PEPTIDE RECEPTORS

This section will identify those receptor populations that have been shown to be transported in the vagus nerve, outline the vagal components in which transport has been identified and specify the characteristics of transport. Included in Table 1 are the those receptors which have been shown to be present in and be transported along the vagus nerve. These are two types, peptide and nonpeptide receptors. We will begin with a discussion of nonpeptide receptors.

The axonal transport of muscarinic cholinergic receptors in the rat vagus nerve was initially outlined by Zarbin et al.[28] Figure 3 demonstrates the time course of muscarinic cholinergic binding site accumulation around a cervical vagal ligation. In this case, a clear accumulation of binding sites occurred on both the proximal and distal ends of the ligation indicating the presence of both anterograde and retrograde receptor transport. Further experiments which utilized a double ligature demonstrated that there was an accumulation of receptors observed proximally to both ligatures. The accumulation proximal to the distal ligature (that furthest from the nodose ganglion) was about 50% of that at the

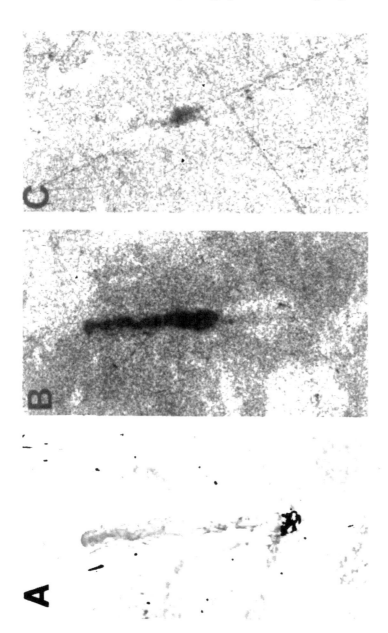

FIGURE 2. Photomicrographs of autoradiographs and stained section of vagal segments demonstrating CCK receptor transport as demonstrated by a buildup of labeled binding sites proximal to a ligature site. A: Stained section, B: Autoradiograph demonstrating total binding, C: Autoradiograph demonstrating nonspecific binding.

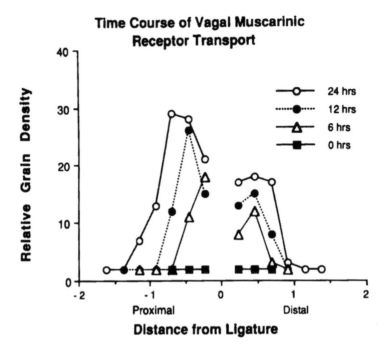

FIGURE 3. Time course of muscarinic cholinergic binding site accumulation. Vagal nerve trunks were ligated for various times from 0–24 hrs. Proximal indicates x coordinates proximal to the ligation point. The x coordinate O is assigned to the point at which the ligation was placed. (Adapted with permission by *Journal of Neuroscience*, from Zarbin *et al.*[28])

proximal ligature site. In contrast, while there was an accumulation of receptors distal to the distal ligature, there was no detectable accumulation distal to the proximal ligature. At no point between the ligature sites did the binding site density decrease to background levels. This result implied that only a portion of the binding sites found within the axon undergo transport. The calculated rate of anterograde receptor accumulation was almost two times greater than the calculated rate for retrograde accumulation. These data appear to be in agreement with the generally accepted view that the anterograde transport of other molecules occurs at about twice the rate of retrograde transport. This difference in transport rates could also explain why the accumulation of receptors proximal to ligature sites is consistently greater than that found distal to ligature sites.

Another difference in the binding sites found proximal and distal to the ligatures was a pharmacological one. It has been demonstrated that most cholinergic agonists bind to a multiplicity of receptor sites in brain, each site distinguished by its affinity for the various agonists. On the other hand, antagonists seem to bind with all sites with about equal affinity.[1,7] For example, carbachol, a cholinergic agonist, binds with a much greater potency to a high affinity muscarinic cholinergic receptor. This difference has allowed the

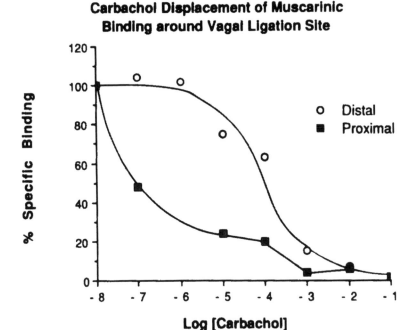

FIGURE 4. Carbachol displacement of [3](H-NMS) binding to ligated rat vagi. Tissue sections ligated for 22 hrs were used in experiment. Consecutive tissue sections were incubated in [3](H-NMS) plus varying concentrations of carbachol. Binding was assayed immediately proximal and distal to the ligature site. (Adapted with permission by *Journal of Neuroscience*, from Zarbin *et al.*[28])

audioradiographic localization of both high and low affinity binding sites in the brain. By incubating tissue sections from the ligated vagi in the presence of ^{3}H-N-methyl scopolamine [3](H-NMS) along with various concentrations of unlabeled carbachol, the authors were able to demonstrate that the binding sites undergoing anterograde transport (those found proximal to the ligature) contained a much higher proportion of the high affinity binding sites than those being transported retrogradely (found distal to the ligature sites). This difference is shown in Figure 4. For binding sites found immediately proximal to the point of ligation, carbachol is a potent inhibitor of [3](H-NMS) binding, displacing the radioligand with an IC_{50} of 9×10^{-8} M. In contrast, distal to the ligature site, carbachol was significantly weaker in inhibiting binding, having an IC_{50} of 1.3 $\times 10^{-4}$. This result was interpreted to suggest that the binding sites being transported anterogradely and retrogradely differ. The fact that the majority of the receptors exported from the soma exist primarily in the high affinity state while most of those returning toward the cell body exist in the low affinity state may explain this phenomenon. The anterogradely transported population may undergo an alteration in binding properties in response to insertion in membrane either at the synaptic terminal or along the axon or in response to being activated while membrane bound. The low affinity state may be maintained because the membrane is then recycled at retrograde transport. Since the majority of nontransported, axonally located, receptors seem to exist in the low affinity state, it is likely that conversion from high to low affinity may take place as the receptors become membrane bound rather than in response to their activation.

The particular limb of the vagus which contains and transports these muscarinic cholinergic receptors has not been investigated. The simple presence of transport does not speak to the issue of whether these binding sites are contained in efferent or afferent fibers.

While beta adrenergic[29] and nicotinic receptors[6,17,21] have been demonstrated to be transported in other systems, this has not been shown to take place in the vagus nerve (Table 1). The properties of transport of these receptor populations appear similar to those described above for the muscarinic cholinergic receptor in the vagus.

VAGAL TRANSPORT OF PEPTIDE RECEPTORS

The peptide receptors for which axonal transport has been demonstrated are shown in Table 1. These vagal receptors have received degrees of study ranging from single reports to more extensive analyses of the nature of the transport and the particular vagal components in which transport takes place. In the following sections, we will review the available information on these peptide receptors.

Opiate Receptors

Opiate receptors were the first receptors for which transport was characterized in the vagus nerve. In the initial report by Young, *et al.*,[26] the phenomenon of receptor transport was examined by ligating the vagus approximately 1.5 cm below the nodose ganglion and sacrificing the rats at various intervals after ligation. A segment of the nerve, consisting of at least 3 or 4 mm on each side of the ligation site was dissected out, mounted in brain paste and sectioned on a microtome. Slide mounted tissue sections were incubated in the presence of labeled opiate ligand and opposed to emulsion coated cover slips to generate autoradiographs. Examination of the autoradiographs demonstrated that there was a time-dependent buildup of binding sites proximal to the ligation. That is, the greater the densities of silver grains, the longer the time between ligation and sacrifice. Pharmacological studies demonstrated that these sites were opiate receptor sites rather than some nonspecific binding sites for the radiolabeled peptide. The sites bound agonist and antagonist radiolabeled drugs, the binding was displaced by unlabeled naloxone, and the binding sites were stereospecific in that only levallorphan but not dextrallorphan displaced binding. Also, binding was decreased in the presence of GTP. In the initial report, the flow of receptors seemed to be unidirectional. Increases in binding were found only proximal and not distal to the ligation site.

In contrast to these results obtained by *in vitro* autoradiography, when opiate receptors were labeled *in vivo* with ^{3}H lofentanil, an accumulation of binding

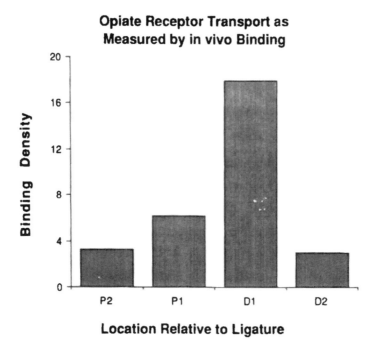

FIGURE 5. Accumulation of labeling in proximal and distal segments of ligated vagus nerves 16 hrs after ligation and *in vivo* injection of ³H lofentanil. (Adapted from Laduron and Janssen.[16])

sites was present on both sides of the ligature.[15] In these studies the ligatures were placed approximately 1.5 cm below the level of the nodose ganglion and 10 μcurries of ³H lofentanil were injected intravenously into rats at different time intervals prior to sacrifice. Nerve segments above and below the ligature were removed and counted for radioactivity. The results demonstrated that there was a buildup of ³H lofentanil in the nerve on both sides of the ligature and, as demonstrated in Figure 5, the magnitude of accumulation was significantly greater distal rather than proximal to the ligature site. Four hours after the *in vivo* ³H lofentanil injection, labeling was maximal proximal to the ligature site. A delay of 16-24 hours between ³H lofentanil injection and sacrifice was necessary to reach a maximum accumulation distal to the site. The rapid appearance in the proximal part was ascribed to the short distance between the ligature and the nodose ganglion. The long distance between the ligature and the nerve terminal located in the gut, heart and lung were thought to explain the delayed accumulation in the distal segment. In rats in which a ligature was not used there was an accumulation of ³H lofentanil in the nodose ganglion. This accumulation was maximal 16 hours following injection and gradually fell off. This accumulation was blocked by vagotomy or capsaicin treatment.

While most studies have examined axonal transport using *in vitro* labeling techniques, the Laduron and Janssen study attempted to do so with an *in vivo* injection of the radioligand at various times before sacrifice. This difference in technique accounts for the very different pattern of results. In the *in vitro* experiments, the investigator looks at the interaction of the radioligand with binding sites which are at particular points along the nerve. The ligation provides a point of binding site accumulation for this interaction. In contrast, in the *in vivo* experiments, interaction between receptor and radioligand occurs at membrane bound receptor sites, and the investigator looks directly at the transport of the injected radioligand in the nerve segment. There is the assumption that the ligand is attached to a receptor and that one is seeing the transport of a ligand/receptor complex. These experiments, however, cannot discount the unlikely possibility that the ^{3}H lofentanil is being transported in the axons unbound to a receptor site. Rather, the inability to detect opiate binding site transport in the *in vitro* situation when transport can apparently be demonstrated in the *in vivo* experiment raises the possibility that retrogradely transported opiate receptors are in some way changed by their interaction with the endogenous ligand. That is, the receptor peptide is being transported but no longer has the ability to bind its usual ligands. Interaction of the receptor with its endogenous ligand at the synapse may then in some way structurally change the receptor protein so that it no longer has an affinity for endogenous or exogenous ligands. A final potential explanation is that once activated by endogenous or exogenous ligand, some receptors become internalized and are transported as a unit back to the soma. This internalization may not take place for other receptors, and the receptor complex may be transported without the ligand. As in the case of cholinergic receptors,[28] some structural change in the receptor may have occurred in response to activation but this structural change is not sufficient to completely prevent binding in an *in vitro* situation.

The data suggesting that the opiate receptor is being retrogradely transported in the vagal axon has been taken as evidence that this retrograde transport to the perikaryan may play an important role in regulation or synaptogenesis.[12,15] The rate at which retrograde transport may occur could provide the cell with feedback signals for the production of further receptor complexes, or it may provide some signal promoting the synthesis of other molecules at the site of the cell body.

Of interest here is the reported inability of antagonists to label transported receptor sites when administered *in vivo*.[13] This may imply that only agonist compounds are able to induce receptor internalization. While the antagonist has a high affinity for the receptor sites, as demonstrated by competitive inhibition, the antagonist may not fully activate the receptor in terms of internalization mechanisms.

Capsaicin treatment has been demonstrated to prevent retrograde receptor transport as measured in response to *in vivo* ^{3}H lofentanil administration.[13] Capsaicin has been shown to cause destruction of non-myelinated small-diameter afferent fibers.[8] Since capsaicin destroys this population and eliminates retrograde opiate receptor transport, it is likely that this transport occurs in this

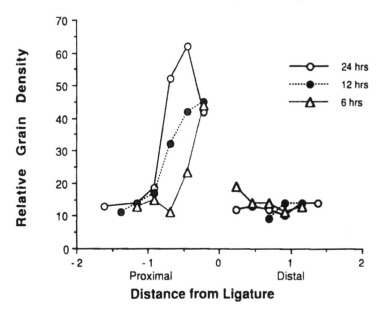

FIGURE 6. Time course of CCK binding site accumulation. Vagi were ligated for various times from 0–24 hrs. Values along the abscissa are distances from the ligation point. Negative values are proximal and positive values distal to the ligature. (Adapted with permission by Pergamon Press, from Zarbin *et al.*[27])

population of vagal afferent fibers. The effect of capsaicin on anterograde transport, as measured by *in vitro* techniques, has not been assessed. It seems likely, however, that anterograde and retrograde transport would occur in the same population of vagal fibers.

Cholecystokinin Receptors

Another peptide receptor whose presence and axonal flow in the vagus nerve has been demonstrated is the receptor for the brain-gut peptide cholecystokinin (CCK). Utilizing the techniques of vagal ligation and *in vitro* autoradiography, Zarbin *et al.*[27] demonstrated both the presence and axonal transport of CCK binding sites in the rat cervical vagus. The time course of CCK binding site accumulation is demonstrated in Figure 6. At all three time points there was a buildup of binding sites proximal to the ligature. The rate of buildup and the distance of buildup from the ligature site appear to be time dependent. In contrast, there was no accumulation of binding sites distal to the ligature site. The use of double ligature experiments demonstrated a significant buildup proximal to the proximal ligature site, some buildup proximal to the distal ligature site, but no significant accumulation distal to either site. The buildup of receptors proximal to the ligature site was dependent on microtubules in that

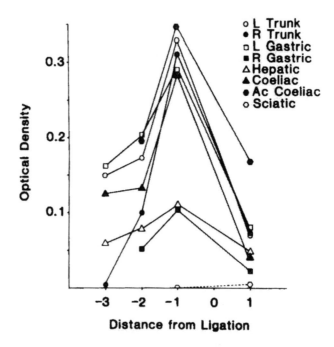

FIGURE 7. Mean specific binding site accumulation (total-nonspecific) around ligations on various vagal segments. Values along the abscissa indicate distance from the ligature (mm). Negative values correspond to areas proximal to the ligature while positive values correspond to distal. Increases in optical density correspond to increases in binding density. (Reprinted with permission by Elsevier Science Publishers, from Moran *et al.*[20])

pretreatment of the animals with colchicine eliminated a significant buildup of binding sites proximal to the ligature.

We have extended this initial report of vagal transport of CCK receptors in the cervical vagus to demonstrate that transport of CCK binding sites occurs in all of the branches of the subdiaphragmatic vagus.[20] As shown in Figure 7, ligating the subdiaphragmatic vagus resulted in significant binding site accumulations proximal to the ligatures placed on either the subdiaphragmatic vagal trunks or the individual subdiaphragmatic vagal branches.

We further demonstrated that the binding sites being transported along the vagus both in the trunk and in the subdiaphragmatic branches met the criteria for an A type CCK receptor.[20] That is, binding to these receptors was dependent upon the presence of sulfated tyrosine in the CCK. Addition of an excess of unlabeled CCK to the incubation buffer inhibited the binding of I^{125} CCK to the receptors proximal to the ligation site. In contrast, addition of the same concentration of unlabeled unsulfated CCK had no effect on this binding (Figure 8).

This pharmacological profile for transported CCK receptors is identical to that found for CCK receptors in the NTS.[19] Since the NTS is the terminus for

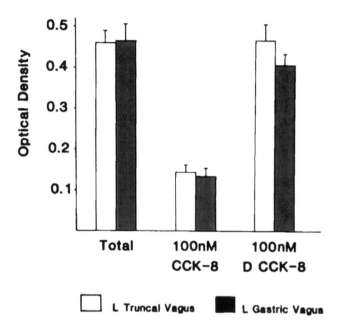

FIGURE 8. Mean optical densities of vagal segments proximal to ligature sites in the left cervical vagus and left gastric branch for total binding and segments incubated in the presence of 100 nM CCK-8 or nonsulfated CCK (d-CCK). (Reprinted with permission by Elsevier Science Publishers, from Moran *et al.*[20])

the central projections of vagal afferents from the nodose ganglion, this similar profile raised the possibility that CCK receptors in the NTS may be localized presynaptically on vagal afferent terminals. Ladenheim *et al.*[10] have demonstrated that unilateral nodosectomy caused a significant reduction in CCK binding in the NTS ipsilateral to the ganglionectomy. This result was consistent with the idea that these receptors were on vagal afferents, since CCK receptors in other hindbrain regions which do not receive a direct vagal input did not show changes in binding in response to this procedure. We have replicated their finding in animals who received unilateral supraganglionic vagotomies.[18] Furthermore, a specific unilateral afferent vagal rootlet transection results in a significant unilateral decrease in CCK binding in the NTS. Together these findings support the idea that a significant portion of CCK binding in the NTS occurs on presynaptic vagal afferent terminals. The disappearance of the binding sites in response to the vagotomy procedures also suggests that the NTS is a site for the terminus of central vagal CCK receptor transport.

We have also addressed the issue of whether the peripheral transport of CCK binding sites occurs in afferent or efferent fibers by examining the effect of unilateral supra- or infraganglionic vagotomy on the vagal transport of CCK receptors.[3] The logic of these experiments was that both supraganglionic and infraganglionic vagotomy disconnect cervical efferent vagal fibers from their

Effect of Vagotomy on Vagal CCK Binding

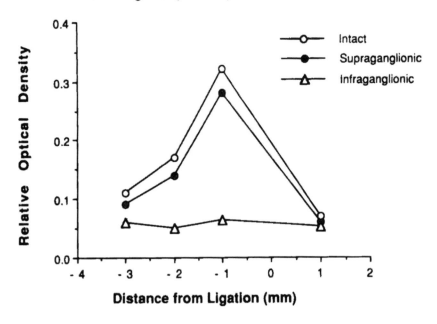

FIGURE 9. Mean CCK binding site accumulation around cervical vagal ligations expressed as relative optical densities in intact rats and rats with either supra- or infra- nodose ganglionic vagotomies. Transection below the level of the nodose ganglionic eliminated the accumulation of binding sites proximal to the ligation while transection above the ganglion did not.

cell bodies in the DMX, and if CCK binding sites were being transported in efferent fibers, both procedures would be expected to eliminate a buildup of CCK binding sites proximal to a ligature site placed along the cervical vagus. If CCK binding sites were being transported in afferent fibers, only the infraganglionic vagotomy would be expected to eliminate this buildup of binding sites proximal to a ligation point. Only this vagotomy would disconnect the cervical afferent axons from their cell bodies in the nodose ganglion.

Analysis of the effects of supra- and infraganglionic vagotomy on the transport of CCK binding sites in the cervical vagus revealed different effects of the two vagotomy procedures proximal but not distal to the vagal ligations. As demonstrated in Figure 9, supraganglionic vagotomy had no effect on vagal CCK receptor transport. There was a significant increase of CCK binding sites proximal to the vagal ligation relative to the binding distal to the ligation. In contrast, infraganglionic vagotomy eliminated the increase in binding density proximal to the ligature site. This result demonstrates that the vagal transport of CCK receptors toward peripheral axon terminals also occurs in afferent fibers. Severing the vagus below the nodose ganglion disconnects axons from both efferent and afferent cell bodies and interrupts this transport. Severing the vagus above the nodose ganglion disconnects axons from only the efferent cell bodies and does not affect transport. This finding, combined with the results of the disappearance of CCK receptors in the NTS following ganglionectomy or supraganglionic vagotomy, suggests that the anterograde transport of CCK binding sites is bidirectional from the afferent cell bodies in the nodose ganglion to vagal afferent terminals in the NTS and toward peripheral target sites. This is the only peptide receptor for which a complete analysis of the vagal limb on which receptor transport occurs has been carried out.

Angiotensin II Receptors

Angiotensin II (ANG II) is another peptide for which the presence and axonal transport of vagal receptors have been demonstrated. ANG II binding sites have been demonstrated in the canine[4] and rat[23] NTS, and DMX and unilateral nodose ganglionectomy produced significant reduction in these receptor populations. The relative disappearance of the ANG II receptor populations from these caudal hindbrain regions following nodosectomy suggested the possibility that these ANG II binding sites were of vagal origin and that they were both contained within the efferent cell bodies in the DMX and transported to afferent terminals in the NTS. To investigate this possibility, the transport of ANG II receptors was directly assessed using vagal ligations.[5] In response to a cervical ligation there was a significant buildup of ANG II binding sites both proximal and distal to the ligature site. Furthermore, when a double ligature was utilized there was a significant accumulation of binding sites distal to the distal ligature. In addition there was very little specific binding in the intermediate region between the two ligature sites indicating that almost all the ANG II binding sites identified by this procedure appear to be undergoing axonal transport. Thus, in contrast to CCK and opiate receptors, the vagal transport of ANG II receptors is bidirectional, and almost all the receptors in the vagal axons undergo transport. Furthermore, in contrast to what has been demonstrated for cholinergic receptors,[28] the receptor sites distal to the distal ligature undergoing retrograde transport and proximal to the proximal ligature undergoing anterograde transport appear to be the same. That is, at least by the techniques used in this study, ANG II receptors do not appear to undergo a change in state between transport from the sensory ganglion or motor neuron and transport back from the vagal terminals. The physiological significance of the similar affinity states for bidirectional transport of the ANG II binding site is unknown.

Thus, the transport of ANG II binding sites demonstrates some properties which are different from those of transported nonpeptide or other peptide receptors. First, bidirectional transport can be demonstrated *in vitro*. This had not been shown for either opiate or CCK receptors. Second, retrograde and anterogradely transported receptors seem to exist in a similar affinity state. ANG II receptor transport contrasts with transport of muscarinic cholinergic receptors, which also is bidirectional, but for which retrograde transport appears to be at a lower affinity state. Finally, the presence of the receptors in both the

NTS and the DMX and the disappearance of these sites in response to the unilateral vagotomy raises the possibility that the ANG II receptors may be present and transported in both afferent and efferent vagal fibers. This possibility has not been directly assessed.

Neurotensin Receptors

The presence and transport of neurotensin binding sites in the rat vagus have also been demonstrated. Neurotensin binding sites are concentrated in both the NTS and the DMX,[22,25] and following a unilateral vagotomy above the level of the nodose ganglion, there is a significant ipsilateral decrease in neurotensin binding both within the NTS and the DMX.[9] As with ANG II binding sites, this suggests that neurotensin binding sites are associated with both primary afferent fibers and with efferent cell bodies. Following vagal nerve ligation, a buildup of NTS binding sites was seen both proximal and distal to the ligation. The buildup of neurotensin binding sites proximal to the ligation was more intense than that found distal to the ligation site. Since there was only a small number of nodose ganglion cells (15%) that exhibited neurotensin binding and a small decrease in NTS binding in response to unilateral supraganglionic vagotomy, it was suggested that the afferent vagus did not contain a sufficient density of receptors to account for the magnitude of the accumulation around a ligation and that some of this transport must be occurring in efferent fibers. This hypothesis has not been directly tested.

Peptide YY Receptors

The vagal transport of peptide YY receptors has recently been reported by Corp and Smith.[2] The results with this peptide receptor are similar to those discussed above for ANG II and neurotensin receptors. Peptide YY receptors are found in both the NTS and the DMX. Placement of a cervical vagal ligature results in a buildup of receptor sites both proximal and distal to the ligation point. There have yet been no reports on the effect of vagal transections above the level of the nodose on peptide YY binding in the NTS or DMX. Also, the particular branch of the vagus in which transport occurs has not yet been demonstrated for this receptor.

GENERAL CHARACTERISTICS OF AXONAL TRANSPORT OF BINDING SITES

In the preceding sections, the specifics of the vagal axonal transport of a variety of binding sites have been presented. There are a number of commonalties among these results and some important differences. Laduron[14] has suggested a number of defining characteristics of the transport of receptors in peripheral nerves. We will use these as organizing points for this discussion.

The first question is whether or not the axonal transport of binding sites is always bidirectional. Although both anterograde and retrograde transport is apparent for a variety of transported binding sites, the retrograde transport of opiate and CCK receptors cannot be demonstrated by *in vitro* techniques. Retrograde transport of opiate receptors can be documented utilizing *in vivo* ligand administration. This has not been attempted with CCK. Laduron suggests that the lack of a demonstrated buildup of binding sites distal to ligation points may simply reflect inadequate technique. He suggests that in some experiments, the lack of retrograde transport was due to the time constants used in those experiments. That is, the accumulation of receptors distal to a ligature may increase only for a very short time after the ligature and then gradually decrease so that if a long period between ligation and sacrifice is utilized, no significant buildup of binding distal to the ligature may be noted. This seems an unlikely explanation for the negative results with opiates and CCK since rats were sacrificed at various times after ligation and retrograde transport in general is slower than anterograde transport. The results with vagal muscarinic receptors and the results with *in vivo* administration of H^3 lofentanil suggest that the inability to demonstrate retrograde transport of some receptors may reflect a change in state between anterograde and retrograde transport. It may be, for example, that vagal CCK receptors are retrogradely transported but they may be transported as a receptor ligand complex (with CCK nonreversibly bound), or it may be that the interaction of CCK with the receptor produced some physical change in the receptor protein resulting in a significantly lowered affinity for CCK such that I^{125} CCK was unable to bind at the concentration used.

A second characteristic of receptor transport is that the rate of transport in the axons is fast. Fast axonal transport appears to depend on microtubules. Colchicine, which has been demonstrated to impair the integrity of microtubules, blocks fast axonal transport. Along this line, Zarbin *et al.*[27] have demonstrated that the transport of CCK receptors is blocked in the presence of colchicine. Furthermore, time course studies have demonstrated that the rate of accumulation of binding sites at a ligature point is consistent with a mechanism of fast axonal transport. Laduron points out that in order to calculate this transport rate a distinction must be made between sites that are being transported and sites which are membrane bound to the axon. For example, in the rat vagus nerve, there are a large number of muscarinic receptors found between two ligations.[28] Binding sites found between two ligatures most likely represent either nonaxonally transported or membrane-bound sites. Therefore, subtracting this value from the total number of sites quantified one can estimate the number of sites flowing down the axons.

A third point is the relationship of receptor transport to the transport of neurotransmitters. The fact that both receptor and neurotransmitter transport occur by fast axonal transport has led to the suggestion that the total transport mechanism for these is similar. Catecholamines have been clearly demonstrated to be transported in synaptic vesicle. Fractionation studies have also provided evidence that muscarinic receptors are associated with vesicles carrying norepinephrine and dopamine beta hydroxylace.[13] This suggests that there is a coexistence of neurotransmitter and receptor in the same vesicle. Just as a neuron may have several coexisting transmitters, a transmitter might coexist with one or more receptor populations in a synaptic vesicle.

Finally, while the function of anterograde receptor transport is clear, the role of retrograde transport is not. Receptors can only be synthesized in the cell body and must be transported to their site of membrane incorporation. Laduron[13,14] has suggested a number of potential roles for retrograde receptor transport from the periphery to the cell body. One role is to provide some recycling of the amino acid components of the receptor protein complex. This may take place either as recycling via the Golgi apparatus or degradation after fusion of lysosomes. The rate at which the retrograde transport and recycling of the components occurs may in some way play an important role in receptor regulation. For example, the synthesis of new receptor proteins may depend upon the rate at which recycled receptor components are returned to the cell body. The presence of these components may serve as a signal for receptor synthesis.

Laduron[14] has further suggested that recycling of receptors and bound ligand may play a role in the regulation of gene expression beyond the synthesis of new receptor proteins. Transport of the ligand to the soma may enable that ligand to bind on nuclear DNA fragments producing a variety of alterations in cellular functions. Laduron suggests that one such alteration may be the formation of new synaptic connections—a mechanism of long-term memory. While these suggestions are speculative, they do point to the potential of axonal receptor transport to serve a variety of functions in nerve cells, functions which are not limited to the simple supply of binding sites to synaptic terminals.

REFERENCES

1. **Birdsall, N.J.M., Burgen, A.S.V., and Hulme, E.C.,** The binding of agonists to brain muscarinic receptors, *Mol. Pharmacol.,* 14, 723-736, 1978.
2. **Corp, E.S., and Smith, G.P,** Axonal transport of peptide Y binding sites in the rat vagus nerve, *Soc. Neurosci. Abstr.,* 15, 346, 1989.
3. **Crosby, R.J., Norgren, R., Moran, T.H., and McHugh, P.R.,** Central and peripheral transport of CCK-A receptors on vagal afferent fibers, *FASEB J.,* 3, A998, 1989.
4. **Diz, D.I., Barnes, K.L., and Ferrario, C.M.,** Functional characteristics of neuropeptides in the dorsal medulla oblongata and vagus nerve, *Fed. Proc.,* 46, 30-35, 1987.
5. **Diz, D.I., and Ferrario, C.M.,** Bidirectional transport of angiotensin II binding sites in the vagus nerve, *Hypertension,* 11 (Suppl I), I139-I143, 1988.
6. **Henley, J.M., Lindstrom, J.M., and Oswald, R.E.,** Acetylcholine receptor synthesis in retina and transport to optic tectum in goldfish, *Science,* 232, 1627-1629, 1986.
7. **Hulme, E.C., Birdsall, N.J.M., Burgen, A.S.V., and Metha, P.,** The binding of antagonists to brain muscarino receptors, *Mol. Pharmacol.,* 14, 737-750, 1978.
8. **Jancsó, G., and Király, E.,** Sensory neurotoxins: Chemically induced selective destruction of primary sensory neurons, *Brain Res.,* 210, 83-89, 1981.
9. **Kessler, J.P., and Beaudet, A.,** Association of neurotensin binding sites with sensory and visceromotor components of the vagus nerve, *J. Neurosci.,* 9(2), 466-472, 1989.
10. **Ladenheim, E.E., Speth, R.C., and Ritter, R.C.,** Reduction of CCK-8 binding in the nucleus of the solitary tract in unilaterally nodosectomized rats, *Brain Res.,* 474, 125-129, 1988.

11. Laduron, P., Axoplasmic transport of muscarinc receptors, *Nature*, 286, 287-288, 1980.
12. Laduron, P.M., Axonal transport of opiate receptors in capsaicin-sensitive neurons, *Brain Res.*, 157-160, 1984.
13. Laduron, P.M., Axonal transport of receptors: Coexistence with neurotransmitter and recycling, *Biochem. Pharmacol.*, 33, 897-903, 1984.
14. Laduron, P.M., Axonal transport of receptors: Characterization, role in receptor regulation and possible involvement in learning, *J. Recept. Res.*, 7, 417-434, 1987.
15. Laduron, P.M., and Janssen, P.F.M., Impaired axonal transport of opiate and muscarinic receptors in streptozocin-diabetic rats, *Brain Res.*, 333, 389-392, 1985.
16. Laduron, P.M., and Janssen, P.F.M., Impaired axonal transport of opiate and muscarinic receptors in streptozocin-diabetic rats, *Brain Res.*, 380, 359-362, 1986.
17. Millington, W.R., Aizenman, E., Bierkamper, G.G., Zarbin, M.A., and Kuhar, M.J., Axonal transport of α bungrotoxin binding sites in rat sciatic nerve, *Brain Res.*, 340, 269-276, 1985.
18. Moran, T.H., Norgren, R., Crosby, R.J., and McHugh, P.R., Central and peripheral transport of vagal cholecystokinin binding sites occurs in afferent fibers, *Brain Res.*, 526, 95-106, 1990.
19. Moran, T.H., Robinson, P.H., Goldrich, M.S., and McHugh, P.R., Two brain CCK receptors: Implications for behavioral actions, *Brain Res.*, 362, 175-179, 1986.
20. Moran, T.H., Smith, G.P., Hostetler, A.M., and McHugh, P.R., Transport of cholecystokinin (CCK) binding sites in subdiaphragmatic vagal branches, *Brain Res.*, 415, 149-152, 1987.
21. Ninkovic, M., and Hunt, S.P., Å bungarotoxin binding sites in sensory neurons and their axonal transport in sensory afferents, *Brain Res.*, 272, 57-69, 1983.
22. Quiron, R., Gaudreau, P., St. Pierre, S., Rioux, F., and Pert, C.B., Autoradiographic distribution of neurotensin receptors in rat brain: Visualization by tritium sensitive film, *Peptides*, 3, 757-763, 1982.
23. Speth, R.C., Dinh, T.T., and Ritter, S., Nodose ganglionectomy reduces angiotensin II receptor binding in the rat brainstem, *Peptides*, 8, 677-685, 1987.
24. Weiss, P., and Hiscoe, H.B., Experiments in the mechanisms of nerve growth, *J. Exp. Zool.*, 107, 315-329, 1948.
25. Young, W.S., and Kuhar, M.J., Neurotensin receptor localization by light microscopic autoradiography in the rat brain, *Brain Res.*, 206, 273-285, 1981.
26. Young, W.S., Wamsley, J.K., Karbin, M.A., and Kuhar, M.J., Opioid receptors undergo axonal flow, *Science*, 210, 76-77, 1980.
27. Zarbin, M.A., Wamsley, J.K., Innis, R.B., and Kuhar, M.J., Cholecystokinin receptors: Presence and axonal flow in the rat vagus nerve, *Life Sci.*, 29, 697-705, 1981.
28. Zarbin, M.A., Wamsley, J.K., and Kuhar, M.J., Axonal transport of muscarinic cholinergic receptors in rat vagus nerve: high and low affinity agonist receptors move in opposite directions and differ in nucleotide sensitivity, *J. Neurosci.*, 2, 934-941, 1982.
29. Zarbin, M.A., Wamsley, J.K., and Kuhar, M.J., Axonal transport of Beta-Adrenergic receptors. Antero- and retrogradely transported receptors differ in agonist affinity and nucleotide sensitivity, *Mol. Pharmacol.*, 24, 341-348, 1983.

Chapter 8

VAGAL AFFERENT MECHANISMS OF MECHANO- AND CHEMORECEPTION

D. Grundy

TABLE OF CONTENTS

INTRODUCTION

Implicit in the title of this chapter are two important questions. First, what is the nature of the afferent information relayed centrally in the vagus nerve? This question takes on added significance when one considers that the vagus is predominantly an afferent nerve. There are about 50,000 fibers in the vagus at the level of the diaphragm. After supranodose vagotomy, only 10% of these degenerate. Therefore, the subdiaphragmatic vagus has about 5,000 motor fibers.[2] Clearly, there is an enormous volume of information being relayed centrally. These afferent lines can be "tapped" using a variety of neurophysiological techniques in both anesthetized and conscious animals in order to establish the nature of the afferent traffic passing to the central nervous system (see Grundy and Scratcherd[22]). The vagal afferent signals rarely impinge on consciousness, being more involved in reflex regulation of gastrointestinal function and in behavioral responses like feeding, satiety, nausea and vomiting.

The second question concerns the transduction mechanism in mechanoreceptor and chemoreceptor endings. This is difficult to study directly because visceral sensory nerve terminals, with the exception of the Pacinian corpuscle, are not readily identifiable. Both vagal and splanchnic afferent nerve endings are unencapsulated, unmyelinated and lacking in morphological specialization. The vagal afferents are distributed in the layers of the gut wall to the muscle and mucosa where they are relatively inaccessible. These problems are compounded further by the fact that these primary afferents are not the only "afferents" supplying this gastrointestinal muscle and mucosa (Figure 1). Most neural elements in the gut wall are intrinsic as part of the enteric innervation.[18] Intrinsic sensory neurons enable the enteric nervous system to function independently of the extrinsic innervation, a property that has led to its description as the "brain of the gut."[41] Other enteric neurons project to the prevertebral ganglia where they mediate peripheral reflexes through sympathetic post-ganglionic neurons.[40]

An added complication is the presence of neuropeptides like substance-P, CCK, VIP and somatostatin, which are transported from the site of synthesis in the cell bodies in the nodose ganglia, against the flow of impulse afferent traffic, to the periphery where they can be released from nerve terminals.[14] The function of these neuropeptides is not fully established but clearly the potential is there for local regulation via axon reflexes. Thus, while autoradiographic techniques can be used to visualize afferent terminations in muscle and close to the mucosa which may play a receptive function, other terminations in the myenteric and sub-mucosal plexuses suggest axon-collaterals which may mediate local reflex responses.[39] Reflexes (local and otherwise), together with endocrine and paracrine agents released from the GI mucosa can alter secretion, motility and blood flow, making the application of controlled stimuli to the gut difficult to maintain and nearly impossible to reproduce. Moreover, when recording from the afferent fiber itself at some distance from its peripheral terminals, one has

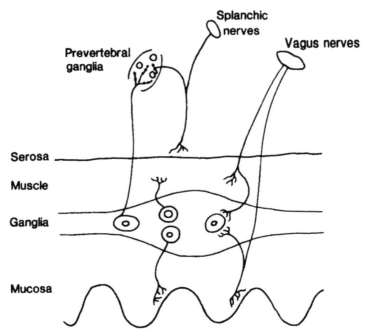

FIGURE 1. Schematic diagram showing the different types of "sensory" nerve endings in the gastrointestinal wall. For simplicity, only one muscle layer and one nerve plexus is illustrated. From left to right: An intramural ganglion cell projecting to the prevertebral ganglia; intrinsic sensory nerves supplying muscle and mucosa; primary afferents in the splanchnic and vagal nerves terminating in the serosa, muscle and mucosa. Note axon collaterals of the primary afferents projecting to the ganglia.

to use rigorous criteria to ensure that a response to a particular stimulus is not an indirect result of local reflex action. Many of the uncertainties regarding gastrointestinal sensory mechanisms result from the failure to exclude indirect activation.

CHARACTERISTICS OF VAGAL AFFERENT DISCHARGE

The response characteristics of individual vagal afferent fibers have recently been reviewed[22] and are briefly summarized below.

Vagal afferent fibers have been classified into three main groups according to the location of their endings in the serosa, muscularis or mucosa. Afferent fibers with endings in the serosa are found predominantly in splanchnic nerves, and in addition to activating sympathetic reflexes, are considered to mediate visceral pain.[9] Vagal afferents do not generally supply the serosa of the GI tract. However, a small number of mechanoreceptors have been identified in the serous membrane of the lower esophageal sphincter.[10] These were silent at physiological levels of stimulation but responded to strong stretch and distension. The authors speculate that such afferents may be active only under certain special circumstances, such as vomiting.

Muscle Receptors

Muscle afferents are sensitive to tension generated by stretch or contraction. Spontaneous activity in these afferents reflects current levels of tone in the muscle (Figure 2). However, the vagal afferent response to distension and the sensitivity to stretch and contraction differ from one gut region to another. In the esophagus, muscle mechanoreceptors respond maximally at small luminal volumes, with pressures < 10 mmHg. This range of sensitivity may be a reflection of activity in an organ with low residual volume. Contractions are also a potent stimulus to these afferent endings,[38] which signal to the brainstem the progress of primary and secondary peristaltic waves. This afferent feedback allows the central motor program to be adjusted according to the effectiveness of the peristaltic contraction and moreover is responsible for triggering secondary peristalsis if the bolus becomes lodged in the esophagus or if reflux of gastric contents occurs.

Contraction is a potent stimulus to tension receptors in other regions of the GI tract, such as the gastric antrum and small intestine (Figure 2). Through these afferent fibers the brainstem is kept informed of the amplitude and waveform of every contraction that occurs. Convergence of inputs from adjacent afferent endings provide information on the rate and direction of contractions which may be important in the regulation of gastric emptying. In the case of the retrograde giant contractions (RGC) seen in the prodromal phase of vomiting,

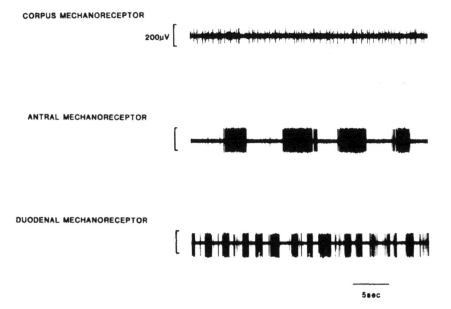

FIGURE 2. Mechanosensitivity of vagal afferent fiber supplying different regions of the gastrointestinal tract. Spontaneous discharge of three muscle mechanoreceptors supplying the corpus, antrum and duodenum are illustrated. Note the phasic patterns of discharge in the antral and duodenal afferents which reflects ongoing contractile activity in these regions. In the corpus the muscle mechanoreceptor discharge is more tonic (Blackshaw and Grundy, unpublished data).

afferent feedback may be important for the coordination of visceral and somatic events such that retching occurs after the RGC has invaded the antrum.[26]

Afferent fibers innervating a distensible region like the gastric corpus, while capable of responding to contraction, are more sensitive to distension.[3] They monitor the degree of gastric filling. The feeling of fullness after a heavy meal may, in part, be mediated by such distension sensitive afferents. Their involvement in satiety is indicated by the negative correlation between gastric volume and food intake.[27] Moreover, neurons in the lateral hypothalamus receive input from distension sensitive gastric afferents.[1] In addition to its potential role in ingestive behavior, gastric distension serves as a trigger for many motor and secretory responses to food intake, including gastric secretion[20] and postprandial patterns of motility.[8]

This ability of muscle mechanoreceptors to respond to tension generated passively by stretch and actively during contraction has led to their description as "in-series tension receptors."[23] The in-series concept was developed in skeletal muscle to distinguish between the "in-parallel" muscle spindle and the tendon organ. However, the in-series location of receptors in the gastrointestinal musculature has not been universally accepted. There are two reasons for skepticism with regard to in-series tension receptors. First, there is no morphological data to support the existence of such receptors. Second, in a hollow viscus, contraction of one region can cause stretch in another and lead to concomitant changes in tension in the mesentery. Consequently, some splanchnic afferents with endings in the mesentery, at some distance from the bowel wall, respond to both contraction and distension, with no possibility of an in-series location.[32]

We recently attempted to resolve this issue by looking at the response of vagal afferent fibers in the gastric corpus and considering not only their response to contraction under isovolumetric and isotonic conditions but also their response during relaxation induced by electrical stimulation of the vagal nonadrenergic, non-cholinergic (NANC) pathway.[6] The rationale for this approach is that because the relaxations are slow in onset and, in the ferret corpus, last for several minutes, inertia of the fluid becomes less of a problem and it is possible to achieve near isotonic conditions.

Under isovolumetric conditions the discharge in the corpus afferents mirrored the increase and decrease in intragastric pressure during contraction and relaxation (Figure 3). Under isotonic conditions, achieved by connecting the corpus cannula to a fluid reservoir of large cross-sectional area, the pressure response especially during relaxation was attenuated. In most cases the afferent discharge followed the pressure profile despite large changes in corpus volume.

Observations that the afferent fibers do not respond during isotonic increases in length would indicate that tension is indeed the primary stimulus to these endings, and by analogy with the skeletal muscle, one would put the endings in the tendon. However, in smooth muscle the role of tendon is played by the laminar septa of connective tissue which run parallel to and separate the

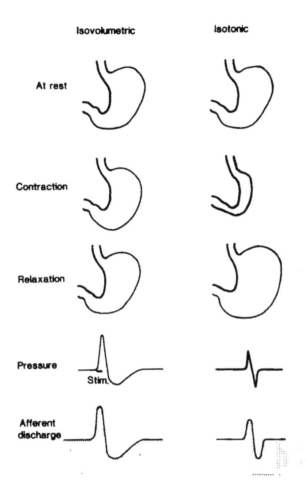

FIGURE 3. The use of isotonic and isovolumetric recordings of gastric pressure during electric vagal stimulation to investigate the role of muscle length vs. muscle tension as the determinant of afferent discharge. Under isovolumetric conditions when intragastric volume is fixed the contractions and relaxations give rise to large pressure changes. When gastric volume is allowed to change, the pressure response is attenuated as fluid flows in and out of the reservoir. Afferent discharge mimics pressure under both conditions indicating that tension and not length is the major determinant of afferent sensitivity.

neighboring bundles of smooth muscle.[19] One might postulate that this would be the site of the muscle receptor and, if this is the case, the muscle tension receptors behave functionally as in-series receptors from an in-parallel location.

Mucosal Receptors

Muscle receptors are relatively homogeneous in their response to tension, although they differ in the levels of discharge and thresholds for activation. Mucosal receptors, on the other hand, are a more heterogeneous population and fall into one of two main groups (see Grundy and Scratcherd[22]). Multimodal receptors respond to mechanical and/or chemical stimulation of the mucosal epithelium. Their mechanical sensitivity is primarily to mucosal deformation, experimentally in the form of mucosal stroking (Figure 4, top). The exquisite sensitivity to mucosal stroking indicates that this is likely to be a primary sensitivity of these endings which have therefore been postulated to function as contact receptors detecting the particulate nature of luminal contents.[12] In addition, many (but not all) mucosal endings show chemosensitivity, responding to the luminal application of a variety of chemicals. The responses are generally non-specific with individual mucosal afferents responding whenever luminal contents differ appreciably from neutral pH, isotonicity or contain nutrients (Figure 4, bottom).

Multimodal mucosal receptors have been described in a variety of species by several research groups. Quality specific chemoreceptors, on the other hand, have been described only in the cat and only by Mei's group in Marseilles. These chemoreceptors are insensitive to mechanical stimulation and respond only to a narrow range of luminal chemicals. Thus, glucoreceptors (or more accurately, carbohydrate receptors),[29] amino acid receptors,[24] receptors to short and long chain fats,[31] acid,[15] and thermoreceptors[16] have all been described.

The mucosal receptors keep the brainstem informed about the luminal environment and may be responsible for the reflex adjustments in motor and secretory activity in response to the physical and chemical nature of gastric and intestinal chyme (for example, feedback regulation of gastric emptying from chyme in the duodenum; see Raybould, chapter 9 of this volume).

In addition, however, vagal afferents play a role in behavioral responses such as satiety (see R.C. Ritter *et al.*, chapter 10 of this volume) and vomiting. In the case of the latter, gastrointestinal afferents may form part of a toxin-detecting system to protect the body against the ingestion of harmful material.[11]

Under normal circumstances the events signaled by vagal mechano- and chemoreceptors continue without any conscious awareness. However, these afferents may contribute to some of the symptoms associated with a variety of gastrointestinal disorders.[21] There is little known about the way afferent sensitivity is affected by local irritation, inflammation or changes in blood flow.

TRANSDUCTION

Despite the lack of any direct studies of impulse generation in vagal afferent endings, it is probably safe to assume that mechanosensitivity arises following deformation of the receptor ending and the generation of a receptor potential. With chemoreceptors, several possibilities exist and have been discussed previously.[30] These include acceptor molecules on the receptor membrane, mechanical deformation caused by obligatory water movements across the mucosa and secondary sense cells. Here, in light of recent studies, the latter hypothesis will be developed.

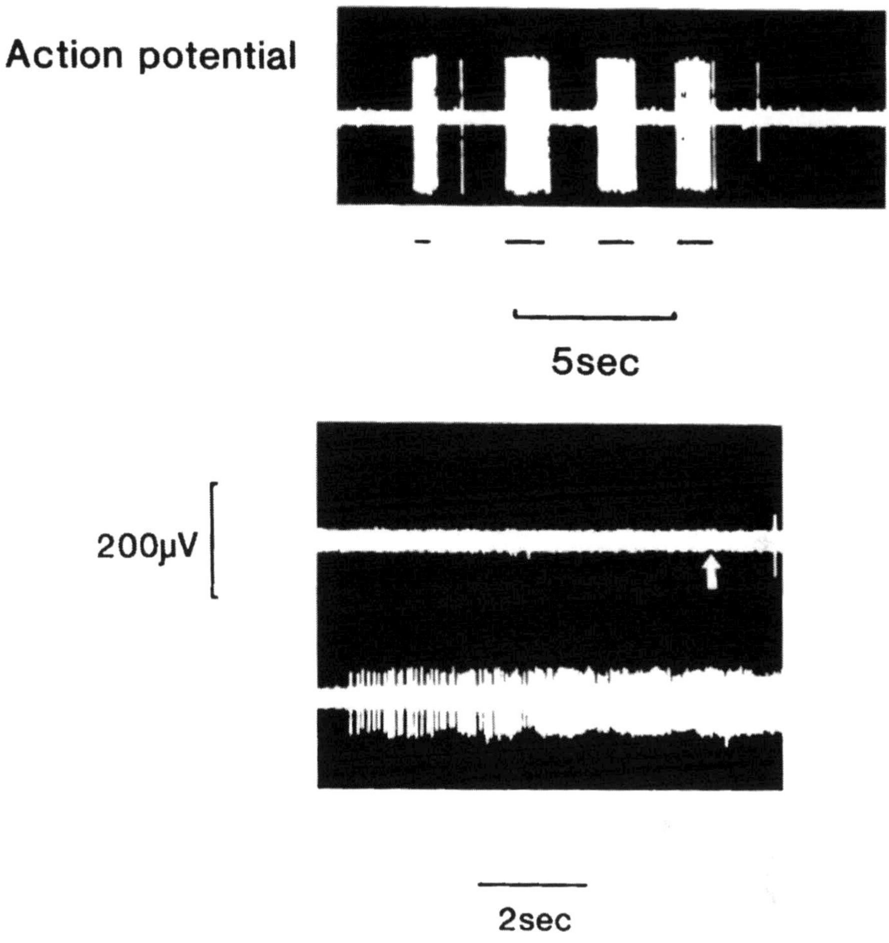

Action potential

5sec

200µV

2sec

FIGURE 4. Discharge of a vagal mucosal afferent in response to (*top*) stroking the mucosa overlying the receptive field in the duodenum (bars) and (*bottom*) perfusion of the duodenum with 500 mM sodium chloride (from arrow, upper and lower traces are continuous) (Blackshaw and Grundy, unpublished data).

A secondary sense cell, in the context of the present discussion, is any cell in the mucosa that samples the luminal contents and releases from the basolateral membrane a neuromodulator which causes activation or augmentation of receptor discharge (Figure 5). Such neuromodulation could be specific for afferent activity or could mediate more general effects via paracrine or endocrine actions elsewhere. As such, gut endocrine cells (or at least some of them) could be envisaged as playing a role as chemoreceptors.[17] Alternatively, there may be specific secondary sense cells as proposed by Newson *et al.*[33,34] on the basis of morphological investigations of the intestinal mucosa. They described some cells in the crypt region which they argue resemble the gustatory taste cells and thus referred to them as epithelial "taste cells."

This analogy with gustatory afferents is an interesting one. The study of transduction in gustatory afferents is considerably more developed than that in the GI tract. The various modalities of taste are proposed to involve a diversity of transduction mechanisms from receptor-mediated stimulation of adenylate cyclase and release of intracellular calcium to direct effects on apical ion channels.[25] A parallel exists between gustatory and GI afferents, if a little contrived. The four modalities of taste–sour, salt, sweet and bitter–have their counterparts in the gut as acid, sodium chloride, carbohydrate and amino-acid receptors, although there are obvious differences in the milieu of the receptors

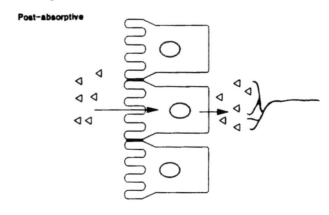

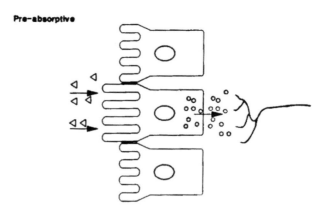

FIGURE 5. Schematic diagram illustrating pre-absorptive and post-absorptive mechanisms of mucosal afferent transduction. For a post-absorptive mechanism the stimulus interacts with the afferent ending following absorption across the enterocyte. With pre-absorptive mechanisms the stimulus interacts with a specialized mucosal cell which monitors luminal conditions and releases a neuromodulator from the basolateral aspects of the cell to influence afferent discharge.

and their relative sensitivities. However, even in this more accessible tissue the neurotransmitter involved in gustatory taste cell synapses is poorly understood.

In the gut there is evidence for serotonin (5HT) as a stimulus for afferent activation. This comes from studies in which a number of emetic stimuli, including radiation and cytotoxic drugs, have been shown to act via vagal afferents and that a new class of 5HT receptor antagonists (5HT$_3$) can abolish such emetic responses.[4,5] These observations indicate that vagal afferents respond not only to luminal stimuli but also to substances released from the mucosa itself.

A similar situation arises in the case of CCK and satiety. Compelling evidence suggests that CCK action on gastric emptying and satiety is mediated by vagal afferents[28,35,36,37] and it has been suggested that mechanoreceptors in the corpus have a unique sensitivity to CCK.[13] These receptors are therefore proposed to signal not only the degree of gastric distension but also, following CCK released into the bloodstream, nutrient delivery to the intestines and thus mediate satiety. In contrast, preliminary studies from my laboratory show that in the ferret it is the mucosal receptors rather than muscle mechanoreceptors that are sensitive to intra-arterial CCK.[7] The implication of these findings relates to the mechanism by which luminal stimuli give rise to afferent discharge and raises the possibility that rather than luminal stimuli acting directly on the receptor ending following absorption across the mucosa, they act on a mucosal cell strategically placed to sample luminal contents. In response to an effective stimulus, they release a paracrine or endocrine substance, with the latter giving rise to the discharge.

CONCLUSION

Gastrointestinal afferents provide afferent information on the level of activity in the muscle wall and on the physical and chemical nature of the changing luminal environment. In addition, these endings are subjected to an ever changing chemical environment from paracrine agents within the internal structure of the gut wall and hormones from the bloodstream. Unraveling this range of sensitivity will provide a greater understanding of the autonomic control mechanisms which serve to adjust gastrointestinal function to the needs of the individual.

REFERENCES

1. **Anand, B.K., and Pillai, R.V.,** Activity of single neurones in the hypothalamic feeding centers: Effects of gastric distension, *J. Physiol.*, 192, 63-77, 1967.
2. **Andrews, P.L.R.,** Vagal afferent innervation of the gastrointestinal tract, in *Progress in Brain Research,* Vol. 67, Cervero, F., and Morrison, J.F.B., Eds., Elsevier Science Publishers, Amsterdam, 1986, 65-86.
3. **Andrews, P.L.R., Grundy, D., and Scratcherd, T.,** Vagal afferent discharge from mechanoreceptors in different regions of the ferret stomach, *J. Physiol.*, 289, 513-524, 1980.

4. **Andrews, P.L.R., and Hawthorn, J.,** The neurophysiology of vomiting, in *Balliere Clinical Gastroenterology 2(1)*, Grundy, D., and Read, N.W., Eds., Balliere Tindall, London, 1988, 141-168.

5. **Andrews, P.L.R., Rapeport, W.G., and Sanger, G.J.,** Neuropharmacology of emesis induced by anti-cancer therapy, *TIPS*, 9, 334-341, 1988.

6. **Blackshaw, L.A., Grundy, D., and Scratcherd, T.,** Vagal afferent discharge from gastric mechanoreceptors during contraction and relaxation of the ferret corpus, *J. Auton. Nerv. Syst.*, 18, 19-24, 1987.

7. **Blackshaw, L.A., Grundy, D.,** Different effects of CCK 8 on two classes of gastroduodenal vagal afferent fiber—a novel mechanism for gastric relaxation, *J. Gastrointest. Motil.*, 1(1), A63, 1989.

8. **Bull, J.S., Grundy, D., and Scratcherd, T.,** Disruption of the jejunal migrating motor complex by gastric distension and feeding in the dog, *J. Physiol.*, 394, 381-392, 1987.

9. **Cervero, F.,** Visceral nociception: Peripheral and central aspects of visceral nociceptive systems, *Philos. Trans. R. Soc. Lond. B. Biol. Sci.*, 308, 325-337, 1985.

10. **Clerc, N., and Mei, N.,** Vagal mechanoreceptors located in the lower oesophageal sphincter of the cat, *J. Physiol. Lond.*, 336, 487-498, 1983.

11. **Davies, C.J., Harding, R.K., Leslie, R.A., and Andrews, P.L.R.,** The organisation of vomiting as a protective reflex, in *Nausea and Vomiting: Mechanisms and Treatment*, Davies, C.J., Lake-Bakaar, G.B., and Graham-Smith, D.G., Eds., Springer-Verlag, Berlin, 1986, 65-75.

12. **Davison, J.S.,** The electrophysiology of gastrointestinal chemoreceptors, *Digestion*, 7, 312-317, 1972.

13. **Davison, J.S., and Clarke, G.D.,** Mechanical properties and sensitivity to CCK of vagal gastric slowly adapting mechanoreceptors, *Am. J. Physiol.*, 255, G55-G61, 1988.

14. **Dockray, G.J., and Sharkey, K.A.,** Neurochemistry of visceral afferent neurones, in *Progress in Brain Research*, Cervero, F., and Morrison, J.F.B., Eds., Elsevier Science Publishers, 1986, 133-148.

15. **El Ouazzani, T., and Mei, N.,** Acido- et glucorecepteurs vagaux de la region gastro-duodenale, *Exp. Brain Res.*, 42, 442-452, 1981.

16. **El Ouazzani, T., and Mei, N.,** Electrophysiologic properties and role of the vagal thermoreceptors of lower esophagus and stomach of cat, *Gastroenterology*, 83, 995-1001, 1982.

17. **Fujita, T., Kobayashi, S., Muraki, S., Sato, K., and Shimojo, K.,** Gut endocrine cells as chemoreceptors, in *Gut Peptides: Secretion, Function and Clinical Aspects*, Miyoshi, A., Ed., Kodansha/Elsevier, Tokyo, 1979, 47-52.

18. **Furness, J.B., and Costa, M.,** *The Enteric Nervous System*, Churchill Livingstone, Edinburgh, 1987, 290.

19. **Gabella, G.,** Structure of muscles and nerves in the gastrointestinal tract, in *Physiology of the Gastrointestinal Tract*, Vol. 1, 2nd edition, Johnson, L.R., Ed., Raven Press, New York, 1987, 335-382.

20. **Grossman, M.I.,** Secretion of acid and pepsin in response to distension of vagally innervated fundic gland area in dogs, *Gastroenterology*, 42, 718-721, 1962.

21. **Grundy, D.,** Involvement of extrinsic nerves in functional disorders of the bowel, in *The Neurotic and Demented Bowel*, Read, N.W., Ed., Blackwells, Oxford, 1991, 51-57.

22. **Grundy, D., and Scratcherd, T.,** Sensory afferents from the gastrointestinal tract, in *Handbook of Physiology*, Section 6, Vol. 1, Part 1, Wood, J.D., Ed., American Physiological Society, Bethesda, Maryland, 1989, 593-620.

23. **Iggo, A.,** Gastrointestinal tension receptors with unmyelinated afferent fibres in the vagus of the cat, *Q. J. Exp. Physiol.*, 42, 130-143, 1957.

24. **Jeanningros, R.,** Vagal unitary responses to intestinal amino acid infusions in the anaesthetized cat: A putative signal for protein induced satiety, *Physiol. Behav.*, 28, 9-21, 1982.

25. **Kinnamon, S.C.,** Taste transduction: A diversity of mechanisms, *TINS,* 11 (11), 491-496, 1988.

26. **Lang, I.M., and Sarna, S.K.,** Neural control of initiation and propagation of retrograde giant contradictions associated with vomiting, in *Nerves and the Gastrointestinal Tract,* Falk Symposium 50, Singer, N.V., and Goebell, H., Eds., Kluer Academic Publishers, Lancaster, 1989, 726-731.

27. **Le Magnen, J.,** Control of eating behaviour, in *Gastrointestinal Neurophysiology,* Grundy, D., and Read, N.W., Eds., Balliere Tindall, London, 1988, 169-182.

28. **McCann, M.J., Verbalis, J.G., and Stricker, E.M.,** Capsaicin pre-treatment attenuates multiple responses to cholycystokinin in rats, *J. Auton. Nerv. Syst.,* 23, 265-272, 1988.

29. **Mei, N.,** Vagal glucoreceptors in the small intestine of the cat, *J. Physiol.,* 282, 485-506, 1978.

30. **Mei, N.,** Intestinal chemosensitivity, *Physiol. Rev.,* 65, 211-237, 1985.

31. **Melone, J.,** Vagal receptors sensitive to lipids in the small intestine of the cat, *J. Auton. Nerv. Syst.,* 17, 231-241, 1986.

32. **Morrison, J.F.B.,** The afferent innervation of the gastrointestinal tract, in *Nerves and the Gut,* Brooks, F.P., and Evers, P.W., Eds., Slack, Thorofare, N.J., 1977, 297-326.

33. **Newson, B., Ahlman, H., Dahlstrom, A., Das Gupta, T.K., and Nyhus, L.M,** On the innervation of the ileal mucosa in the rat—a synapse, *Acta Physiol. Scand.,* 105, 387-389, 1979.

34. **Newson, B., Ahlman, H., Dahlstrom, A., and Nyhus, L.M.,** Ultrastructural observations in the rat ileal mucosa of possible epithelial "taste cells" and submucosal sensory neurones, *Acta Physiol. Scand.,* 114, 161-164, 1982.

35. **Raybould, H.E., Gayton, R.J., and Dockray, G.J.,** CNS effects of circulating CCK 8: Involvement of brain stem neurones responding to gastric distension, *Brain Res.,* 342, 187-190, 1985.

36. **Raybould, H.E., Gayton, R.J., and Dockray, G.J.,** Mechanisms of action of peripherally administered cholycystokinin octa-peptide on brain stem neurones in the rat, *J. Neurosci.,* 8, 3018-3024, 1988.

37. **Raybould, A.G., and Tashe, Y.,** Cholycystokinin inhibits gastric motility and emptying via capsaicin sensitive vagal pathway in the rat, *Am. J. Physiol.,* 255, G242-G246, 1988.

38. **Satchell, P.M.,** Canine oesophageal mechanoreceptors, *J. Physiol. Lond.,* 346, 287-300, 1984.

39. **Sato, M., and Koyano, H.,** Autoradiographic study of the distribution of vagal afferent nerve fibers in the gastroduodenal wall of the rabbit, *Brain Res.,* 440, 101-109, 1987.

40. **Szurszewski, J.H. and King, B.F.,** Physiology of prevertebral ganglia in mammals, with special reference to inferior mesenteric ganglian, in *Handbook of Physiology,* Section 6, Vol. 1, Part 1, Wood, J.D., Ed., American Physiological Society, Bethesda, Maryland, 1989, 519-592.

41. **Wood, J.D.,** Physiology of the enteric nervous system, in *Physiology of the Gastrointestinal Tract,* Vol. 1, 1st ed., Johnson, L.R., Ed., Raven Press, New York, 1981, 1-38.

Chapter 9

VAGAL AFFERENT INNERVATION AND THE REGULATION OF GASTRIC MOTOR FUNCTION

H.E. Raybould

TABLE OF CONTENTS

LIST OF ABBREVIATIONS

CCK = cholecystokinin
CCK-8 = cholecystokinin octapeptide
CGRP = calcitonin gene-related peptide
CRF = corticotropin-releasing factor
NTS = nucleus tractus solitarius
SBTI = soya bean trypsin inhibitor
SP = substance P
VIP = vasoactive intestinal polypeptide

INTRODUCTION

The control of gastric motility by neuronal mechanisms is integrated in a hierarchy of reflexes. The enteric nervous system is capable of initiating and coordinating complex reflexes along the gastrointestinal tract. The second level of control consists of afferent neurons whose cell bodies lie in the enteric plexuses of the gut wall and fibers that pass to the prevertebral ganglia in the mesenteric nerves. These afferent neurons are capable of generating reflex effects on gastrointestinal function mediated entirely through the prevertebral ganglia. In addition, reflexes controlling motility are transmitted through long extrinsic reflexes mediated through the central nervous system. The afferent fibers pass to the central nervous system either with the parasympathetic or sympathetic nerves which also contain the efferent limbs of these reflex pathways.

This chapter will review the control of gastric motility via vago-vagal pathways. The emphasis will be placed on the role of these reflexes in the intestinal feedback regulation of gastric motor function. Many of the reflexes mediated in this way have been described for some time, but recent evidence suggests that signals arising from the intestine have powerful effects on gastric motility and that these reflexes are mediated by the vagus nerve. In addition, it is becoming evident that hormones, released postprandially, may also act on the vagal afferent pathway and initiate reflex activity which modulates gastric motor function.

HISTORICAL PERSPECTIVE

At the turn of the century, the vagus nerve was considered to be primarily a motor nerve. It was recognized that many movements of the stomach were independent of the extrinsic innervation but that gastric tone and contractions could be modified through these nerves. Many early studies concentrated on the sensations arising from the viscera as a means to study the afferent innervation. However, as Ranson pointed out in his 1921 review, "the majority of the afferent impulses from the viscera never rise to the level of consciousness at all but expend themselves in the production of reflexes."[54]

Visceral Reflexes

Experiments using electrical stimulation of the peripheral cut stumps of the vagus nerve to activate efferent fibers had been shown to produce both inhibition and excitation of gastric motility (see McSwinney[44]). In 1904, Page May used electrical stimulation of the central cut end of the vagus nerve, together with an intact contralateral vagus, to demonstrate vago-vagal reflex effects on gastric motility. He reported that electrical stimulation of the central cut end of the vagus nerve inhibited ongoing gastric contractions in several species including dog, cat, rabbit and monkey.[52] In contrast, in decerebrate

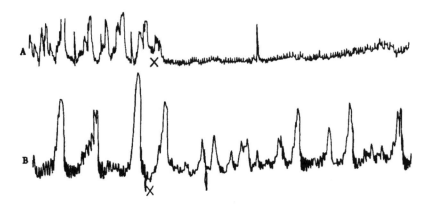

FIGURE 1. Original records of gastric motility measured using an intragastric balloon inserted through a gastric fistula in conscious dogs. Introduction of brandy into the stomach of an intact dog is associated with inhibition of gastric contractions, termed hunger contractions (A). Following vagal and splanchnic section (B), the response to chemical stimulation of the mucosa with alcohol is greatly reduced. The same response was obtained with alkali, acid and other alcohols (wine and beer). (Used with permisson by *Am. J. Physiol.,* from Carlson.[13])

dogs, electrical stimulation of the central cut end of the vagus nerve caused contraction of the whole stomach.[61] Thus vagal efferent fibers excitatory or inhibitory to gastric motor function could be activated by afferent stimulation, although it was not clear whether the two fiber populations could be selectively activated.

Other studies used more physiological methods to evoke visceral reflexes. Carlson[13] found that stimulation of the gastric mucosa by acid, alcohol and alkali inhibited both gastric tone and contractions in conscious dog and man. This inhibition was diminished in dogs by section of the vagus nerve alone and by combined vagal and splanchnic section (Figure 1).

During his studies on the peristaltic activity of the stomach and intestine in conscious cats, Cannon recognized that the stomach acted as a reservoir. "Whatever the amount of food sent to the stomach, the organ has a wonderful ability to adapt itself with precision to the volume of its contents."[12] Furthermore, he stated that the stomach achieved this without large increases in intraluminal pressure. In 1911, Cannon demonstrated that this receptive relaxation was mediated via a vago-vagal reflex.[12] Cannon and Lieb placed esophageal fistulas in cats and inserted a balloon in the stomach to measure gastric volume. Whenever the cat took a piece of meat and swallowed, the volume of the balloon increased representing a gastric relaxation (Figure 2). The onset of the response was rapid, within 2 sec, and did not occur when the vagus was cut, thus Cannon concluded it was a reflex mediated by the vagus nerves. Cannon also demonstrated the phenomenon in man.

During the next 20-30 years, little progress was made on the reflex control of gastric motility as the emphasis shifted to the role of hormones and intrinsic

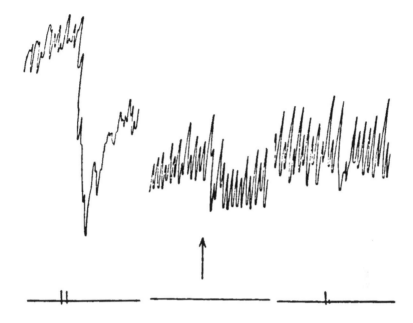

FIGURE 2. Original records of gastric motility recorded in conscious cats by an intragastric balloon inserted through an esophageal fistula. The animals were trained to sit quietly on the experimenter's lap and accept a piece of raw beef. The meat did not pass to the stomach but passed out through the esophageal fistula. A few seconds after swallowing the meat, intragastric pressure fell sharply. This inhibition of gastric tone after swallowing was reduced by cutting one vagus (middle trace) and abolished after bilateral vagal section (third trace). (Used with permission by *Am. J. Physiol.*, from Cannon and Lieb.[12])

reflexes mediated through the enteric nervous system. However, in the 1950s, two important observations were made concerning the vagal afferent innervation of the viscera. The work of light microscopists revealed that in the vagus, considered primarily a motor nerve, afferent fibers were present in far greater numbers than were efferent fibers. Also, electrophysiological studies by Iggo and Paintal independently showed that afferent C-fibers in the vagus carried signals from the stomach to the central nervous system concerning the level of tension developed in the gastric wall (see Leek[39]). In 1959, Harper returned to the technique of electrical stimulation of the cut end of the central vagal stump to demonstrate the existence of vago-vagal reflexes controlling gastric motility and secretion.[29] This was the first study to clearly demonstrate that reflex alteration in gastric motor function could be obtained by stimulation of the abdominal vagal branches. In the majority of cats (80%) spontaneous gastric motility, measured manometrically, was inhibited by stimulation of the abdominal vagal trunks (Figure 3); however, in the remaining animals the response to electrical stimulation consisted of increased phasic contractions superimposed on a background of decreased basal tone. These responses were unaffected by splanchnic section but abolished by section of the contralateral vagus nerve.

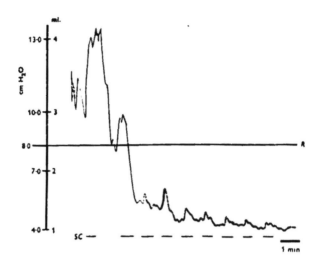

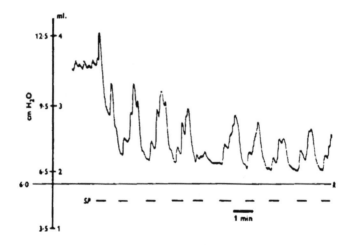

FIGURE 3. Records of gastric motility measured manometrically in anesthetized cats in response to antidromic stimulation of vagal afferent fibers. In 80% of cats, electrical stimulation of the central cut end of the right vagus nerve (SC and each —) resulted in inhibition of ongoing gastric contractions and a large decrease of gastric tone (upper trace). In the remaining cats, electrical stimulation produced a decrease in gastric tone on which was superimposed large phasic contractions in response to each period of vagal stimulation. These reflex changes in gastric motor function were abolished by contralateral vagal section. (Used with permission by *J. Physiol.*, from Harper et al.[29])

Gastric responses were obtained during stimulation of either the ventral or dorsal vagal branches of the subdiaphragmatic vagus, but it was not clear whether stimulation of a particular branch was associated with the production of excitatory or inhibitory responses.

These observations were later confirmed by Martinson and co-workers[32,43] and others.[50] In some species, these two groups of efferent fibers can be differentiated on the basis of the threshold to electrical stimulation, although in other species the inhibitory effect is seen only after blockade of the excitatory pathway with atropine.[62] The excitatory pathway consists of preganglionic cholinergic fibers that synapse with myenteric cholinergic neurons, releasing acetylcholine that contracts gastric smooth muscle. The vagal inhibitory fibers consist of a cholinergic preganglionic neuron that synapses onto a non-adrenergic, non-cholinergic myenteric neuron; recent evidence suggests that vasoactive intestinal peptide might be the transmitter used by these neurons.[46]

VAGAL AFFERENT INNERVATION OF THE GI TRACT

Although recently reviewed,[28] the vagal afferent innervation of the GI tract will be summarized here in order to clairfy the characteristics of the afferent arm producing the reflexes under consideration.

The abdominal vagus innervates the esophagus, stomach, all parts of the small intestine and the proximal two-thirds of the colon. Electrophysiological studies recording the impulse activity in single fibers have provided evidence that vagal afferent fibers show sensitivity to a variety of stimuli, including mechanical, chemical, thermal and osmotic. The majority of gastrointestinal sensory receptors do not show any morphological specialization and are considered to be free nerve endings; the response characteristics of the afferent fibers to a stimulus is dependent on the position of the receptor ending within the gut wall.[28,39]

Receptors that are sensitive to stimuli applied to the visceral lumen have been described throughout the gastrointestinal tract, in particular the gastric antrum and duodenum. The receptors are located in the mucosa or submucosa and are especially sensitive to stroking of the mucosa. These mucosal mechanoreceptors are relatively insensitive to distension, contraction or compression except when distortion of the mucosa occurs. The majority of mucosal receptors respond to various chemicals, applied either to the lumen or in the blood, and have been termed multimodal receptors. It is unclear whether this chemical sensitivity is secondary to reflex or local contractions of smooth muscle or to direct effects on nerve endings.[26] Some receptors, such as those sensitive to glucose or acid, are specific for that particular stimulus, while others appear to act as nonspecific or polymodal receptors.[45] Vagal afferent fibers responding to acid, alkali, glucose, amino acids and hypo- and hypertonic solutions have been described in several species. In addition, the intestine is innervated by thermal receptors.

Receptors located in the muscle layers of the viscera are activated by distension, contraction or compression of the viscus. The responses slowly adapt to a maintained stimulus. Because of the mechanical sensitivity these receptors have to tension developed in the viscus wall, they are termed in-series tension receptors. Isometric contractions will stimulate visceral mechanorecep-tors even at low volumes. The rate of distension may also be an important determinant of the afferent response. The same type of receptor exists through-out the gastrointestinal tract, although there are differences in the response characteristics in different regions of the bowel. For example, with mechano-receptors in the gastric corpus, which accommodates most of the intragastric volume, the afferent response is in proportion to the distending volume, whereas the response of mechanoreceptors located in the antrum show phasic activity occurring with each antral wave.

REFLEX MODULATION OF VAGAL EFFERENT FIBER ACTIVITY

Effective stimuli of vagal afferent fiber discharge have been used to deter-mine reflex activation of vagal efferent fiber discharge in single unit studies of the cervical vagus. Most studies describe reflex responses to gastric or intestinal distension, in part because of the readiness with which this stimulus can be applied reproducibly, but also because of the number of reflex changes in gastric motility and other gastrointestinal functions that are known to occur following distension or contraction of the viscera.

In the anesthetized rat and ferret, efferent units can be classified according to their response to gastric distension or active contraction.[9,19,27] The discharge of single efferent units was either excited or inhibited by gastric distension or contraction (Figure 4). Patterns of modulation indicate that the efferent fibers receive an input from gastric in-series mechanoreceptors.[27] The reciprocal organization supports the possibility that activation of vago-vagal reflexes involves reciprocal inhibition of the antagonistic (excitatory and inhibitory) pathways.[19] In contrast to the strong mechanoreceptor representation, little evidence for reflex vagal efferent discharge by intestinal chemical stimulation with nutrients was obtained in the anesthetized ferret.[9] Fewer units responded and in general the efferent responses were weak, of gradual onset and long latency, unlike afferent responses to the same stimuli or efferent responses to distension. It is worth noting that many efferent units responding to gastric distension also responded to distension of the intestine;[9,27] at least some of these responses were mediated by the vagus nerve.

The discharge pattern of vagal efferent fibers has been studied in conscious dogs using the cross innervation technique by Miolan and Roman.[48] During proximal gastric relaxation, caused by swallowing, esophageal distention or antral contractions, the discharge frequency in vagal efferent fibers was in-creased or decreased, again confirming the reciprocal control of vagal efferent pathways. In addition, the discharge of vagal efferent units was modified by introduction of hydrochloric acid into the duodenum or by moderate duodenal distension.[48]

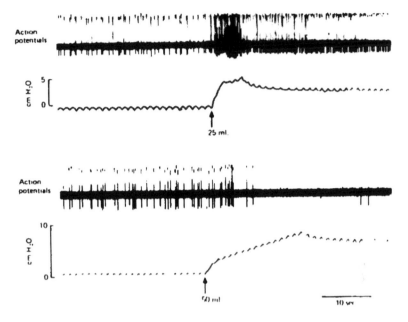

FIGURE 4. Responses of two vagal efferent fibers to gastric distension. A single fiber technique was used to record action potentials in single vagal efferent units in the anesthetized ferret. In the each record, the upper trace shows action potentials and the lower trace intragastric pressure measured manometrically. Gastric distension (marked by the arrows) caused either increase (upper record) or decrease (lower record) in efferent fiber discharge. Bilateral vagotomy abolished the response to gastric distension in 68% of the units tested. (Used with permission by *J. Physiol.*, from Grundy *et al.*[27])

REFLEXES INITIATED FROM THE STOMACH

Jansson[32] had clearly demonstrated that the inhibitory vagal efferent pathway to the stomach could be reflexly activated by esophageal distension, pharyngeal touch or swallowing; this corresponded to the receptive relaxation termed by Cannon in the early part of the century. In 1973, Abrahamsson demonstrated that a reflex inhibition of gastric motility similar to that due to esophageal stimulation can be initiated from the stomach. Stimulation of gastric mechanoreceptors by transient, graded distension (by increase in intragastric pressure) produced a long-lasting gastric relaxation (Figure 5). Cooling the vagus nerves to block neurotransmission impeded inflow into the stomach as it was distended, and distension did not produce a long-lasting gastric relaxation.[2] It was also demonstrated that antral distension alone, or close arterial injection of acetylcholine, produced gastric relaxation.[1]

Excitatory vago-vagal reflexes can also be initiated from the stomach, thus extending the work of Harper *et al.*[29] In the anesthetized ferret, inflation of the whole stomach or corpus pouch produced antral contractions which were abolished by vagal section[4] (Figure 6). The threshold intragastric pressure required

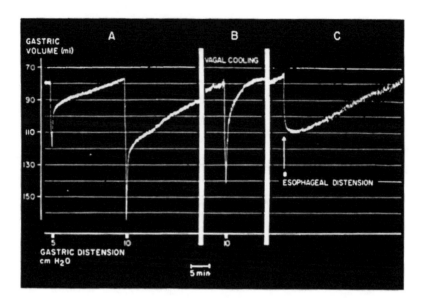

FIGURE 5. Original records of gastric motility recorded in the anesthetized cat. Gastric motility was monitored by recording the volume of an intragastric balloon attached to a large reservoir to keep intragastric pressure constant. Gastric distension was produced by elevating the reservoir over the control level thereby causing inflow of water into the intragastric balloon. Increasing gastric pressure by 5 and 10 cmH$_2$O (A) for 30 sec caused a long-lasting gastric relaxation which was absent in the presence of vagal cooling (B). The response to gastric distension showed similarity with that produced by esophageal stimulation (C). (Used with permission by *Acta Physiol. Scand.*, from Abrahamsson and Jansson.[2])

to initiate this reflex was around 3 cmH$_2$O; above 6 cmH$_2$O distension decreased intraluminal pressure.

Despite the absence of reflex vagal efferent fiber discharge induced by mucosal stimulation in the ferret, application of acid, alkali and hypertonic saline to the antral mucosa produce a reflex decrease in intragastric pressure.[5] The response was abolished by vagal section and was mediated by a non-adrenergic and non-muscarinic pathway. In conscious dogs, chemical stimulation of the gastric mucosa decreased gastric electrical activity.[36]

Functional Significance of Gastric Vago-vagal Reflexes

It is plain that the stomach's ability to accommodate volumes by relaxation of the walls will aid ingestion of a meal, and several types of stimulation have been shown to initiate this reflex. Abrahamsson[1] suggested that activation of tension receptors in the antrum to produce a decrease in gastric intraluminal pressure would also prevent excessive distension of the antrum by controlling delivery of food from the corpus. These reflexes are long acting and slowly adapting and thus would remain active during a prolonged gastric distension, such as after ingestion of a meal. Stimulation of antral mucosal receptors by the chemical constituents of a meal could also achieve the same end. Andrews and

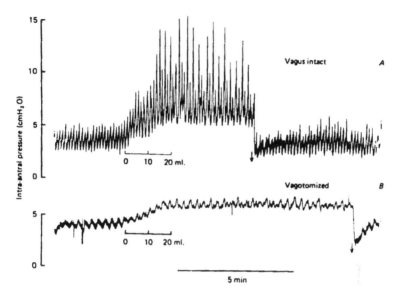

FIGURE 6. The effect of corpus distension on antral motility in the anesthetized ferret. The stomach was divided into a separate antral and corpus pouch by placing two ligatures around the stomach 1 cm orad of the incisura angularis. The stomach was then transected between the two ligatures. Antral motility was recorded manometrically. Corpus distension was associated with large antral contractions (A) which returned to baseline levels on removal of the distension (arrows). After bilateral cervical vagotomy (B) corpus distension was without effect on the antrum suggesting that this is a reflex mediated by the vagus nerves. (Used with permission by *J. Physiol.*, from Andrews *et al.*[4])

Wood[5] have suggested that these reflexes may be involved in producing some of the changes in gastric motility associated with vomiting. Sensing of the antral contents would result in inhibition of gastric motility as part of the emetic reflex, thus providing protection of the duodenal lumen from toxins. Stimulation of antral activity by gastric distension could also be involved in initiating the process of gastric mixing and emptying after a meal or in initiation of other reflexes, such as gastric acid or pancreatic secretion.

REFLEXES INITIATED FROM THE INTESTINE

Boldireff reported in 1904 that placing acid in the intestine inhibited the periodic activity of the emptying stomach and that this inhibition is not obtained by water or alkaline solutions (see Davenport[17]). Brunnemeier and Carlson[10] made some interesting observations showing the powerful effects of stimulating the intestinal mucosa on gastric motility. Stimulation of the intestinal mucosa with acid, peptone, glucose and mechanical stimulation consisting of light stroking produced a long-lasting inhibition of ongoing gastric contractions, termed hunger contractions. The stimuli produced the same effect, and although they were still effective after vagal and splanchnic section, the response latency was greatly increased and the magnitude and duration of the response greatly reduced (Figure 7). In 1934, Thomas *et al.* confirmed these findings and found that after severing the vagus nerves in the neck of dogs, the response to moderate stimuli was abolished while the response to stronger stimuli was markedly attenuated. Thomas designated this effect on gastric motility as the enterogastric reflex.[67] He recognized that this mechanism could be very important in the regulation of gastric emptying. The threshold for activation of this reflex was less than that required to cause closure of the pyloric sphincter, and therefore, Thomas concluded that inhibition of gastric motility by acid in the duodenum is of prime importance in the control of gastric emptying.

Recently, Malagelada provided evidence for reflex control of gastric motility from the duodenum in conscious dogs. Duodenal acid perfusion[15,63,67] or duodenal distension[22,38] decreases proximal gastric motility measured by strain gauges, manometrically and by a gastric barostat. There is good evidence in the conscious dog that these reflexes are mediated solely by the vagus nerve through a non-adrenergic non-muscarinic reflex pathway similar to that mediating the inhibition of proximal gastric motility in response to esophageal and gastric distension.[22] Duodenal infusion of different components of a meal also produce changes in proximal gastric motility[6] (Figure 8). In conscious dogs, intestinal perfusion with an isotonic mixture of protein, fat and carbohydrate into the jejunum decreased gastric tone measured with a barostat via a vago-

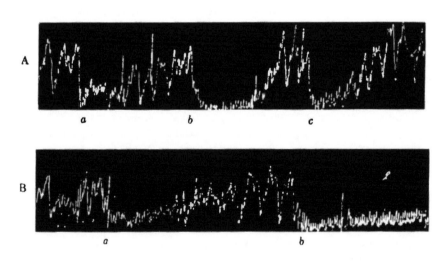

FIGURE 7. Original records of gastric motility from a conscious fasted dog. Dogs had intestinal fistulas through which the lumen could be mechanically or chemically stimulated and gastric fistulas for insertion of the recording balloon. Mechanical stimulation (A.*a*, moving a rubber tube over the mucosa), introduction of water (A.*b*), alkali (A.*c*), peptone (B.*a*) or milk (B.*b*) into the intestine all decreased gastric tone and inhibited "hunger contractions" of the stomach. Following vagal section, the responses had a much longer latency, a decreased degree of inhibition and shorter duration. (Used with permission by *Am. J. Physiol.*, from Brunemeier and Carlson.[10])

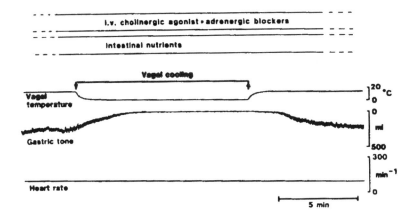

FIGURE 8. Gastric motility recorded in conscious dogs using an electronically controlled gastric barostat. Cholinergic agonists were infused to suppress the effects of vagal cooling on gastric tone. Adrenergic antagonists were infused to block sympathetic inhibitory reflex activity to the stomach. Vagal cooling during intestinal perfusion with a mixed nutrient meal resulted in blockade of the gastric relaxation induced by the nutrients, suggesting that nutrients induce gastric relaxation by a non-adrenergic, non-cholinergic pathway. (Used with permission by *Am. J. Physiol.*, from Azpiroz and Malagelada.[6])

vagal non-adrenergic, non-muscarinic reflex pathway. Antral contractions are inhibited by duodenal infusion of oil, glucose or acid into the duodenum of conscious pigs; these effects were largely mediated by the vagus nerve.[63] The afferent and efferent reflex pathways are summarized in Figure 9.

GASTRIC MOTOR FUNCTION AND REGULATION OF GASTRIC EMPTYING

The significance of these intestino-gastric reflexes is in the regulation of gastric emptying. The emptying of meals from the stomach is regulated by chemoreceptive mechanisms in the duodenum. These mechanisms are capable of producing selective responses to meal components and are quantitatively capable of regulating the number of calories emptied from the stomach despite wide variations in nutrient density of meals. The action of different nutrients to delay gastric emptying seems to be mediated by hormonal or neural mechanisms or by a combination of both.

Postprandial Changes in Gastroduodenal Motor Function

The search for the controlling mechanisms in intestinal inhibition of gastric emptying has been based on the study of the nutrient infusion effects on motor function of different gastroduodenal regions. These studies have revealed that the control of gastric emptying results from pressure changes at different gastroduodenal sites, namely the proximal stomach, antrum, pylorus and duo-

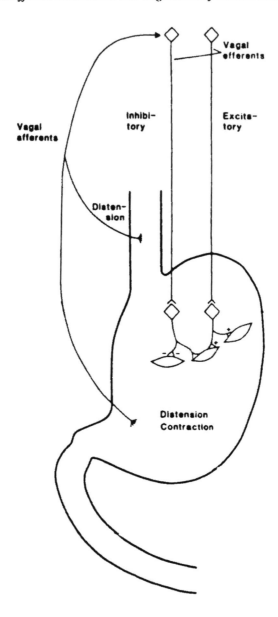

FIGURE 9. Summary of the vago-vagal reflexes to the upper gastrointestinal tract. (Adapted from Abrahamsson.[1])

denum, and that the extrinsic innervation plays a significant role in these control mechanisms.

There is evidence that changes in proximal gastric tone and the resultant change in the gastroduodenal pressure gradient will modify the rate of gastric emptying. Strunz and Grossman[66] studied canine gastric emptying of liquids while holding intragastric pressure constant with a barostat; they found that gastric emptying increased linearly with increasing proximal intragastric pressure. The influence of intestinal nutrients on gastric motility has already been discussed, and there is good evidence that these effects are mediated via the vagus nerve. This fits well with the hypothesis that the proximal stomach plays a role in the regulation of gastric emptying.

However, there is evidence that the proximal stomach does not exclusively provide the driving force for the emptying of liquids and that distal sites are also involved in the regulation of gastric emptying. If fundic and duodenal pressures are held constant by a barostat, the stomach can still expel liquids and emptying can be modified by the presence of nutrients.[47] In conscious dogs, no difference in intragastric pressure was found after meals of saline, glucose or oleate despite the saline meal emptying twice as fast as the nutrient meal. By measuring flow across the antropyloric segment under barostatically controlled pressure gradients, antropyloric resistance increased when oleate or acid perfused the duodenum; this increase was abolished by pyloric myotomy.[47] In a radiographic study, pyloric and antral diameter were smaller after nutrient than non-nutrient meals.[33] Stimuli such as intraduodenal acid, amino acids and lipid stimulate pyloric contractions; the rapidity of onset of the response suggests a neurally mediated event which may be mediated by local reflex pathways across the pylorus or by long vago-vagal pathways.[46]

Thus there is evidence that more than one gastroduodenal region is involved in the regulation of gastric emptying and that the extrinsic innervation plays a role in the control of gastric outflow. However, this does not exclude the possibility of hormonal mechanisms that require an intact neural pathway for their release or for the expression of their effects on target tissue.

REFLEX MODULATION OF GASTRIC MOTOR FUNCTION BY PEPTIDES

Many peptides, when administered exogenously into animals and man, inhibit gastric emptying and alter gastroduodenal motor function. Administration of cholecystokinin (CCK), gastrin, bombesin, somatostatin, glucagon, secretin, peptide YY, pancreatic polypeptide, calcitonin gene-related peptide (CGRP), corticotropin-releasing factor (CRF) and vasoactive intestinal peptide lower proximal intragastric pressure and delay gastric emptying.[34] Of the hormones shown to inhibit gastric emptying, there is evidence that the action of CCK may be physiological.

CCK decreases proximal gastric motility[59,68] (Figure 10). Until recently, the mechanism by which CCK inhibits proximal gastric tone was unclear; it seems to depend partially on the integrity of the vagus nerve.[51] However, evidence is accumulating to suggest that CCK may alter gastric motility and emptying via a vago-vagal reflex pathway. Exogenous administration of sulphated cholecystokinin octapeptide (CCK-8) in urethane-anesthetized rats decreases intragastric

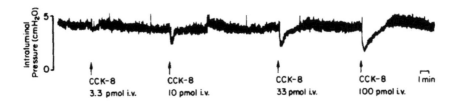

FIGURE 10. Original records of the CCK action on intraluminal pressure in the gastric corpus of anesthetized rats. CCK decreases both tonic intraluminal pressure and the height of phasic gastric contractions. (Used with permission by CRC Press, from Raybould.[56])

pressure in the proximal stomach by pathways involving both the vagal and splanchnic nerves; the vagal pathway is non-adrenergic and hexamethonium-sensitive, suggesting CCK is acting via a vago-vagal reflex[59] (Figure 10).

Vagal Afferent Pathway and the Gastric Motor Response to CCK

Nerve section not only removes the pathway of potential reflexes but also disrupts motor activity and may alter the sensitivity of the gastrointestinal tract to other non-neural influences. Thus, the role of vagal afferent fibers in mediating the effects of CCK on gastroduodenal motor function have been studied using the sensory neurotoxin, capsaicin.

Capsaicin is becoming widely used to investigate the role of afferent C-fibers in a number of physiological processes.[11] In most studies, capsaicin is administered systemically to neonatal or adult rats; in both cases, the lesion extends to all somatic and visceral capsaicin-sensitive fibers. In addition, capsaicin crosses the blood-brain barrier, and systemic treatment will therefore result in largely undefined central actions. There is evidence that capsaicin acts on nerve fibers;[31] the application of capsaicin directly to the nerve pathway of interest has the advantage of defining the nerve pathway and of avoiding direct effects on afferent terminals in the central nervous system. Capsaicin application to the sciatic nerve in rats produces a long-lasting increase in thresholds to mechanical and chemical stimuli, a depletion of peptides and other markers for afferent C-fibers in the central and peripheral terminal fields[3,24] and produces alterations in postsynaptic responses to C-fiber activation in the spinal cord.[69] Perivagal application of capsaicin has been shown to inhibit axonal transport of peptides, including substance P (SP) and somatostatin.[24] Efferent autonomic nerves seem to be unaffected by capsaicin.[14]

Perivagal treatment with capsaicin attenuates the CCK-induced decrease in intraluminal pressure in anesthetized rats[60] (Figure 11). Sympathetic denervation completely abolishes the residual response to CCK, suggesting that perivagal capsaicin treatment has removed the vago-vagal reflex pathway by which CCK decreases proximal gastric motility.

CCK decreases proximal gastric motility but enhances antral and pyloric contractions.[34] In dogs, both of these effects seem to be important for CCK to inhibit gastric emptying.[71] Pyloroplasty and antrectomy inhibit the action of low

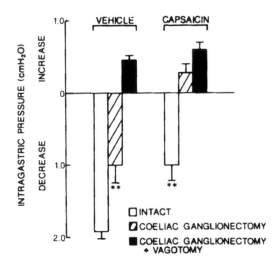

FIGURE 11. Effect of sympathectomy and vagotomy on the CCK-induced decrease in gastric motor function. Responses to CCK were obtained in rats in which the vagus nerves have been pretreated with either vehicle or capsaicin 7-10 days before experiments. Removal of the celiac/superior mesenteric ganglion in vehicle-treated rats decreased the response to CCK; subsequent vagal section abolished the decrease in intraluminal pressure in response to CCK. In contrast, in capsaicin-treated rats, removal of the celiac/superior mesenteric ganglion alone completely abolished the response to CCK. This result suggests that CCK decreases proximal gastric motility in part by a capsaicin-sensitive vagal pathway. (Used with permission by *Am. J. Physiol.*, from Raybould and Taché.[60])

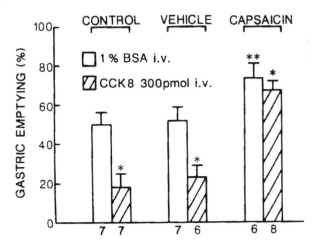

FIGURE 12. Effect of perivagal capsaicin treatment on the CCK-induced delay in gastric emptying in conscious rats. CCK was administered 5 min prior to oral administration of a non-nutrient meal and gastric emptying measured after 20 min. CCK significantly reduced emptying in both control and vehicle-treated rats. Perivagal capsaicin treatment abolished the CCK-induced delay in gastric emptying. In addition, this treatment alone significantly increased gastric emptying. (Used with permission by *Am. J. Physiol.*, from Raybould and Taché.[60])

doses of CCK, but higher doses are still effective, and this is abolished only by vagotomy. However, in the rat, the action of CCK on gastric emptying was unimpaired by pyloric resection or pyloroplasty.[65] Removal of the vagal sensory pathway by pretreatment with perivagal capsaicin completely abolished the ability of intravenously administered CCK to delay gastric emptying in the conscious rat[60] (Figure 12). Taken together, these results suggest that CCK acts via a vagal afferent pathway to decrease gastric motility and that this pathway is important in mediating the CCK-induced delay in gastric emptying. It is interesting to note that perivagal capsaicin treatment alone significantly increased the rate of gastric emptying; this suggests a tonic action of vagal afferent fibers to delay gastric emptying. Electrophysiological studies of vagal efferent fiber discharge showed that these fibers were found to be spontaneously active. Azpiroz and Malagelada[7] found that in conscious dogs, gastric tone was maintained by a vagal cholinergic input. It is possible that vagal afferent fibers are important for maintaining this gastric tone, and in their absence, intraluminal pressure is higher and therefore gastric emptying is more rapid.

Electrophysiological Evidence for Action of CCK

Visceral afferent fibers are sensitive to a variety of peptides and other neuroactive agents.[30] Of particular interest is the sensitivity of intestinal and gastric mechanoreceptive afferent fibers to exogenous CCK. In ferret and sheep, the action of CCK on polymodal receptive endings (i.e., endings responding to both mechanical and chemical stimuli) is secondary to changes in smooth muscle tone.[8,16] Increased afferent fiber discharge in response to CCK in an *in vitro* preparation of the sheep intestine is abolished when smooth muscle contraction is inhibited by hexamethonium and atropine. However, rat gastric mechanoreceptors seem to be directly stimulated by exogenous CCK.[18,35,57] Intravenous administration of CCK stimulates the discharge of gastric mechanoreceptors despite the decreased intraluminal pressure.[18,57] In the dorsal vagal complex, neurons receiving an input from gastric mechanoreceptors responded to intravenous CCK-8 and the changes in neuronal discharge evoked by CCK and gastric distension were in the same direction, suggesting that the two stimuli act through a common or convergent neural pathway[58] (Figure 13). Moreover, CCK was more potent in eliciting changes in neuronal discharge when administered intra-aortically close to the stomach than when administered intravenously, suggesting that CCK acts in the splanchnic bed. These responses were abolished by vagal section but unaffected by prior removal of the celiac/superior mesenteric ganglion. In animals in which the antrum had been resected, units still responded to gastric distension and CCK, suggesting that at least some of the responses come from afferent fibers terminating in the proximal stomach. Intravenous noradrenaline and VIP have effects similar to those of CCK on intragastric pressure but evoked different patterns of responses from brainstem neurons (Table 1). These results are consistent with the idea that CCK acts directly on vagal mechanoreceptive endings in the gastric corpus wall.

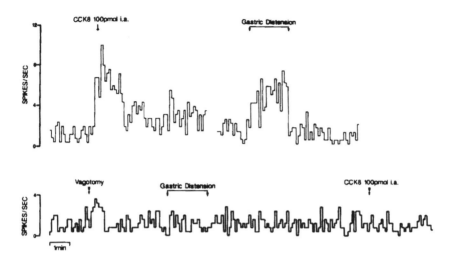

FIGURE 13. Extracellular recording of neuronal activity in the dorsal vagal complex of anesthetized rats. Gastric distension was produced by instillation of 2 ml of physiological saline. Intraaortic injections close to the splanchnic bed were made via a catheter in the aorta. The discharge of this neuron was increased by gastric distension and CCK. Response to both stimuli was abolished by vagal section. (Reprinted with permission by *Journal of Neuroscience*, from Raybould *et al.*[58])

TABLE 1

Response to Gastric Distension	% Concordant Responses with Gastric Distension		
	CCK-8	**Noradrenaline**	**VIP**
gE, (n = 16)	100	43	33
gl, (n = 15)	100	75	18
gN, (n = 18)	0	44	44

Reprinted with permission by *Journal of Neurosci.*, from Raybould *et al.*[58]

Physiological Role for CCK

CCK is a potent inhibitor of gastric emptying of both liquids and solids in several species including man. In man, reproduction of postprandial plasma levels of CCK by infusion of the exogenous peptide delayed gastric emptying.[41] In the dog, the dose of CCK-8 required to inhibit gastric emptying was the same as the ED_{50} for stimulation of pancreatic secretion and gallbladder contraction.[20] These observations are consistent with a physiological role for CCK in the regulation of postprandial gastric emptying.

Antagonists

Recently, this hypothesis has been directly tested with the use of specific and potent CCK antagonists. Administration of L364,718, a potent CCK receptor antagonist for the peripheral type receptor (the "A" receptor),[42] reverses the inhibition of gastric emptying following intragastric protein in the rat.[25] The effects of a mixed nutrient or glucose meal on gastric emptying was reversed by administration of the CCK antagonist loxiglumide in man.[23]

Location

CCK is located in both endocrine cells and neurons within the GI tract. The endocrine cells are scattered evenly throughout the crypts and villi of the duodenum and proximal jejunum, with a few cells present in the ileum.[70] The endocrine cells are in direct contact with the lumen of the intestinal glands and therefore will have direct access to nutrients. Fibers showing immunoreactivity for CCK are found in the mucosa, and the cell bodies are in the overlying submucosa and myenteric plexus.[64] Immunoreactive fibers for CCK are rare in the stomach and there are no reports of cell bodies.

Release

Increased CCK plasma levels would suggest that release of CCK from endocrine cells, rather than from nerve endings, is important in postprandial gastric motility. In rats, intragastric instillation of a mixed meal increased plasma levels of CCK from 0.3 to 6 pM.[40] When different nutrients were administered orogastrically, intact proteins were the only stimulants of CCK release. Hydrolysed protein, amino acids (L-tryptophan and L-phenylalanine), starch, glucose or fat had no effect on plasma levels of CCK. Administration of soya bean trypsin inhibitor (SBTI), thought to release CCK by inhibition of intraluminal trypsin which in turn inhibits release of CCK, resulted in up to 30-fold increases in plasma levels of CCK.

Receptors

Candidate CCK receptor populations for the mediation of changes in gastric motility and emptying have been identified on the circular muscle layer of the pyloric sphincter and the vagus nerve. CCK binding sites have been demonstrated on the vagus nerve and to be transported toward the periphery.[72] More importantly, these binding sites occur on all subdiaphragmatic branches of the vagus.[49] These receptor sites are of the peripheral subtype (A receptors) as binding with CCK-8(s) is not displaced by the desulfated peptide.[49] It is interesting to note that CCK binding sites were relatively specific to the vagus nerve since no sites were found on the rat sciatic nerve. High affinity binding sites for CCK have been demonstrated in the caudal subnucleus of the NTS, the site of central termination of vagal afferent fibers.[37] Unilateral nodose ganglionectomy produced a marked reduction in the density of CCK binding sites in the medial NTS on the ipsilateral side. This suggests that these putative CCK receptors may be located on vagal afferent fibers. Since the inhibition of gastric emptying by CCK is not abolished by resection of the pylorus but is abolished by perivagal capsaicin, it is suggested that CCK binding sites on vagal afferent fibers are important for mediating its action on gastric motor function. The

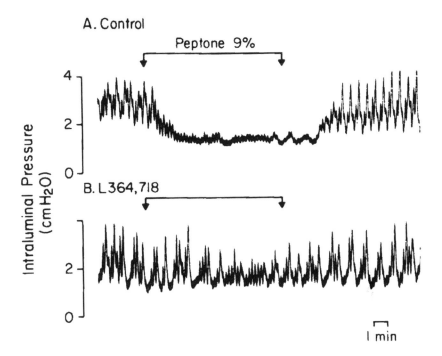

FIGURE 14. Original records of intraluminal pressure of the gastric corpus in anesthetized rats showing the decrease during intestinal infusion of peptone. Similar to administration of exogenous CCK, the response consists of both a decrease in tone and height of phasic contractions. The response to peptone was significantly attenuated by administration of the CCK "A" receptor antagonist, L364,718. (Used with permission by *Peptides*, from Raybould.[55])

decrease in proximal gastric motility in the urethane-anesthetized rat is mediated via a CCK action at an "A" type receptor site since administration of the CCK "A" receptor antagonist, L364,718, abolished the action of low doses of CCK and markedly reduced higher doses.[55] The effect of exogenous administration of CCK on gastric emptying is also abolished by CCK "A" receptor antagonists.[25,42,53]

Endogenous Release of CCK

The effect of release of endogenous CCK from endocrine cells and subsequent increases in plasma levels of CCK on proximal gastric motility was studied using intraduodenal infusion of nutrients.[55] Nutrients that should increase CCK plasma levels (casin, peptone and SBTI) and nutrients that do not (glucose and acid) were infused. Intraduodenal infusion with peptone, casein, acid, glucose or SBTI decreased baseline gastric intraluminal pressure and decreased the height but not the frequency of phasic contractions of the gastric corpus; this response is similar to the effect seen after intravenous injection of CCK (Figure 14). The response to duodenal peptone, casein, and SBTI were

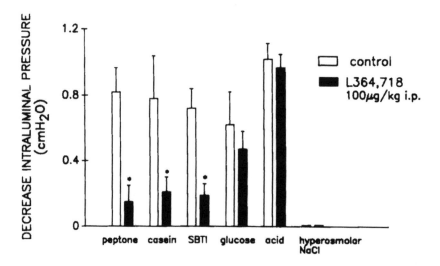

FIGURE 15. Effect of the CCK "A" receptor antagonist on the decrease in tonic proximal gastric motility produced by intraduodenal infusion of nutrient shown to increase plasma levels of CCK (peptone, casein, soya bean trypsin inhibitor [SBTI]) and those that do not (glucose, acid). the response to those nutrients that release CCK was significantly reduced by administration of the CCK receptor antagonist, L364,718. (Used with permission by CRC Press, from Raybould.[56])

inhibited following administration of the CCK "A" receptor antagonist L364,718. However, the response to glucose and acid were unaltered by administration of the antagonist. Thus, nutrients shown to increase plasma levels in the rat (protein and SBTI) act to decrease gastric motility via a CCK-sensitive mechanism (Figure 15).

The afferent pathway that mediates the effects of intraduodenal nutrients was studied by perineural application of the sensory neurotoxin capsaicin. Perivagal application of capsaicin significantly reduced the effects of peptone, glucose and SBTI on gastric motility but had no effect on the inhibition of gastric motility produced by intraduodenal infusion of acid. Thus it seems that intraduodenal peptone and glucose, but not acid, inhibit gastric motility by a capsaicin-sensitive vagal afferent pathway (Figure 16).

SUMMARY AND SPECULATIONS

Evidence has been presented that the vagus nerves mediate reflexes arising from both the stomach and at least the first part of the duodenum; many of these reflexes result in decreased proximal gastric motility. These inhibitory reflexes to the stomach are mediated by non-adrenergic, non-cholinergic pathways, although they may also involve reciprocal inhibition of the vagal cholinergic pathway. It has been suggested that the vagus plays only a permissive role in the generation of reflex control of motility, providing tone upon which enteric reflexes produce reflex activity. However, there is evidence that intraduodenal

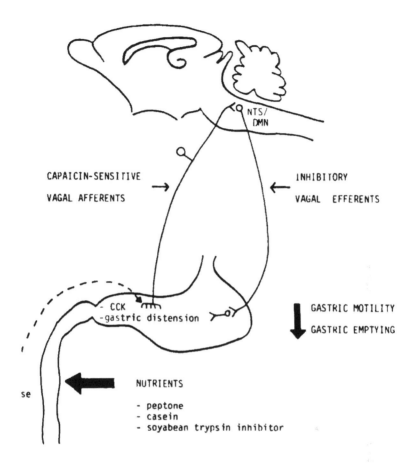

FIGURE 16. Diagram of possible pathways by which CCK inhibits gastric motility. Exogenous administration of CCK stimulates capsaicin-sensitive vagal afferent fibers, resulting in a vago-vagal inhibition of proximal gastric motility. Intraduodenal protein increases circulating levels of CCK which in turn stimulates vagal afferent endings. These changes in proximal gastric motility may well contribute to the delayed gastric emptying after a meal. Thus, CCK released after ingestion of a meal may stimulate vago-vagal reflex pathways to alter gastric motor function and transit.

glucose, which acts to decrease proximal gastric motility, involves the vagal capsaicin-sensitive afferent pathway, at least in the rat. The response to duodenal protein is more complex, but involves both the capsaicin-sensitive vagal afferent pathway and release of CCK. It is suggested that the CCK so released acts on the sensory pathway to produce a decrease in motility. CCK directly stimulates gastric mechanoreceptors and indirectly stimulates duodenal mechanoreceptors through changes in smooth muscle tone. It is not clear which population of afferent fibers is involved in mediating these reflex responses to CCK and protein in the duodenum. The response of the proximal stomach to protein is very rapid; it is possible that release of CCK from fibers in the duodenum stimulates motor function that then stimulates afferent fiber discharge to produce reflex inhibition of proximal gastric motility.

Another property of the sensory innervation of the gastrointestinal tract is the possibility that the afferent endings may also subserve local effector functions. These functions may be mediated by the release of peptides from the peripheral terminals. There is both morphological and functional evidence that capsaicin-sensitive, peptidergic neurons innervate the gastrointestinal tract. However investigations into the role of these afferent fibers in regulation of gastrointestinal function is hampered by the localization of peptides to both afferent fibers and to enteric neurons. It is fortunate, therefore, that the sensory neurotoxin capsaicin seems to be without effect on these neurons and thus becomes an important tool for probing the role of sensory fibers in the functioning of the gastrointestinal tract. Delbro *et al.*[21] demonstrated that electrical stimulation of the vagus caused gastric contractions that were hexamethonium resistant, supporting the concept for antidromic activation of vagal afferent fibers to evoke changes in gastric motility. It is also possible that afferent endings terminate on enteric neurons, and these changes in function may be brought about by the enteric nervous system. It is possible that SP may be involved in the response described by Delbro because the response to electrical stimulation was attenuated by SP antagonist and there was cross tachyphylaxis between electrical stimulation and SP.[21] However, less than 1% of vagal afferents to the stomach contain CGRP or SP, a marked contrast to the spinal afferent innervation to the stomach which contains over 80%. Over 90% of the CGRP in the stomach is of extrinsic sensory origin. It is possible that the small proportion of vagal afferents containing the known sensory peptides may constitute an important functional population. Alternatively, it is possible that there remains an as yet unidentified sensory peptide projecting to the stomach in vagal afferents.

REFERENCES

1. Abrahamsson, H., Studies on the inhibitory nervous control of gastric motility, *Acta Physiol. Scand. [Suppl]*, 390, 1-50, 1973.
2. Abrahamsson, H., and Jansson, G., Vago-vagal gastro-gastric relaxation in the cat, *Acta Physiol. Scand.*, 88, 289-295, 1973.
3. Ainsworth, A., Hall, P., and Wall, P.D., Effects of capsaicin applied locally to adult peripheral nerve, II, Anatomy and enzyme and peptide chemistry of peripheral nerve and spinal cord, *Pain*, 11, 379-388, 1981.
4. Andrews, P.L.R., Grundy, D., and Scratcherd, T., Reflex excitation of antral motility induced by gastric distension in the ferret, *J. Physiol.*, 298, 79-84, 1980.
5. Andrews, P.L.R., and Wood, K.L., Vagally mediated gastric motor and emetic reflexes evoked by stimulation of the antral mucosa in anesthetized ferrets, *J. Physiol.*, 395, 1-16, 1988.
6. Azpiroz, F., and Malagelada, J.R., Vagally mediated gastric relaxation induced by intestinal nutrients in the dog, *Am. J. Physiol.*, 251, G727-G735, 1986.
7. Azpiroz, F., and Malagelada, J.R., Importance of vagal input in maintaining gastric tone in the dog, *J. Physiol.*, 384, 511-524, 1987.

8. **Blackshaw, L.A., Grundy, D., and Scratcherd, T.,** Vagal afferent discharge from gastric mechanoreceptors during contraction and relaxation of the ferret corpus, *J. Auton. Nerv. Syst.,* 18, 19-24, 1987.

9. **Blackshaw, L.A., Grundy, D., and Scratcherd, T.,** Involvement of gastrointestinal mechano- and intestinal chemoreceptors in vagal reflexes: An electrophysiological study, *J. Auton. Nervous Syst.,* 18, 225-234, 1987.

10. **Brunemeier, E.H., and Carlson, A.J.,** Contributions to the physiology of the stomach: Reflexes from the intestinal mucosa to the stomach, *Am. J. Physiol.,* 36, 191-195, 1914.

11. **Buck, S.H., and Burks, T.F.,** The neuropharmacology of capsaicin: Review of some recent observations, *Pharmacol. Rev.,* 38, 179-250, 1986.

12. **Cannon, W.B., and Lieb, C.W.,** The receptive relaxation of the stomach, *Am. J. Physiol,* 29, 267-273, 1911.

13. **Carlson, A.J.,** Contributions to the physiology of the stomach, VII: The inhibitory reflexes from the stomach, *Am. J. Physiol,* 32, 389-397, 1914.

14. **Cervero, F., and McRitchie, M.A.,** Neonatal capsaicin does not affect unmyelinated fibers of the autonomic nervous system, *Brain Res.,* 239, 283-288, 1982.

15. **Cooke, A.R., and Clark, E.D.,** Effect of first part of duodenum on gastric emptying in dogs: Response to acid, fat, glucose, and neural blockade, *Gastroenterology,* 70, 550-555, 1976.

16. **Cottrell, D.F., and Iggo, A.,** The responses of duodenal tension receptors in sheep to pentagastrin, cholecystokinin and some other drugs, *J. Physiol.,* 354, 477-495, 1986.

17. **Davenport, H.W.,** Gastrointestinal physiology, 1895-1975: Motility, in *Handbook of Physiology,* Sec. 6, Schultz, S.G., Ed., American Physiology Society, Bethesda, MD, 1989, Chapter 1.

18. **Davison, J.S., and Clarke, G.D.,** Mechanical properties and sensitivity to CCK of vagal gastric slowly adapting mechanoreceptors, *Am. J. Physiol.,* 255, G55-G61, 1988.

19. **Davison, J.S., and Grundy, D.,** Modulation of single vagal efferent fiber discharge by gastrointestinal afferents in the rat, *J. Physiol.,* 284, 69-82, 1978.

20. **Debas, H.T., Farooq, O., and Grossman, M.I.,** Inhibition of gastric emptying is a physiological action of cholecystokinin, *Gastroenterology,* 68, 1211-1217, 1975.

21. **Delbro, D., Fandriks, L., Rosell, S., and Folkers, K.,** Inhibition of antidromically induced stimulation of gastric motility by substance P receptor blockade, *Acta Physiol. Scand.,* 118, 309-316, 1983.

22. **De Ponti, F., Azpiroz, F., and Malagelada, J.R.,** Reflex gastric relaxation in response to distention of the duodenum, *Am. J. Physiol.,* 252, G595-G601, 1987.

23. **Fried, M., Lochner, C., Erlacher, U., Beglinger, J., Jansen, C., Lamers, J., and Stadler, G.A.,** Role of CCK in the regulation of gastric emptying and pancreatic secretion in man, *Gastroenterology,* 96, A159, 1989.

24. **Gamse, R., Petsche, U., Lembeck, F., and Jansco, G.,** Capsaicin applied to peripheral nerve inhibits axoplasmic transport of substance P and somatostatin, *Brain Res.,* 239, 447-462, 1982.

25. **Green, T., Dimaline, R., and Dockray, G.J.,** Neuroendocrine control mechanisms of gastric emptying in the rat, in *Nerves and the Gastrointestinal Tract,* Singer, M.V., and Goebell, H., Eds., Kluwar, Netherlands, 1989, 433-446.

26. **Grundy, D.,** Speculations on the structure/function relationship for vagal and splanchnic afferent endings supplying the gastrointestinal tract, *J. Auton. Nerv. Syst.,* 22, 175-180, 1988.

27. **Grundy, D., Salih, A.A., and Scratcherd, T.,** Modulation of vagal efferent fiber discharge by mechanoreceptors in the stomach, duodenum and colon of the ferret, *J. Physiol.,* 319, 43-52, 1981.

28. **Grundy, D., and Scratcherd, T.,** Sensory afferents from the gastrointestinal tract, in *Handbook of Physiology,* Sec. 6, Schultz, S.G., Ed., American Physiology Society, Bethesda, MD., 1989, Chapter 10.

29. **Harper, A.A., Kidd, C., and Scratcherd, T.,** Vago-vagal reflex effects on gastric and pancreatic secretion and gastrointestinal motility, *J. Physiol.,* 148, 417-436, 1959.

30. Higashi, H., Pharmacological aspects of visceral sensory receptors, *Prog. Brain Res.*, 67, 149-162, 1986.

31. Jancsó, G., Király, E., and Jancsó-Gábor, A., Direct evidence for an axonal site of action of capsaicin, *Naunyn Schmiedebergs Arch. Pharmacol.*, 313, 91-94, 1980.

32. Jansson, G., Extrinsic nervous control of gastric motility: An experimental study in the cat, *Acta Physiol. Scand. [Suppl]*, 326, 1969.

33. Keinke, O., Schemann, M., and Ehrlein, H.J., Mechanical factors regulating gastric emptying of viscous nutrient meals in dogs, *Q. J. Exp. Physiol.*, 69, 781-795, 1984.

34. Kelly, K.A., Gastric emptying of liquids and solids: Roles of proximal and distal stomach, *Am. J. Physiol.*, 239, G71-G76, 1980.

35. Klimov, P.K., Nozdrachev, A.D., Chubarova, N.I., Barachkova, G.M., Martin, A., Murat, J.E., and Nikolov, N.A., Afferent impulses from the autonomic nerves of the stomach during treatment with pentagastrin, cholecystokinin-pancreozymin, serotonin, thyrotropin and glucagon, *Agressologie*, 23, 249-251, 1982.

36. Kuwahara, A., Changes in gastric motility by chemical and mechanical stimulation in the dog, *Jpn. J. Physiol.*, 33, 29-40, 1983.

37. Ladenheim, E.E., Speth, R.C., and Ritter, R.C., Reduction of CCK-8 binding in the nucleus of the solitary tract in unilaterally nodosectomized rats, *Brain Res.*, 474, 125-129, 1988.

38. Lalich, J., Meek, W.J., and Herrin, R.C., Reflex pathways concerned in inhibition of hunger contractions by intestinal distension, *Am. J. Physiol.*, 115, 410-414, 1936.

39. Leek, B.F., Abdominal visceral receptors, in *Handbook of Sensory Physiology: Enteroceptors*, Neil, E., Ed., Springer-Verlag, Berlin, 1972, 131-160.

40. Liddle, R.A., Green, G.M., Conrad, C.K., and Williams, J.A., Proteins but not amino acids, carbohydrates, or fats stimulate cholecystokinin secretion in the rat, *Am. J. Physiol.*, 251, G243-G245, 1986.

41. Liddle, R.A., Morita, E.T., Conrad, C.K., and Williams, J.A., Regulation of gastric emptying in humans by cholecystokinin, *J. Clin. Invest.*, 77, 992-996, 1986.

42. Lotti, V.J., Pendleton, R.G., Gould, R.J., Hanson, H.M., Chang, R.S., and Clineschmidt, B.V., *In vivo* pharmacology of L-364,718, a new potent nonpeptide peripheral cholecystokinin antagonist, *J. Pharmacol. Exp. Ther.*, 241, 103-109, 1987.

43. Martinson, J., The effect of graded stimulation of efferent vagal nerve fibers on gastric motility, *Acta Physiol. Scand.*, 62, 256-262, 1964.

44. McSwinney, B.A., Innervation of the stomach, *Physiol. Rev.*, 11, 478-514, 1931.

45. Mei, N., Intestinal chemosensitivity, *Physiol. Rev.*, 65, 211-237, 1985.

46. Meyer, J.H., Motility of the stomach and gastroduodenal junction, in *Physiology of the Gastrointestinal Tract*, Johnson, L.R., Ed., Raven Press, New York, 1987, 613-629.

47. Miller, J., Kauffman, G., Elashoff, J., Ohashi, H., Carter, D., and Meyer, J.H., Search for resistances controlling canine gastric emptying of liquid meals, *Am. J. Physiol.*, 241, 403-415, 1981.

48. Miolan, J.P., and Roman, C., The role of oesophageal and intestinal receptors in the control of gastric motility, *J. Auton. Nerv. Syst.*, 10, 235-241, 1984.

49. Moran, T.H., Smith, G.P., Hostetler, A.M., and McHugh, P.R., Transport of cholecystokinin (CCK) binding sites in subdiaphragmatic vagal branches, *Brain Res.*, 415, 149-152, 1987.

50. Ohga, A., Nakazato, Y., and Saito, K., Considerations of the efferent nervous mechanisms of the vago-vagal reflex relaxation of the stomach in the dog, *Jpn. J. Pharmacol.*, 20, 116-130, 1970.

51. Okike, N., and Kelly, K.A., Vagotomy impairs pentagastrin-induced relaxation of canine gastric fundus, *Am. J. Physiol.*, 232, E504-E509, 1977.

52. Page May, W., The innervation of the sphincters and musculature of the stomach, *J. Physiol.*, 31, 261-271, 1904.

53. Pendleton, R.G., Bendesky, R.J., Schaffer, L., Nolan, T.E., Gould, R.J., and Clineschmidt, B.V., Roles of endogenous cholecystokinin in biliary, pancreatic and gastric function: Studies with L-364,718, a specific cholecystokinin receptor antagonist, *J. Pharmacol. Exp. Ther.*, 241, 110-116, 1987.

54. **Ranson, S.W.,** Afferent paths for visceral reflexes, *Physiol. Rev.,* 1, 477-522, 1921.
55. **Raybould, H.E.,** Cholecystokinin and capsaicin-sensitive afferent fibers mediate changes in gastric motility following intraduodenal infusion of protein in the rat, *Gastroenterology,* 96, A410, 1989.
56. **Raybould, H.E.,** Vagal afferent modulation of gastric motor functions by neuropeptides, in *Brain-Gut Interactions,* Taché, Y., and Wingate, D., Ed., CRC Press, Boca Raton, 1991, 133-146.
57. **Raybould, H.E., and Davison, J.S.,** Perivagal application of capsaicin abolishes the response of vagal gastric mechanoreceptors to cholecystokinin, *Soc. Neurosci. Abstr.,* 15, 973, 1989.
58. **Raybould, H.E., Gayton, R.J., and Dockray, G.J.,** Mechanism of action of cholecystokinin on brainstem neurons in the rat, *J. Neurosci.,* 8, 3018-3024, 1988.
59. **Raybould, H.E., Roberts, M.E., and Dockray, G.J.,** Reflex decreases in intragastric pressure in response to cholecystokinin in rats, *Am. J. Physiol.,* 253, G165-G170, 1987.
60. **Raybould, H.E., and Taché, Y.,** Cholecystokinin inhibits gastric motility and emptying via a capsaicin-sensitive vagal afferent pathway in rats, *Am. J. Physiol.,* 255, G242-G246, 1988.
61. **Rogers, F.T.,** Reflex control of gastric vagus-tonus, *Am. J. Physiol.,* 42, 605-606, 1917.
62. **Roman, C., and Gonella, J.,** Extrinsic control of digestive tract motility, in *Physiology of the Gastrointestinal Tract,* Johnson, L.R., Ed., Raven Press, New York, 1987, 507-553.
63. **Roze, C., Couturier, D., Chariot, J., and Debray, C.,** Inhibition of gastric electrical and mechanical activity by intraduodenal agents in pigs and effects of vagotomy, *Digestion,* 15, 526-539, 1977.
64. **Schultzberg, M., Hökfelt, T., Nilsson, G., Terenius, L., Fehfeld, J.F., Brown, M., Elde, R., Goldstein, M., and Said, S.,** Distribution of peptide and catecholamine neurons in the gastrointestinal tract of the rat and guinea pig: Immunohistochemical studies using antisera to substance P, VIP, enkephalins, somatostatin, gastrin, neurotensin and dopamine-b-hydroxylase, *Neuroscience,* 5, 689-723, 1980.
65. **Smith, G.P., Falasco, J., Moran, T.H., Joyner, K.M.S., and Gibbs, J.,** CCK-8 decreases food intake and gastric emptying after pylorectomy or pyloroplasty, *Am. J. Physiol.,* 255, R113-R117, 1988.
66. **Strunz, U.T., and Grossman, M.I.,** Effect of intragastric pressure on gastric emptying and secretion, *Am. J. Physiol.,* 235, E552-E555, 1978.
67. **Thomas, J.E., Crider, J.O., and Morgan, C.J.,** A study of reflexes involving the pyloric sphincter and antrum and their role in gastric evacuation, *Am. J. Physiol.,* 108, 683-700, 1934.
68. **Valenzuela, J.E., and Grossman, M.I.,** Effect of pentagastrin and caerulein on intragastric pressure in the dog, *Gastroenterology,* 69, 1383-1384, 1975.
69. **Wall, P.D., and Fitzgerald, M.,** Effects of capsaicin applied locally to adult peripheral nerve, I, Physiology of peripheral nerve and spinal cord, *Pain,* 11, 363-377, 1981.
70. **Walsh, J.H.,** Gastrointestinal hormones, in *Physiology of the Gastrointestinal Tract,* Johnson L.R., Ed., Raven Press, New York, 1987, 181-253.
71. **Yamagishi, T., and Debas, H.T.,** Cholecystokinin inhibits gastric emptying by acting on both proximal stomach and pylorus, *Am. J. Physiol.,* 234, E375-E378, 1978.
72. **Zarbin, M.A., Wamsley, J.K., Innis, R.B., and Kuhar, M.J.,** Cholecystokinin receptors: Presence and axonal flow in the rat vagus nerve, *Life Sci.,* 29, 697-705, 1981.

Chapter 10

PARTICIPATION OF VAGAL SENSORY NEURONS IN PUTATIVE SATIETY SIGNALS FROM THE UPPER GASTROINTESTINAL TRACT

R.C. Ritter, L. Brenner and D.P. Yox

TABLE OF CONTENTS

LIST OF ABBREVIATIONS

AP = area postrema
CCK = cholecystokinin
D-Phe = D-phenylalanine
Fosli = fos-like immunreactivity
L-Phe = L-phenylalanine
NST = nucleus tractus solitarius

INTRODUCTION

The Roman physician, Galen, during the second century B.C., described the vagus nerve. However, he did not distinguish the vagus as separate from the sympathetic chain, which he suggested interacted with the muscles of the back.[25] In the 16th and 17th centuries, Vesalius[85] and later Willis (see Pick[61]) recognized the vagi as discrete nerves that innervated the abdominal viscera. Visceromotor function of the vagus was appreciated through the work of Langley[49] and Gaskell[26] at the beginning of the 20th century. However, little attention was given to the potential sensory properties of the vagus until the 1930s, when the anatomical studies of Du Bois and Foley[18] demonstrated that vagal sensory fibers far outnumber vagal motor fibers and Adrian[1] provided electrophysiological data documenting the existence of cardiopulmonary vagal afferents. Subsequent electrophysiological experiments by Iggo[36,37,38] Paintal[59] and others[7,8] established that the abdominal vagi contain afferent fibers that respond to a variety of gastrointestinal stimuli, both mechanical and chemical. More recently, the elegant work of Powley, Berthoud and their co-workers[3,4,62] has demonstrated that the vagus innervates the entire gastrointestinal tract as far caudal as the descending colon, much, perhaps most, of this innervation being provided through contacts with the ganglia and connectives of the enteric plexes.

To what use may the sensory information from the GI tract be applied? One very plausible hypothesis is that some vagal sensory information is used to control food intake. Appreciation of the peripheral sensations associated with the fasting and fed states led 18th, 19th and early 20th century physiologists to view the control of food intake as entirely gastrointestinal in origin (for review see Grossman[33]). This view of the control of ingestion is no longer tenable. It remains clear, however, that food in the upper GI tract is one of several factors that influences the subsequent course of ingestion.

Perhaps the most compelling evidence that entry of food into the GI tract is important for the control of food intake comes from experiments in which food-related stimulation of the upper GI tract is prevented or reduced by continuously removing ingested material through an open gastric fistula. In such experimental preparations, animals are fed a liquid diet. With the fistula closed, ingesta enters the stomach and is emptied to the intestine. When the fistula is open, ingested diet drains from the stomach and none passes to the intestine. Young et al.[88] found that rats with open gastric fistulas ate almost continuously during a 2.5 hr test period, consuming nearly five times as much liquid diet as they did when their fistulas were closed. Gibbs et al.[27] subsequently replicated this phenomenon in the rhesus monkey. Since differences in intake between animals with open and closed gastric fistulas are apparent within the first 15 min after presentation of food, it seems likely that the GI tract is the source of signals contributing to the termination of eating.

The stomach, upper small intestine, lower small intestine, the liver and the colon, have all been suggested as exercising control over food intake. Although, all of these organs may receive vagal sensory innervation, there is no compelling evidence for participation of the vagus in proposed lower small intestine or colonic effects on feeding. The possibility of hepatic vagal involvement in the metabolic control of food intake is discussed by S. Ritter *et al.* in chapter 11 of this volume. Therefore, the remainder of this chapter will focus on vagal participation in the control of food intake by the stomach and small intestine.

GASTRIC CONTROL OF FOOD INTAKE

Sensory Modalities from the Stomach

Recordings from gastric mechanoresponsive fibers in the vagus were among the first data supporting the vagal role in gastrointestinal sensation. For example several studies in the 1950s reported vagal fibers that increased their firing in response to gastric distension.[36,37,58] Subsequent experiments by many groups confirm that the stomach is mechanosensitive and demonstrate the existence of mechanosensation from both the fundus/corpus and the gastric antrum (for review see Grundy and Scratchard[34]). It appears that both the fundic and antral mechanoreceptors are "in series," stretch receptors, responding to increases in tension rather than muscle fiber length (for review, see Grundy, chapter 8 in this volume). However, considering the nature of discharge of antral and fundic receptors during physiological stimulation and the physiological functions of the antral and fundic gastric regions, it would appear that tonically discharging fundic receptors are likely to provide information on gastric fullness, while antral receptors telegraph the phasic activities of the antral mill to the brain. Thus, information from the fundic, capacitance, region of the stomach might be expected to be more important for the control of food intake. "In series" stretch receptors are adapted to monitor tension, regardless of its cause, rather than to monitor muscle fiber length, as is the case with parallel receptors, such as the muscle spindle. In other words, the gastric mechanoreceptors are adapted to monitor intragastric pressure.

In addition to muscle stretch receptors, the stomach also is innervated by vagal sensory fibers that respond to mucosal stimulation. Many of these mucosal receptors respond to mechanical stimulation of the mucosa as well as to stimulation with strong acids or bases.[8,11,37] Also, there are some of the mucosal receptors that appear to be specifically thermosensitive.[21,22] Finally, El Ouazzami and Mei,[22] have reported the existence of specific HCl receptors and specific carbohydrate receptors in the cat stomach. Therefore, it is possible that the stomach may apprise the brain of gastric nutrient content as well as volume or pressure.

Gastric Stimuli that Reduce Food Intake

Ingesta in the stomach is capable of reducing food intake in the absence of intestinal stimulation. The evidence for this assertion comes from experiments in which the pylorus is reversibly occluded using an inflatable cuff[14,15,16] or noose.[46] When rats eat with the pylorus patent, some of the ingesta empties to the small intestine. On the other hand, if the pylorus is occluded by cuff or noose, the ingesta remains in the stomach. The small intestine should not be stimulated. Interestingly, animals consume the same amounts, in short tests, with the pylorus occluded as they do with the pylorus patent. Furthermore, in the Deutch *et al.*[16] work, if liquid food is syphoned from the stomach, the animal will resume eating to replace the material that has been removed. Two conclusions have been drawn from these results, but only one is valid. First, it may be concluded that gastric stimulation alone is capable of terminating food intake; this is a valid conclusion. A second conclusion, drawn by some, is that small intestinal stimulation does not participate in meal termination under the conditions of the pyloric occlusion experiments. This conclusion is premature, however. When the pylorus is patent, a very significant proportion of ingesta leaves the stomach during a meal. For example, Paul Tracy, in my lab, has found that rats eating 15% sucrose consume 8 to 12 mls in the first 12 min of a 30 min sucrose presentation. During this period of time 40–60% of the ingesta empties to the intestine and rate of ingestion is substantially reduced, often to zero. Assuming a similar emptying profile for other studies using liquid diets, one can easily see that the process of satiation occurs with only half as much ingesta in the stomach when the pylorus is patent as when it is occluded. Thus while gastric stimulation may be sufficient to terminate ingestion, it is erroneous to conclude that it is the only source of alimentary signals for meal termination.

As discussed above, the stomach appears to contain sensory receptors for a variety of specific stimuli. There is evidence that both mechanoreception and chemoreception may participate in meal termination. First it is clear that during large meals gastric distension contributes to meal termination. For example, Pappas *et al.*[60] reported that, in dogs with open esophageal fistulas, physiological levels of gastric distension with inert Karaya liquid or liquid diet reduced food intake by similar amounts during a 7.5 min test. Although they did not report measurements of gastric emptying, they concluded that distension of the stomach with either nutrient or non-nutrient material was a physiological satiety signal. Some other investigators have asserted, however, that gastric distension, *per se*, is not an important stimulus for termination of small meals. In this regard, Deutch[15] has suggested that gastric chemosensation may be an important signal for meal termination. Using a pyloric cuff preparation, they found that when ingesta was siphoned from the stomach, rats replaced the lost ingesta by consuming an approximately equal number of calories. If, during the meal, a small volume of saline or fresh corn oil emulsion was infused into the stomach, this preload did not reduce subsequent intake. However, if the preload consisted of "predigested" emulsion from a donor's stomach, the size of the ensuing meal was reduced. These results might indicate the existence of gastric chemosensitive control of ingestion. However, since the pylorus was not occluded during syphoning or intragastric infusion experiments, it is equally plausible that caloric compensation occurred in response to chemical stimuli acting in the intestine and interacting with chemical or mechanical signals from the stomach.

Deutch[15] has suggested that the vagus controls intake in response to gastric distension only when intake is very high. He suggests that splanchnic afferents participate in control of food intake by gastric chemical stimuli. Kraly and co-workers[46] also failed to find evidence for vagal participation in satiation, during intake of small meals of solid food. Thus the role of the vagus nerve in the control of food intake by gastric signals requires clarification.

While the results of experiments designed to minimize interaction of different GI stimuli, such as gastric distension and chemosensation, are useful to understanding control of ingestion, we must not ignore the fact that expression of some controls may depend on interaction of several distinct signals from different parts of the GI tract. Indeed, Moran and McHugh[55] reported that in the presence of low doses of the gut peptide, cholecystokinin (CCK), small intragastric loads of isotonic saline, which alone did not reduce food intake, suppressed food intake in monkeys. Thus the suppression of intake via the interaction of CCK with gastric distension appears to require vagal neurons. The effect of CCK and gastric distension on feeding might result from convergence of separate populations of CCK responsive and mechanoresponsive vagal afferents, as suggested by the electrophysiological results of Ritter *et al.*[71] On the other hand, recent recordings from teased vagal fibers by Schwartz *et al.*[77] suggest that responses of some vagal mechanoresponsive vagal afferents are enhanced by CCK, suggesting that CCK also might influence control of food intake by acting directly on gastric mechanoreceptors or the vagal sensory fibers innervating them. Definition of vagal participation in gastric control of food intake awaits more compelling experimental analyses of the interaction of gastric and non-gastric stimuli in control of ingestion.

Another mechanism by which gastric distension and intestinal chemosensation may interact to control ingestion is via intestinal inhibition of gastric emptying. It is well demonstrated that nutrients entering the intestine slow the rate of gastric emptying, presumably allowing greater distension of the stomach.[53,54] At least some intestinal nutrients inhibit gastric emptying via a vagal reflex.[63] Thus the intestine, via the vagus, could exert control on ingestion, in part, via a gastric servomechanism. It is probable, however, that the intestine also contributes to the control of food intake by mechanisms that do not depend of a gastric interaction.

INTESTINAL CONTROL OF FOOD INTAKE

Sensory Modalities of the Intestine

Intraintestinal infusions of mixed nutrient solutions probably present multiple stimuli to the intestine. In fact, intestinal infusion of a variety of substances elicit neuronal responses from the vagus nerve or responses from brain neurons that depend upon an intact vagus nerve. In early work Paintal[59] demonstrated intestinal receptors that fire during stimulated contractions of the intestinal muscularis mucosa. In addition several investigators have reported vagal fibers that discharge in response to brushing or stroking the intestinal mucosa.[5,8] It is noteworthy that many of the vagal fibers that respond to mechanical stimulation of the intestine also increase their discharge in response to introduction of acid, base, osmotically active solutions and changes in temperature.[6,21,22,23,34,38] The apparent variety of stimuli to which some vagal afferents respond has led to the suggestion that these fibers comprise polymodal sensory receptors.[34] While polymodal sensory receptors may exist, it is also possible that the receptive units themselves are enteric sensory neurons or non-neuronal cells (e.g., enterocytes or interstitial cells of Cajal) and that some vagal fibers receive convergent input from more than one type of receptor. This possibility has not yet been investigated experimentally. Nevertheless, recent anatomical studies by Berthoud and colleagues,[3,4] indicate that enteric ganglia of both the myenteric and submucous plexes are penetrated by large numbers of highly arborized vagal sensory fibers. Furthermore, it appears that some submucous neurons that project to the myenteric plexus exhibit both anatomical and electrophysiological qualities that suggest they are sensory in nature.[40,45] Both these observations make the possibility that enteric neurons serve as primary sensory neurons innervating vagal afferents anatomically plausible.

With regard to chemical stimulation of the intestine, a variety of nutrient-related responses have been observed. Mei[51] has reported afferent fibers that increase their firing rate in response to intraluminal oligosaccharides, especially glucose. Likewise, hindbrain neurons that receive afferent vagal projections also respond to intestinal glucose infusion.[24] Jeanningros[44] has reported intestinal afferents that respond rather selectively to amino acids. Although a few of these units also responded to glucose, they were not responsive to osmotic or mechanical stimuli. Vagal afferents responding to fatty acids have been recorded by Melone.[52] The fatty acid response is greater to long-chain than short-chain fatty acids and is not mimicked by other organic acids or mineral acids.

The gastrointestinal tract may be the largest endocrine organ in the body. In addition, it contains a population of resident enteric neurons, equal in number to the neuronal population of the spinal cord.[9] Since peptides and amines are released from gut endocrine cells by nutrients and may also be released from enteric neurons,[9] it is plausible that they may translate luminal stimulation into signals that activate vagal afferent neurons. Of particular relevance to the discussion to follow is that several investigators, recording from the hindbrain[64,71] or from teased vagal fibers of the rat[11,77] and ferret[5] have reported afferents that respond to CCK. In most of these studies fibers or hindbrain cells that responded to CCK also responded to gastric distension. At least in the rat, however, CCK-induced firing of mechanoreceptive units appears to result from direct sensitivity of vagal afferents to CCK, because while distension stretches the gastric wall activating mechanoresponsive fibers, CCK causes gastric relaxation while still increasing firing in distension responsive units.[64] Thus the mechanoreceptors themselves are unloaded by gastric relaxation, but are firing in response to CCK. Ritter *et al.*[71] have demonstrated that firing by dorsal vagal complex neurons in response to near coeliac artery infusion of CCK is reduced in rats previously treated with capsaicin, a neurotoxin that damages some small unmyelinated primary sensory cells and fibers.[41,42,43,73] Interestingly, capsaicin did not reduce the response of hindbrain units to gastric distension or the peptide bombesin.[71] These data suggest that while CCK and other neuroactive substances may act in part by activating mechanoresponsive fibers, the CCK-responsive population(s) of vagal afferents does not encompass all mechanoreceptive neurons. Indeed, Blackshaw and Grundy[5] recently characterized a population of intestinal vagal afferents responding to mucosal stimulation and CCK but not to mechanical stimulation. In fact these investigators found that changes in firing of gastric and intestinal mechanoresponsive fibers always were attributable to changes in intraluminal pressure caused by CCK administration, whereas responses by mucosal receptors apparently were the result of direct CCK sensitivity.

Intraintestinal Stimuli that Reduce Food Intake

The hypothesis that signals from the small intestine may participate in the control of food intake derives from experiments in which solutions infused into the intestine produce rapid reductions of ongoing or subsequent food intake. Such experiments have been performed in several mammalian species including humans.[27,30,66,67,86,87,90] Particularly compelling are studies that couple intraintestinal infusion with sham feeding, because in this experimental preparation the effect of intestinal infusion on food intake can be dissociated from its effects on gastric emptying. For example, Gibbs *et al.* demonstrated that infusions of liquid diet into the duodenum suppressed sham feeding in monkeys[27] (Figure 1). The latency for suppression of intake was very short (minutes). Suppression of intake was not produced by isotonic saline infusion. These results implied that intestinal stimulation with liquid diet was detected by luminal elements capable of communicating a signal for inhibition of further ingestion to the brain. The nature of the intestinal stimulus and the substrates responsible for its communication were not specified in this experiment. However, subsequent work indicates that intestinal stimulation by multiple components of diet, both chemical and colligative, are capable of suppressing sham food intake.

Houpt *et al.* showed that intestinal infusion of hyperosmotic solutions reduced food intake in pigs.[35] In addition, they found that when ingesta emptied from the stomach after a meal, there was a rise in the osmolality of the intestinal contents that was equal to or greater than the changes produced by their infusions. Thus, they concluded that intestinal osmotic stimulation may be one of the physiological determinants of satiation in pigs. Houpt *et al.*[35] also investigated the neural substrates responsible for suppression of food intake by osmotically active intraintestinal infusions. They found that subdiaphragmatic

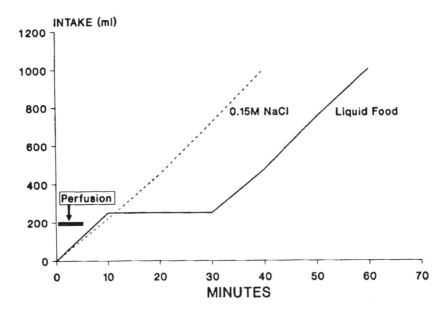

FIGURE 1. Sham feeding following intraintestinal infusion of liquid diet in a rhesus monkey. (Redrawn from Gibbs *et al.*[27])

vagotomy attenuated but did not abolish suppression of feeding by osmotic stimuli. Although they also found that ingestion of hypertonic solutions prior to a meal reduced intake in proportion to solute concentration, the solute they chose was glucose. Hence, it is not certain that the suppressive effects on feeding were entirely due to osmotic properties of the glucose solutions. Some of the feeding inhibitory effects of their solutions may have been due to chemical as well as colligative properties of the ingestate.

In our laboratory we have examined suppression of sham feeding by isotonic, isocaloric solutions of a variety of nutrients and digestive products. From this work it has become clear that nutrients can suppress food intake, independent of osmotic stimulation or alterations in gastric emptying. Furthermore, it is clear that not all nutrients are equally effective in activating intestinal mechanisms that suppress food intake (Figure 2). For example, we have examined suppression of sham feeding by intraintestinal infusions of glucose or the oligoglucosides, maltose and maltotriose.[72] Using infusions of each of these substances at a 180 mM concentration, we found that maltotriose suppressed sham feeding more than maltose which in turn produced greater suppression than glucose. It is important to note that equimolal infusions of these three sugars produce gradations of intestinal caloric stimulation, the caloric concentration of 180 mM maltotriose being three times the caloric concentration of 180 mM glucose. Figure 3A illustrates that suppression of feeding by these three sugars is proportional to the intestinal caloric load.

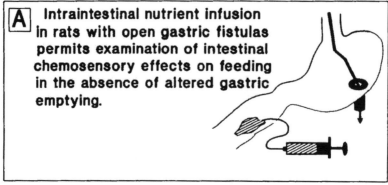

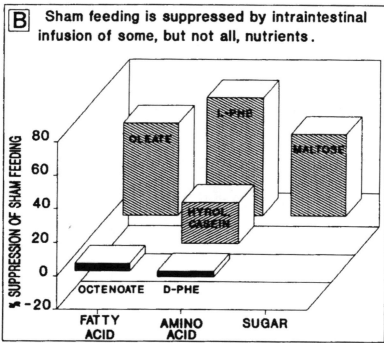

FIGURE 2A. Schematic depiction of preparation used to study the behavioral effects of intraintestinal nutrient infusions in freely moving rats with open gastric fistulas (sham feeding). In our studies, intestinal infusions (1 ml/min) are begun 5 min before presentation of a liquid food (15% sucrose) and terminated after a total infusion time of 10 min. Consumption is measured over 30 min, while all of the solution consumed drains from the open gastric fistula into graduated cylinders. B. Some nutrients markedly suppress sham feeding, while others are much less effective. In general, fatty acids and oligosaccharides of longer chain length are more effective than those of shorter chain length. L-phenylalanine (L-PHE) is more effective than d-phenylalanine (D-PHE), suggesting suppression of intake by this amino acid is stereo specific. Also, a mixture of many different amino acids (hydrolyzed casein) is much less effective for suppression of food intake than L-PHE, indicating that not all amino acids are equivalent with regard to suppression of food intake.

Maltose and maltotriose are hydrolyzed to glucose at the brush border. If there was instantaneous hydrolysis of these oligosaccharides, without absorption of glucose or water, then the maltose and maltotriose infusates could produce intestinal osmotic concentrations of 480 mOsm and 660 mOsm respectively. It is possible, therefore, that suppression of intake by these oligosaccharides is due to increased osmotic stimulation. This is unlikely, however, because suppressions of food intake by glucose, maltose and maltotriose[71] are all markedly attenuated when these sugars are coinfused with phloridzin, a glycoside that blocks sodium linked intestinal glucose transport. By monitoring plasma glucose concentrations, we verified that phloridzin indeed inhibited transport of glucose derived from infused oligosaccharides. Therefore, intestinal osmotic concentrations should have been higher in the presence of phloridzin than in its absence. Yet significant suppression of intake occurred only in the absence of phloridzin, indicating 1) that suppression of intake was probably specific for glucose generated by oligosaccharide hydrolysis and 2) that binding and/or transport of glucose was necessary for suppression of food intake by all three sugars. Thus, most of the suppression of sham feeding by isotonic solutions of oligoglucosides is probably due to glucose sensitivity rather than osmosensitivity.

The fact that phloridzin antagonized suppression of feeding by glucoe and its oligosaccharides raises the possibility that effects on feeding may be mediated by glucoreceptors remote from the intestine. However, others have found that while intraintestinal glucose infusions reduce food intake, intrahepatic vein or intrajugular infusions are much less effective.[84] Furthermore, in a regression analysis, we have plotted the peak glucose concentration during the 30 min post infusion against the calories infused as glucose, maltose or maltotriose. Whereas, suppression of food intake increases linearly with oligosaccharide chain length (caloric concentration; Figure 3A), the blood glucose concentration achieved during the 30 min period actually is negatively correlated with oligosaccharide chain length (Figure 3B). Therefore, it appears that oligosaccharides suppress sham feeding by acting on glucoreceptors in or near the intestine.

Several investigators have reported that amino acids reduce food intake when infused into the small intestine. Gibbs *et al.*[28] reported that intraintestinal L-phenylalanine (L-PHE) but not D-phenylalanine (D-PHE) suppressed food intake by monkeys. Our own work indicates that L-PHE but not D-PHE also suppresses sham feeding in rats (Figure 2B). The fact that L-PHE inhibits sham feeding indicates that suppression of intake by this amino acid is not merely a result of altered gastric emptying. Furthermore, both Gibbs *et al.*[28] and our own results[90] indicated that the receptors that suppress feeding in response to PHE are stereo specific. Infusion of D-PHE does not suppress sham feeding. We also have compared the efficacy of infusions of L-PHE, mixed amino acids (casein hydrolysate) and unhydrolyzed protein (casein) on suppression of sham feeding in rats (Figure 2B). Whereas L-PHE reduced sham feeding by 70%, intraintestinal infusion of mixed amino acids and peptides or unhydrolyzed casein had much less effect on suppression of sham feeding (11-15% suppression).[90] These

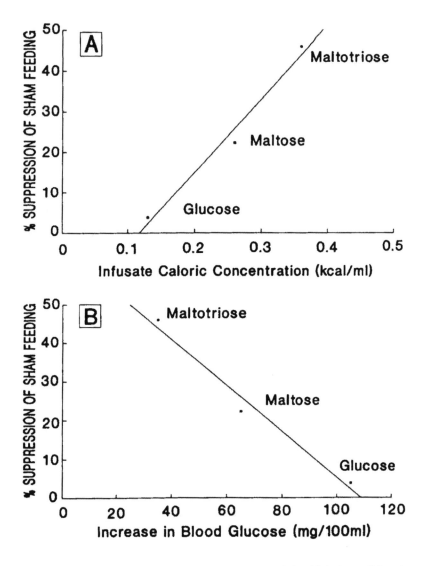

FIGURE 3A. Caloric concentration of 180 mM sugar solutions infused into the small intestine, plotted against suppression of sham feeding produced by these solutions. There was a significant, positive correlation ($r = 0.978$) between caloric concentration of the infusate and suppression of intake. Suppression of sham feeding by all three sugars was attenuated by coinfusion of phloridzin, a blocker of the intestinal Na^+/glucose cotransporter. B. Blood glucose concentration plotted against suppression of sham feeding by 180 mM sugar solutions. There was a significant negative correlation between blood glucose level and suppression of food intake. It appears that suppression of sham feeding by glucose and its oligosaccharides is not correlated with digestion, absorption and blood glucose levels, but is related to the caloric concentration or form sugar in the infusate.

findings suggest that suppression of food intake may only occur with certain amino acids and that an adequate concentration of effective amino acid may not be reached during digestion of a protein such as casein.

Intraintestinal infusion of either triglyceride or fatty acids have been reported to suppress food intake in rats[30,58,90] and people.[86,87] Greenberg *et al.*[31] reported that suppression of food intake by triglyceride occurred prior to absorption of labeled triglyceride. Furthermore, in a recent report[32] these investigators demonstrated that, unlike intraintestinal triglyceride infusion, intra-hepatic-portal infusion failed to reduce sham feeding in rats. Thus intraintestinal triglyceride probably suppresses food intake by acting prehepatically—perhaps on luminal receptors.

Triglyceride is hydrolyzed to fatty acids and 2-monoglycerides prior to uptake into enterocytes. Therefore, we have examined the ability of two fatty acids oleic (C-18) and octanoic (C-8) to suppress sham feeding when infused at low concentrations (0.065-0.13 kcal/ml) in isotonic solutions.[90] At these concentrations, only oleic acid suppressed sham feeding. Octanoic acid had no effect (Figure 2B). These results indicate that while medium-chain fatty acids might suppress food intake at high concentrations, long-chain fatty acids are more potent for suppressing feeding. This conclusion is reinforced when one considers the fact that at equicaloric concentrations, the molar concentration of octanoic acid is more than twice that of oleic acid.

Clearly, representatives of all three macronutrient groups are capable of suppressing food intake when infused into the small intestine under conditions that minimize the possibility that their effects are due to osmotic stimulation. It is also clear, however, that suppression of food intake by intestinal nutrient stimulation is not merely the result of detection of caloric content. For, as previously mentioned, some metabolizable substances produce little or no suppression of food intake, while others dramatically reduce intake. Thus, it is probable that nutrients in the intestine alter ingestion through actions on *nutrient specific* receptors.

Vagal Substrates for Suppression of Food Intake by Intestinal Stimuli

The extrinsic sensory innervation of the GI tract is from two sources: the spinal cord and the vagus nerve. It is possible, of course, that sensory fibers of both vagal and spinal destinies participate in suppression of food intake by intestinal nutrients. We have assessed the role of the vagus in suppression of food intake by examining nutrient-induced suppression of sham feeding in subdiaphragmatically vagotomized rats. We found that suppression of sham feeding by intraintestinal maltose or oleic acid was abolished in vagotomized rats[93] (Figure 4). Suppression of sham feeding by L-PHE was attenuated, but was not abolished. Thus, at least at low caloric concentrations, suppression of sham feeding by oleic acid and maltose, and perhaps other fats and carbohydrates, is mediated entirely by the vagus nerve. The picture for L-PHE appears more complex, with non-vagal participation apparently playing an important role in the effects of this amino acid on food intake.

Assessing the neural substrate responding to intestinal stimulation is somewhat complex because digestive processes modify some chemical stimuli as they are applied to the intestine. Such stimulus modification occasionally may explain disparate results from apparently similar experiments. For example, in pioneering work by Novin et al.,[58] vagotomy only slightly attenuated suppression of real feeding in rats given intraintestinal infusions of peanut oil emulsion. In contrast to our findings using oleate,[93] these investigators suggested that intraintestinal fat suppresses feeding, at least in part, by non vagal mechanisms. We feel, however, that the peanut oil emulsion used by Novin et al. constituted a compound stimulus that was likely to suppress intake by more than one mechanism. For example, Novin et al. performed their experiments in real feeding animals. That is, the food consumed by their rats accumulated in the stomach. On the other hand, our experiments were performed in rats with open gastric fistulas, sham feeding. It is possible that, during real feeding, intestinal infusion of fat may interact with the accumulation of ingesta in the stomach to initiate gastric motility changes[53,54] that may be communicated to the brain via non-vagal routes (see preceding section). Our animals were not subject to changes in gastric emptying or distension produced by intraintestinal infusions, via neural or humoral enterogastric reflexes. Another possible explanation for differences between our findings and those of Novin et al. concerns the amount of fat infused and the concentration of fatty acids that might be generated in the

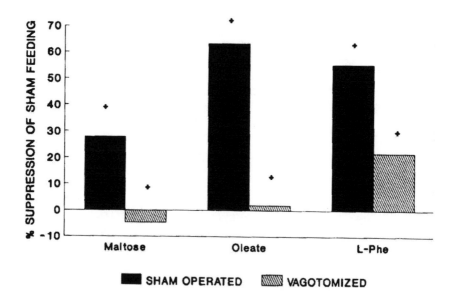

FIGURE 4. Suppression of food intake by 0.13 kcal/ml maltose, oleate or L-Phe in intact rats and rats with total subdiaphragmatic vagotomies. Note that suppression of sham feeding by oleate and maltose is eliminated by vagotomy. Suppression of sham feeding by L-Phe is attenuated but not eliminated.

intestinal lumen via the action of pancreatic lipase. Our infusions never exceeded a total of 1.3 kcal whereas Novin *et al.*[58] infused approximately 4.5 kcal. Furthermore, hydrolysis of this amount of peanut oil triglyceride by pancreatic lipase could result in intestinal concentrations of lipolytic products 3.5 to 9 times higher than those produced by our oleate infusions. Such high intestinal calorie or fatty acid concentrations might influence food intake by activating both vagal and non vagal substrates. For example, it is possible that lipolytic products of peanut oil triglycerides could produce a hypertonic intestinal stimulus. Houpt *et al.*[35] demonstrated that vagotomy attenuates, but does not abolish, the suppression of feeding induced by hypertonic intestinal stimuli in the pig. Thus, the suppression of feeding by the oil suspension in vagotomized rats could be the result of a response to a stimulus not directly related to the chemical properties of the lipolytic products. The oleate solution that we infused was isotonic (300 mOsm/l) and probably would not have increased the osmolality of the intestinal contents because oleate is not subject to hydrolysis prior to absorption.

Surgical vagotomy causes vagal deefferentation as well as deafferentation of the GI tract. The deleterious effects of this procedure for gastrointestinal motility and secretion are well documented. In an effort to assess the role of sensory fibers, as opposed to motor fibers, in suppression of feeding by intestinal nutrients, we have studied the behavioral effects of intestinal nutrient infusion in sham feeding rats previously treated with capsaicin. Capsaicin damages or destroys small unmyelinated sensory neurons in the peripheral nervous system, including those of the vagal and spinal innervations to the GI tract.[41,42,73] Vagal motor neurons do not appear to degenerate following capsaicin.[73] Our experiments revealed that rats treated systemically with capsaicin no longer reduced their sham feeding when given intraintestinal infusions of maltose or oleic acid[90] (Figure 5). Suppression of sham feeding by L-PHE was also diminished but not abolished. These results, taken together with the results of our vagotomy studies, suggest that suppression of food intake by maltose and oleic acid is mediated by capsaicin-sensitive vagal sensory fibers. Suppression of sham feeding by L-PHE, on the other hand, depends in part, but not entirely, on capsaicin-sensitive fibers.

In an effort to target capsaicin's action on vagal afferent projections, we treated animals with microgram doses of the toxin via the fourth cerebral ventricle.[92] Our rationale was that this route of application was close to the nucleus of the solitary tract (NST), where the vagal sensory fibers terminate. Silver stain studies of capsaicin-induced nerve degeneration reveal that both systemic and intracisternal capsaicin administration cause vagal sensory degeneration in the NST and do not produce signs of vagal motor cell damage.[41,74] Vagal sensory degeneration produced by fourth ventricular capsaicin appears slightly less intense than that produced by high dose systemic treatment.[74] However, neither silver stain[74] nor immunohistochemical assessment[82] reveals evidence of degeneration in the spinal cord or forebrain following fourth

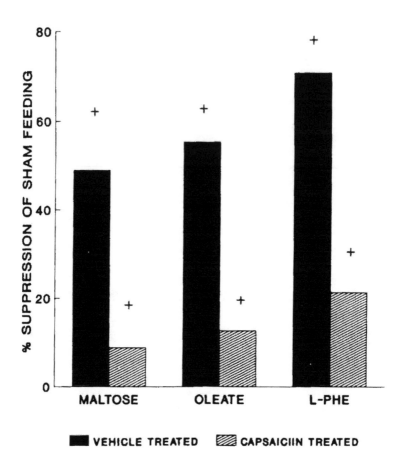

FIGURE 5. Suppression of food intake by 0.13 kcal/ml maltose, oleate or L-PHE in intact rats and rats pretreated with the neurotoxin capsaicin approximately one month prior to the beginning of sham feeding experiments. Capsaicin destroys a subpopulation of small-caliber, unmyelinated, sensory neurons in the vagus and other nerves. Suppression of sham feeding by all three nutrients was attenuated in capsaicin-pretreated rats.

ventricle capsaicin application. Thus any effects of fourth ventricular capsaicin on suppression of feeding by intestinal nutrients are likely due to capsaicin action on vagal sensory terminals in the NST.

We found that fourth ventricular capsaicin treatment abolished maltose-induced suppression of sham feeding and attenuated suppression of sham feeding by oleic acid. Fourth ventricular capsaicin had no effect, however, on suppression of sham feeding by intraintestinal L-PHE. Apparently, capsaicin-sensitive vagal sensory fibers participate in suppression of sham feeding by maltose and oleic acid. However, if there are any vagal sensory fibers that participate in suppression of sham feeding by L-PHE, they are not capsaicin-sensitive.

Suppression of sham feeding by intestinal nutrients may be mediated by capsaicin-sensitive vagal fibers in the intestinal wall or may be relayed to vagal fibers by enteric neurons. Findings supporting this hypothesis were recently reported by Tamura and Ritter.[83] In that study we found that low doses of capsaicin infused into the intestine suppressed sham feeding and caused a transient desensitization of suppression of sham feeding by oleate. Intraintestinal capsaicin did not cause neuropathology associated with systemic capsaicin injection of the toxin, suggesting that the effect of intestinal capsaicin was indeed a local one. Furthermore, the fact that suppression of sham feeding by oleate was only transiently abolished and was fully recovered by 48 hr post capsaicin, suggests that the effect of intestinal capsaicin is not due to neuronal degeneration. Intestinal capsaicin infusions may be useful in determining the mechanism by which luminal signals are transmitted to vagal afferents.

Peptide Participation in Vagally Mediated Satiety Signals

Although many peptides appear to have effects on ingestive behavior, the most extensively studied is CCK. CCK was originally identified as a hormone released by gastrointestinal endocrine cells.[39] However, CCK also is produced by subpopulations of enteric neurons,[65] primary sensory neurons[50,65] and central nervous system neurons.[50]

In 1973 Gibbs *et al.*[29] demonstrated that systemic administration of exogenous CCK suppresses food intake and, under appropriate circumstances,[2] arouses behavior patterns resembling those observed following food-induced termination of feeding (satiety). Subsequently, the same group demonstrated that section of the abdominal vagi, specifically the gastric branches of the vagi, markedly attenuated suppression of food intake by exogenous CCK.[79]

Work in our laboratory indicated that rats treated with capsaicin, either systemically or via the fourth ventricle, no longer reduced their real feeding or sham feeding in response to systemic CCK injection.[69,82] Capsaicin treatment did not impair suppression of food intake by gastric distension.[69] These data, taken together with the results of vagotomy experiments, suggested that CCK suppressed food intake by acting on capsaicin-sensitive vagal sensory fibers.

The notion that sensory vagal fibers are adapted to mediate suppression of food intake by exogenous CCK is supported by two lines of technically independent investigation. First, the abdominal vagi transport CCK receptor protein both toward the periphery and toward the brain.[17,48,56] CCK receptors appear to be associated specifically with the sensory and not the motor component of the vagus[10,47] (see also Moran in chapter 7 of this volume). Second, electrophysiological data indicate that vagal fibers respond to exogenously administered CCK and that these CCK responsive fibers belong to a subpopulation of neurons that is damaged or destroyed by the neurotoxin capsaicin.[71] At least some of the CCK responsive fibers appear to be distinct from gastric mechanoreceptive fibers (but see also Schwartz *et al.*[77]).

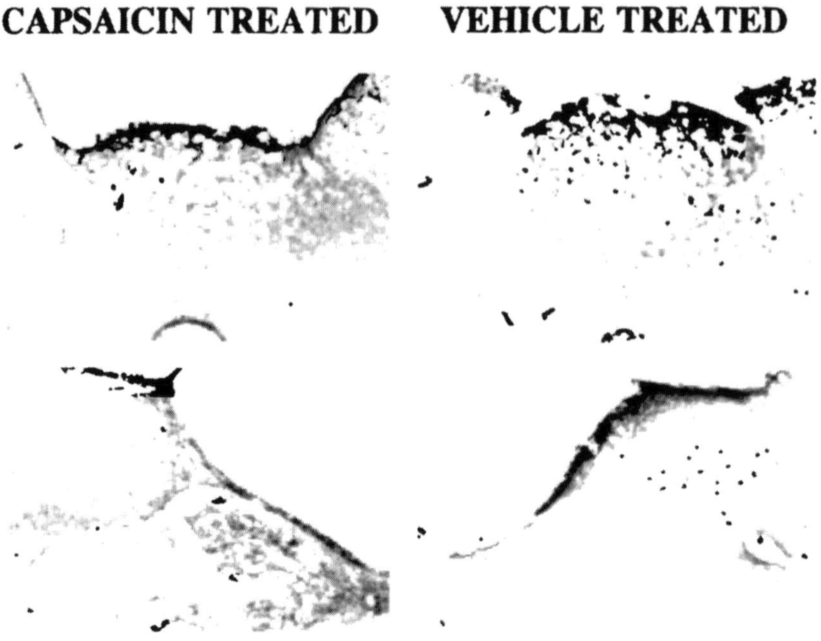

CAPSAICIN TREATED   VEHICLE TREATED

FIGURE 6. Immunohistochemical staining for Fos-like immunoreactive (Fosli) neuronal nuclei in the nucleus of the solitary tract (NTS) and area postrema (AP). *Right Panels*: Following intraintestinal infusion of oleic acid (0.08 kcal/ml) there are numerous immunoreactive nuclei in both the AP and NTS of intact (vehicle treated) rats. *Left Panels*: In rats pretreated with capsaicin, expression of Fosli is markedly reduced or absent. These results, taken together with other experiments using Fos immunohistochemistry, suggest that intestinal nutrients activate capsaicin-sensitive, vagal sensory neurons from the GI tract. The distribution of neurons activated by nutrients is similar to that of neurons activated by exogenous CCK.

Comparing characteristics of the neural substrate mediating suppression of food intake by CCK with those mediating suppression of food intake by some intestinal nutrients reveals marked similarities and suggests that the same fibers might mediate behavioral responses to exogenous CCK and some nutrients. For example, suppression of sham feeding, at least by some nutrients, is abolished by vagotomy as is suppression of food intake by CCK.[78] Likewise, pretreatment with systemic or fourth ventricular capsaicin attenuates suppression of sham feeding by both CCK and intestinal nutrients.

The similarity of neural substrates mediating suppression of food intake by CCK and intestinal nutrients is further supported by recent experiments we have done using Fos protein immunohistochemistry.[70] Fos protein is the product of the protooncogene, c-fos. This gene is believed to be a transcription modulator that is expressed in some neurons following stimulation (for review see Morgan and Curran[57]). The Fos protein, having been translated in the cytoplasm, binds together with another protein, Jun, in the nucleus, where it modulates transcription of mRNAs for other protein products of the cell. The expression of the c-fos thus may represent a part of a long-term adaptive response to stimulation. Since transcription of c-fos mRNA and associated translation of Fos protein begins within minutes of stimulation and is histochemically detectable from 0.5 to several hours following stimulation, the histochemical detection of c-fos appears to be a good marker for activation of neurons that express this gene. Injection of exogenous CCK or intraintestinal infusion of oleate and maltose, the only nutrients we have examined thus far, cause expression of Fos-like immunoreactivity (Fosli) in the NTS. The distribution of Fosli after nutrient infusion is similar to its distribution after exogenous CCK (Figure 6). Moreover, either capsaicin treatment (Figure 6) or vagotomy (data not shown), attenuates expression of Fosli by both CCK or intestinal nutrient infusion. Like our behavioral results, these data suggest that intestinal nutrients and exogenous CCK activate similar or identical vagal sensory pathways.

Could release of endogenous CCK be mediating suppression of sham feeding by intestinal nutrients? To test this hypothesis we examined the ability of CCK receptor antagonists to attenuate suppression of sham feeding by intestinal nutrients.[89,91] We found that two chemically different CCK-A receptor antagonists blocked suppression of food intake by oleic acid or maltose. However, lorglumide, the only CCK-A antagonist tested with L-PHE, did not block suppression of sham feeding by this nutrient (Figure 7). The CCK-B receptor antagonist, L365260, had no effect on suppression of sham feeding by any intestinal nutrient tested. These results suggest that suppression of sham feeding by maltose, oleate and perhaps L-PHE, are mediated by endogenous CCK acting at a CCK-A-like receptor.

This interpretation becomes problematic, however, when one compares the ability of various nutrients to elevate plasma CCK with their ability to suppress sham feeding.[68,89] As can be seen in Figure 8, intestinal maltose, which suppresses sham feeding by a CCK-dependent mechanism, does not elevate plasma CCK concentrations. Likewise, intestinal L-PHE infusion does not cause increased plasma CCK levels. On the other hand, unhydrolyzed casein has only slight effects on sham feeding but markedly elevates plasma CCK concentration. Clearly, the ability of an intestinal infusion to suppress sham feeding does not rely upon its ability to elevate CCK in the plasma. Therefore, the CCK that mediates suppression of sham feeding by intestinal nutrients must not be endocrine. Rather, suppression of sham feeding by oleate or maltose seems likely to depend on CCK of neural or paracrine origin.

As previously mentioned, CCK is found in enteric neurons, vagal sensory neurons and in brain neurons, and any of these neurons might be a source of neuronal CCK-mediating suppression of sham feeding (Figure 9). Della-Fera and colleagues,[12,13] reported that intracranial infusion of CCK decreased feeding in sheep, while infusion of antiserum against CCK increased food intake. Furthermore, Schick et al.[75,76] have reported CCK release from the hypothalamus following eating or gastric distension. Nevertheless, preliminary work

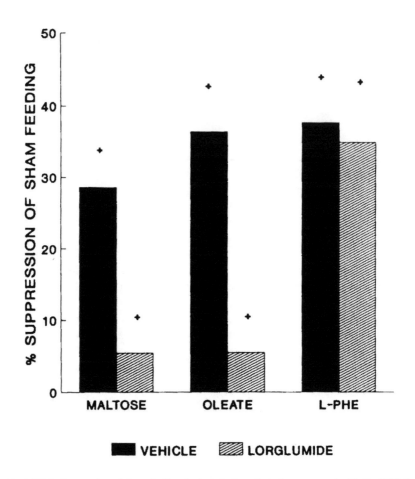

FIGURE 7. Suppression of sham feeding by intestinal nutrients in rats treated with the CCK-A receptor antagonist, lorglumide (CR1409). Similar results have been obtained using MK329. Note that suppression of sham feeding by maltose or oleate is abolished by lorglumide. At the doses we used (300 and 600 μg/kg) lorglumide failed to attenuate suppression of sham feeding by L-PHE.

from our laboratory, using intracranial CCK antagonist administration suggests that brain CCK receptors are not responsible for suppression of sham feeding by intestinal nutrients. For example, when administered into the lateral ventricle, even 300 μg of MK329 fails to abolish suppression of sham feeding by intestinal oleate, whereas 75 μg of MK 329 given intraperitoneally abolishes suppression of sham feeding by the same oleate dose. Taken together with the results outlined in the last two paragraphs, these preliminary findings suggest that peripheral, non-endocrine, CCK mediates suppression of food intake by some intestinal nutrients. Suppression of food intake by both peripherally injected exogenous CCK and by intestinal nutrients is mediated by capsaicin-sensitive vagal neurons. Therefore, it is tempting to speculate that nutrients cause neural or paracrine CCK release in the GI tract and that this locally released CCK, acting via the vagus, suppresses food intake.

Physiological Role of the Vagus in Satiation

Defining the importance of the gastrointestinal vagus in physiological termination of food intake (satiation) will probably depend upon the temporal period

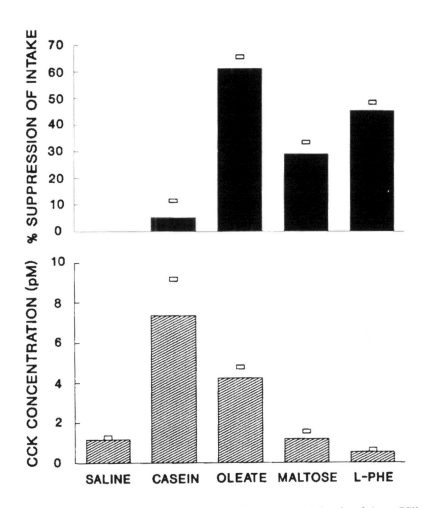

FIGURE 8. Comparison between suppression of sham feeding (top) and elevation of plasma CCK (bottom), following intraintestinal infusion of nutrients. Note that while casein markedly elevates plasma CCK, it does not suppress sham feeding. While maltose and L-PHE suppress sham feeding, they do not elevate plasma CCK. Other results indicate that suppression of sham feeding by maltose is blocked by CCK-A antagonists. However, the lack of correlation between plasma CCK levels and suppression of sham feeding suggests that the CCK involved in nutrient-induced suppression of sham feeding is not endocrine.

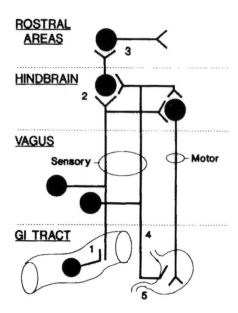

FIGURE 9. Schematic diagram of neural connections between gut and brain. Sites of potential action of neuronal CCK in suppression of feeding are numbered. In a few cases, an action of circulating endocrine CCK is also plausible. (1) Chemical stimulation of intestine might release CCK from enteric neurons and thereby activate vagal sensory terminals. (2) Vagal sensory terminals might release CCK, thereby activating second order neurons in brainstem. (3) CCK may be released by higher order brain neurons in response to GI stimuli, like intestinal nutrients (4) Neuronal or circulating CCK may modulate the activity of gastric mechanoresponsive, vagal afferents (5) By inhibiting gastric emptying, endocrine CCK may enhance gastric mechanoreceptor activation.

over which control of feeding is examined and the sorts of stimuli arising from ingestion. However, if the vagus carries signals that participate in termination of food intake, then one might reasonably expect vagotomy to result in increased food intake or, specifically, increased meal size. In fact, subdiaphragmatic vagotomy has been reported to produce just the opposite effects. For example, Snowdon and Epstein,[80] found that vagotomized rats ate smaller meals than sham vagotomized controls. Unfortunately, surgical vagotomy causes severe impairment of gastric capacitance, emptying and motility as well as changes in gastrointestinal secretory function. These changes are likely to mask any increases in intake brought about by loss of GI sensations.

Intuitively, it seems probable that gastrointestinal controls of ingestion are open loop controls. That is to say they are controls that do not depend on negative feedback from a regulated entity such as body energy stores. Thus the GI stimuli are most likely functions to control meal size in the interest of efficient digestion and absorption and in the interest of avoiding large positive oscillations in the number of calories being presented for storage in body fat depots. Several lines of evidence suggest that vagal sensory signals may serve in such a fashion. First, it is well demonstrated that rats with lesions of the area postrema (AP) and adjacent portions of the NTS over-consume palatable or novel foods during short feeding tests.[20] These lesions typically destroy portions of the primary vagal sensory projections from the GI tract.[19] Therefore, it is conceivable that overeating in these lesioned rats is due in part to loss of vagally communicated gastrointestinal signals. Second, injection of capsaicin into the AP and caudal subnuclei of the NTS also causes animals to overeat when intake is driven by palatability.[81] Since capsaicin destroys small unmyelinated vagal sensory neurons, overeating by capsaicin-treated rats is consistent with loss of vagal satiety cues.

Both the effects of surgical lesions of the AP/NTS and capsaicin treatment were evident only when intake was high, (i.e., driven by palatability). To our knowledge, experiments examining intake in similar preparations during other high-intake conditions have not been reported. However, it should be remembered that the rat is an opportunistic omnivore whose diet may be expected to vary much more than that of our laboratory specimens. Hence, intake during ingestion of familiar yet infrequently available foods may cause many feeding opportunities similar to those caricatured by short laboratory experiments with palatable foods. In this regard it may be interesting to consider the possibility that vagal sensory cues are involved in conditioned satiety. Preliminary observations in our laboratory indicate that when intact and vagotomized rats, familiarized with 15% sucrose solution by repeated presentations of small volumes, are allowed to consume as much 15% sucrose as they want during a 30 min test, both groups consume large volumes (15-18 mls). However, when the sucrose solution is offered again, intact rats reduce their intake by about 50%, while vagotomized rats do not. These observations suggest that vagal cues may be important in terminating ingestion during high intake situations and in providing conditioning stimuli that influence subsequent ingestion when the food is encountered again.

Clearly, gastrointestinal vagal innervation detects and responds to mechanical and chemical properties of ingesta during each meal. It would be surprising, however, if changes in food intake were mediated exclusively by signals from this innervation. In fact we can say with certainty that they are not. Nevertheless, sensory neurons of the vagus nerve respond to a variety of stimuli appropriate as putative satiety signals and it is probable that vagal sensory mechanisms make an important contribution to the process of satiation by relaying information to the brain on chemical and mechanical qualities of ingesta. We expect that continued study will reveal 1) the nature of signal transduction for intestinal stimuli, 2) the site and source of peptide participation in vagal control of ingestion and 3) the central neural pathways that integrate vagal signals with other information, allowing adaptive, physiological control of ingestion.

REFERENCES

1. **Adrian, E.D.,** Afferent impulses in the vagus and their influence on respiration, *J. Physiol.,* 79, 332-358, 1933.
2. **Antin, J., Gibbs, J., Holt, J., Young, R.C., and Smith, G.P.,** Cholecystokinin elicits the complete behavioral satiety sequence in rats, *J. Comp. Physiol. Psychol.,* 89, 784-790, 1975.
3. **Berthoud, H.-R., Jedrzejewska, A., and Powley, T.L.,** Simultaneous identification of afferent inputs and efferent gastrointestinal projections of the dorsal vagal complex in the rat, *J. Comp. Neurol.,* 301(1), 65-79, 1990.
4. **Berthoud, H.-R., and Powley, T.L.,** Morphology and distribution of vagal afferent innervation of rat gastrointestinal tract, *Soc. Neurosci. Abstr.,* 17(2), 1365, 1991.
5. **Blackshaw, L.A., and Grundy, D.,** Effects of cholecystokinin (CCK-8) on two classes of gastroduodenal vagal afferent fibre, *J. Autonom. Nerv. Syst.,* 31, 191-201, 1990.
6. **Cervero, F., and Sharkey, K.A,** An electrophysiological and anatomical study of intestinal afferent fibres in the rat, *J. Physiol. (Lond.),* 401, 381-397, 1988.
7. **Clarke, G.D., and Davison, J.S.,** Tension receptors in the oesophagus and stomach of the rat, *J. Physiol.,* 244, 41P-42P, 1975.
8. **Clarke, G.D., and Davison, J.S.,** Mucosal receptors in the gastric antrum and intestine of the rat with afferent fibers in the cervical vagus, *J. Physiol.,* 284, 55-67, 1978.
9. **Costa, M., Furness, J.B., and Lewellyn-Smith, I.J.,** Histochemistry of the enteric nervous system, in *Physiology of the Gastrointestinal Tract,* Johnson, L.R., Ed., Raven Press, New York, 1987, 1-40.
10. **Crosby, R.J., Norgren, R., Moran, T.H., and McHugh, P.R.,** Central and peripheral transport of CCK-A receptors on vagal afferent fibers, *FASEB J.,* 3, A998, 1989.
11. **Davison, J.S.,** Response of single vagal afferent fibres to mechanical and chemical stimulation of gastric and duodenal mucosa in cats, *Q. J. Exp. Physiol.,* 57, 405-416, 1972.
12. **Della-Fera, M.A., and Baile, C.A.,** Cholecystokinin octapeptide: continuous picomole injections into the cerebral ventricles of sheep suppress feeding, *Science,* 206, 471-473, 1979.
13. **Della-Fera, M.A., Baile, C.A., Shneider, B.S., and Grinker, J.A.,** Cholecystokinin antibody injected in cerebral ventricles of sheep suppress feeding, *Science,* 212, 687-689, 1981.
14. **Deutch. J.A.,** The stomach in food satiation and the regulation of appetite, *Prog. Neurobiol.,* 10, 133-153, 1978.
15. **Deutch, J.A.,** The role of the stomach in eating, *Amer. J. Clin. Nutr.,* 42, 1040-1043, 1985.
16. **Deutch, J.A., Young, W.G. and Kalogeris, T.J.,** The stomach signals satiety, *Science,* 201, 165-167, 1978.
17. **Dockray, G.J., Forster, E.R., and Louis, S.M.,** Peptides and their receptors on afferent neurons to the upper gastrointestinal tract, in *Sensory Nerves and Neuropeptides in Gastroenterology,* Costa, M., Surrenti, C., Gorini, S., Maggi, C.A., and Meli, A., Eds., Plenum Press, New York, 1991, 53-62.
18. **DuBois, F.S., and Foley, J.O.,** Experimental studies on the vagus and spinal accessory nerves in the cat, *Anat. Rec.,* 64, 285-307, 1936.
19. **Edwards, G.L., Ladenheim, E.E., and Ritter, R.C.,** Dorsomedial hindbrain participation in cholecystokinin-induced satiety, *Am. J. Physiol.,* 251, R971-R977, 1986.
20. **Edwards, G.L., and Ritter, R.C.,** Ablation of the area postrema causes exaggerated consumption of preferred foods in the rat, *Brain Res.,* 216, 265-276, 1981.
21. **El Ouazzani, T., and Mei, N.,** Mise en evidence electrophysiologie des thermorecepteurs vagaux dans la region gastrointestinale. Leur role dans la regulation de la moticite digestive, *Exp. Brain Res.,* 39, 419-434, 1979.
22. **El Ouazzani, T., and Mei, N.,** Acido et glucoreptors vagaux de la region gastroduodenale, *Exp. Brain Res.,* 42, 442-452, 1981.
23. **El Ouazzani, T., and Mei, N.,** Electrophysiologic properties and role of vagal thermoreceptor of lower esophagus and stomach of cat, *Gastroenterology,* 83, 995-1001, 1982.

24. **Ewart, W.R. and Wingate, D.L.,** Central representation of arrival of nutrient in the duodenum, *Am. J. Physiol.,* 246, G750–G756, 1984.
25. **Galen, C.,** *De usu partium corporis humani: Liber IX,* Lugduni, Nicolao Regio Calbre, 1550, 129-199.
26. **Gaskell, W.H.,** *The Involuntary Nervous System,* Longmans, Green and Company, London, 1916.
27. **Gibbs, J., Maddison, S.P., and Rolls, E.T.,** Satiety role of the small intestine examined in sham feeding rhesus monkeys, *J. Comp. Physiol. Psychol.,* 95, 1003-1015, 1981.
28. **Gibbs, J., and Smith, G.P.,** The neuroendocrinology of postprandial satiety, in *Frontiers in Neuroendocrinology, vol. 8,* Martini, L., and Ganong, W.F., Eds., Raven Press, New York, 1984, 223-245.
29. **Gibbs, J., Young, R.C., and Smith, G.P.,** Cholecystokinin decreases food intake in rats, *J. Comp. Physiol. Psych.,* 84, 488-495, 1973.
30. **Greenberg, D., Gibbs, J., and Smith, G.P.,** Intraduodenal infusions of fat inhibit sham feeding in Zucker rats, *Brain Res. Bull.,* 17, 599-604, 1986.
31. **Greenberg, D., Kava, R., Wojnar, Z., and Greenwood, M.R.C.,** Satiation following intraduodenal infusion of intralipid occurs prior to appearance of [14C]-Intralipid in plasma, *Soc. Neurosci. Abstr.,* 15, 1280, 1989.
32. **Greenberg, D., Smith, G.P., and Gibbs, J.,** Intravenous triglycerides fail to elicit satiety in sham feeding rats, *Am. J. Physiol.,* 1992.
33. **Grossman, S.P.,** *A Textbook of Physiological Psychology,* John Wiley and Sons, Inc., New York. 1967.
34. **Grundy, D., and Scratchard, T.,** Sensory afferents from the gastrointestinal tract, in *Handbook of Physiology,* vol. 1, section 6, part 1, Wood, J.D., Ed., American Physiological Society, Bethesda, MD., 1989.
35. **Houpt, T.R., Houpt, K.A., and Swan, A.A.,** Duodenal osmoconcentration and food intake in pigs after ingestion of hypertonic nutrients, *Am. J. Physiol.,* 245, R181-R189, 1983.
36. **Iggo, A.,** Gastrointestinal tension receptors in the stomach and the urinary bladder, *J. Physiol.,* 128, 593-607, 1955.
37. **Iggo, A.,** Gastro-intestinal tension receptors with unmyelinated afferent fibres in the vagus of the cat, *Quart. J. Exp. Physiol.,* 42, 130-141, 1957.
38. **Iggo, A.,** Gastric mucosal chemoreceptors with vagal afferent fibres in the vagus, *Quart. J. Exp. Physiol.,* 42, 389-409, 1957.
39. **Ivy, A.C., and Oldenberg, E.,** A hormone mechanism for gallbladder contraction and evacuation, *Am. J. Physiol.,* 86, 599-613, 1928.
40. **Iyer, V., Bornstein, J.C., Costa, M., Furness, J.B., Takahashi, Y., and Iwanga, T.,** Electrophysiology of guinea-pig myenteric neurons correlated with immunoreactivity for a calcium-binding protein, *J. Autonom. Nerv. Sys.,* 22, 141-150, 1988.
41. **Jancso, G.,** Intracisternal capsaicin: selective degeneration of chemosensitive primary sensory afferents in the adult rat, *Neurosci. Lett.,* 27, 41-45, 1981.
42. **Jancso, G., and Kiraly, E.,** Distribution of chemosensitive primary sensory afferents in the central nervous system of the rat, *J. Comp. Neurol.,* 190, 781-792, 1980.
43. **Jancso, G., Kiraly, E., and Jancso-Gabor, A.,** Pharmacologically-induced selective degeneration of chemosensitive primary sensory neurons, *Nature* (Lond.), 270, 741-743, 1977.
44. **Jeanningros, R.,** Vagal unitary responses to intestinal amino acid infusions in the anesthetized cat: a putative signal for protein induced satiety, *Physiol. Behav.,* 28, 9-21, 1982.
45. **Kirchgessner, A.L., and Gershon, M.D.,** Projections of submucosal neurons to the myenteric plexus of the guinea pig intestine: In vitro tracing of mircocircuits by retrograde and anterograde transport, *J. Comp. Neurol.,* 277, 487-498, 1988.
46. **Kraly, F.S., and Gibbs, J.,** Vagotomy fails to block the satiating effect of food in the stomach, *Physiol. Behav.,* 24, 1007-1010, 1980.

47. **Ladenheim, E.E., Speth, R.C., and Ritter, R.C.**, Reduction of CCK-8 binding in the nucleus of the solitary tract in capsaicin treated rats, *Soc. Neurosci. Abstr.*, 12(2), 828, 1986.

48. **Ladenheim, E.E., Speth, R.C., and Ritter, R.C.**, Reduction of CCK-8 binding in the nucleus of the solitary tract in unilaterally nodosectomized rats, *Brain Res.*, 474, 125-129, 1988.

49. **Langley, J.N.,** The autonomic nervous system, *Brain*, 26, 1-26, 1903.

50. **Larson, L.I., and Rehfield, J.F.,** Localisation and molecular heterogeneity of cholecystokinin in the central and peripheral nervous systems, *Brain Res.*, 165, 201-218, 1979.

51. **Mei, N.,** Vagal glucoreceptors in the small intestine of the cat, *J. Physiol.*, 282, 485-506, 1978.

52. **Melone, J.,** Vagal receptors sensitive to lipids in the small intestine of the cat, *J. Auton. Nerv. Sys.*, 17, 231-241, 1986.

53. **Meyer, J.H.,** Motility of the stomach and gastroduodenal junction, in *Physiology of the Gastrointestinal Tract*, Johnson, L.R., Ed., Raven Press, New York, 1987, 613-629.

54. **Miller, L.J., Malagelada, J-R., Taylor, W.F., and Go, V.L.W.,** Intestinal control of human postprandial gastric function: the role of components of jejunoileal chyme in regulating gastric secretion and emptying, *Gastroenterology*, 80, 763-769, 1981.

55. **Moran, T.H., and McHugh, P.R.,** Cholecystokinin suppresses food intake by inhibiting gastric emptying, *Am. J. Physiol.*, 242, R491-R497, 1982.

56. **Moran, T.H., Smith, G.P., Hostetler, A.M., and McHugh, P.R.,** Transport of cholecystokinin (CCK) binding sites in subdiaphragmatic vagal branches, *Brain Res.*, 415, 149-152, 1987.

57. **Morgan, J.I., and Curran, T.,** Stimulus-transcription coupling in neurons: role of cellular immediate-early genes, *Trend in Neuroscience*, 12(11), 459-462, 1989.

58. **Novin, D., Sanderson, J., and Gonzalez, M.,** Feeding after nutrient infusions: Effects of hypothalamic lesions and vagotomy, *Physiol. Behav.*, 22, 107-113, 1979.

59. **Paintal, A.S.,** A study of gastric stretch receptors. Their role in the peripheral mechanism of satiation of hunger and thirst, *J. Physiol.*, 126, 255-270, 1954.

60. **Pappas, T.N., Melendez, R.L., and Debas, H.T.,** Gastric distension is a physiological satiety signal in the Dog, *Dig. Dis. Sci.*, 34, 1489-1493, 1989.

61. **Pick, J.,** *The Autonomic Nervous System, Morphological Comparative and Surgical Aspects*, J.B. Lippincott, Philadelphia, 1970.

62. **Powley, T.L., and Berthoud, H.-R.,** Participation of the vagus and other autonomic nerves in the control of food intake, in *Feeding Behavior: Neural and Humoral Controls*, Ritter, R.C., Ritter, S., and Barnes, C.D., Eds., Academic Press, Orlando, 1986, 67-101.

63. **Raybould, H.E.,** Cholecystokinin and capsaicin-sensitive afferent fibers mediate changes in gastric motility following intraduodenal infusion of protein in the rat, *Gastroenterology*, 96, A410, 1989.

64. **Raybould, H.E., Gayton, R.J., and Dockray, G.J.,** CNS effects of circulating CCK-8: involvement of brainstem neurones responding to gastric distension, *Brain Res.*, 342, 187-190, 1985.

65. **Rehfield, J.F.,** Immunohistochemical studies of cholecystokinin. II. Distribution and molecular heterogeneity in the central nervous system and the small intestine of man and hog, *J. Biol. Chem.*, 253, 4022-4030, 1978.

66. **Reidelberger, R.D., Kalogeris, T.J., Leung, P.M., and Mendel, V.E.,** Postgastric satiety in the sham feeding rat, *Am. J. Physiol.*, 244, R872-R881, 1983.

67. **Rezek, M., and Novin, D.,** Duodenal nutrient infusion: effects on feeding in intact and vagotomized rabbits, *J. Nutr.*, 106, 812-820, 1976.

68. **Ritter, R.C., and Brenner, L.,** Cholecystokinin (CCK) is released by intraintestinal infusion of sodium oleate in the rat, *Gastroenterol.* (GASTAB), 96 (abstract), A417, 1989.

69. **Ritter, R.C., and Ladenheim, E.E.,** Capsaicin pretreatment attenuates suppression of food intake by cholecystokinin octapeptide, *Am. J. Physiol.*, 248, R501-R504, 1985.

70. **Ritter, R.C., and Maundu, J.T.,** c-fos-like immunoreactivity in the caudal hindbrain following feeding suppressive intraintestinal nutrient infusions or exogenous CCK-8 injection, *Soc. Neurosci. Abstr.*, No.81.7, 192, 1991.

71. **Ritter, R.C., Ritter, S., Ewart, W.R., and Wingate, D.L.,** Capsaicin attenuates hindbrain neuron responses to circulating cholecystokinin, *Amer. J. Physiol.,* 257, R1162-R1168, 1989.
72. **Ritter, R.C., and Simon, E.,** Suppression of feeding by intraintestinal maltose is mediated by phloridzin-sensitive mechanism, *Soc. Neurosci. Abstr.,* 16, 646, 1989.
73. **Ritter, S., and Dinh, T.,** Capsaicin-induced neuronal degeneration: Silver impregnation of cell bodies, axons and terminals in the central nervous system of the adult rat, *J. Comp. Neurol.,* 271, 79-90, 1988.
74. **Ritter, S., and Dinh, T.,** Capsaicin: A selective probe for studying specific neuronal populations in brain and retina, in *Methods in Neurosciences, Vol. 8: Neurotoxins.,* Conn, M., Ed., Academic Press, Orlando, Fl., 1992.
75. **Schick, R.R., Reilly, W.M., Roddy, D.R., Yaksh, T.L., and Go, V.L.W.,** Neuronal cholecystokinin-like immunoreactivity is postprandially released from primate hypothalamus, *Brain Res.,* 418, 20-26, 1987.
76. **Schick, R.R., Yaksh, T.L., and Go, V.L.W.,** An intragastric meal releases the putative satiety factor cholecystokinin from hypothalamic neurons in cats, *Brain Res.,* 370, 349-353, 1987.
77. **Schwartz, G.J., McHugh, P.R., and Moran, T.H.,** Vagal afferent responses to gastric loads and cholecystokinin in the rat, *Am. J. Physiol.,* 1992.
78. **Smith, G.P., Jerome, C., Cushin, B., Eterno, R., and Simansky, K.,** Abdominal vagotomy blocks the satiety effect of cholecystokinin in the rat, *Science,* 213, 1036-1037, 1981.
79. **Smith, G.P., Jerome, C., and Norgren, R.,** Afferent axons in abdominal vagus mediate satiety effect of cholecystokinin in rats, *Am. J. Physiol.,* 249, R638-R641, 1985.
80. **Snowdon, C.D., and Epstein, A.N.,** Gastrointestinal sensory and motor control of food intake, *J. Comp. Physiol. Psychol.,* 71, 68-76, 1970.
81. **South, E.H., and Ritter, R.C.,** Overconsumption of preferred foods following capsaicin pretreatment of the area postrema and adjacent nucleus of the solitary tract, *Brain Res.,* 288, 243-250, 1983.
82. **South, E.H., and Ritter, R.C.,** Capsaicin application to central or peripheral vagal fibers attenuates CCK satiety, *Peptides,* 9, 601-612, 1988.
83. **Tamura, C., and Ritter, R.C.,** Transient, selective attenuation of oleate and CCK-induced suppression of sham feeding by intra-intestinal capsaicin infusion, *Soc. Neurosci. Abstr.,* 17, 542, 1991.
84. **Vanderweele, D.A., Novin, D., Rezek, M., and Sanderson, J.D.,** Duodenal or hepatic-portal glucose perfusion: Evidence for duodenally-based satiety, *Physiol. Behav.,* 12, 467-473, 1974.
85. **Vesalius, A.,** *De Humani Corporis,* Fabricia, Basel, 1543.
86. **Welch, I., Saunders, K., and Read, N.W.,** Effects of ileal and intravenous infusions of fat emulsions on feeding and satiety in human volunteers, *Gastroenterol.,* 89, 1293-1297, 1985.
87. **Welch, I.McL., Sepple, C.P., and Read, N.W.,** Comparisons of the effects on satiety and eating behavior of infusion of lipid into the different regions of the small intestine, *Gut,* 29, 306-311, 1988.
88. **Young, R.C., Gibbs, J., Antin, J., Holt, J., and Smith, G.P.,** Absence of satiety during sham feeding in the rat, *J. Comp. Physiol. Psychol.,* 87, 795-800, 1974.
89. **Yox, D.P., Brenner, L., and Ritter, R.C.,** CCK receptor antagonists attenuate suppression of sham feeding by intestinal nutrients, *Amer. J. Physiol.,* 1992.
90. **Yox, D.P., and Ritter, R.C.,** Capsaicin attenuates suppression of sham feeding induced by intestinal nutrients, *Amer. J. Physiol.,* 255, R569-R574, 1988.
91. **Yox, D.P., and Ritter, R.C.,** Suppression of sham feeding induced by oleate: Blockade by a CCK antagonist and reversal of blockade by exogenous CCK, in *The Neuropeptide Cholecystokinin (CCK),* Hughes, J., Dockray, G., and Woodruff, G., Eds., John Wiley and Sons, Chichester and New York, 1989, 218-222.

92. **Yox, D.P., Stokesberry, H., and Ritter, R.C.,** Fourth ventricular capsaicin attenuates suppression of sham feeding induced by intestinal nutrients, *Amer. J. Physiol.*, 260, R263-266, 1991.

93. **Yox, D.P., Stokesberry, H., and Ritter, R.C.,** Vagotomy attenuates suppression of sham feeding induced by intestinal nutrients, *Amer. J. Physiol.*, 260, R503-R508, 1991.

Chapter 11

COOPERATION OF VAGAL AND CENTRAL NEURAL SYSTEMS IN MONITORING METABOLIC EVENTS CONTROLLING FEEDING BEHAVIOR

S. Ritter, N.Y. Calingasan, B. Hutton and T.T. Dinh

TABLE OF CONTENTS

Continued on next page

LIST OF ABBREVIATIONS

AP = area postrema
CNA = central nucleus of the amygdala
DMV = dorsal motor nucleus of the vagus
LPBN = lateral parabrachial nucleus
NTS = nucleus of the solitary tract
PNV = paraventricular nucleus of the hypothalamus
SON = supraoptic nucleus
vLH = ventral lateral hypothalamus

INTRODUCTION

The pivotal role of the subdiaphragmatic vagus nerve in the orchestration of a number of specific ingestive behaviors is now well-established. Ingestive responses mediated at least in part by the vagus nerve include the suppression of feeding by cholecystokinin[68] and PBN pancreatic glucagon,[16,79] by some intraduodenal nutrients[81,82] (see also chapter 10 by R.C. Ritter *et al.*, this volume) and by certain blood-borne metabolic fuels.[28] This chapter will focus narrowly on the cooperative participation of vagal sensory neurons and central nervous system receptors in two specific metabolic controls, the glucoprivic and lipoprivic controls, which stimulate feeding in response to decreased intracellular utilization of glucose or fatty acids, respectively. The role of the vagus nerve in gastric and intestinal controls of feeding will be reviewed by R.C. Ritter *et al.* in chapter 10 of this volume. An excellent comprehensive review of vagal involvement in various aspects of food intake has been provided by Powley and Berthoud.[46]

STIMULATION OF FEEDING BY PHARMACOLOGICALLY-INDUCED BLOCKADE OF GLUCOSE AND FATTY ACID UTILIZATION

Physiological events responsible for triggering food intake have remained elusive throughout the history of ingestive research. However, two distinct metabolic events capable of initiating food intake have been identified with the use of selective antimetabolic drugs. These are decreased glucose utilization (glucoprivation) and decreased fatty acid oxidation (lipoprivation). Glucoprivation can be induced experimentally by injection of antimetabolic glucose analogs, including 2-deoxy-d-glucose (2DG), 5-thioglucose (5TG), 1,5-anhydroglucitol (1DG) and 3-O-methylglucose, or by hypoglycemic doses of insulin[7,35,52,63,67] The glucoprivic control of feeding was first described by Smith and Epstein[67] and has been demonstrated in a number of mammalian species, including humans[22,23,24,35,67,69,72] (for reviews see Epstein *et al.*[12] and Ritter[54]). Lipoprivation can be induced experimentally by administration of beta-mercaptoacetate (MA)[1] or methylpalmoxirate.[27,77] Lipoprivic control of feeding was first demonstrated by Scharrer and Langhans[64] and in the same year by Friedman *et al.*[15]

In the work from my own laboratory to be discussed in this chapter, glucoprivation was induced by systemic administration of 2DG, which blocks phosphohexosisomerase,[8,80] and lipoprivation was induced by systemic administration of MA, which impairs beta oxidation of fatty acids by blocking acyl-CoA dehydrogenases within mitochondria.[1] As shown in the top panels of Figures 1 and 2, both 2DG and MA are potent stimulators of food intake. When administered systemically, both drugs stimulate feeding over a similar time course. Most rats begin to eat within 15 minutes after drug injection. The magnitude and duration of the feeding response is dependent on drug dose.[60]

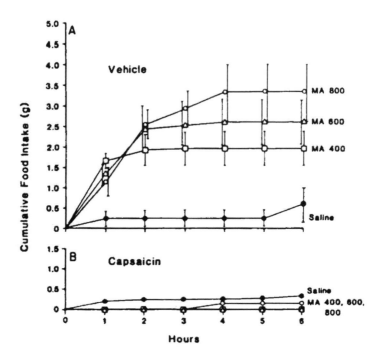

FIGURE 1. Cumulative food intake in a 6-hr test after mercaptoacetate (MA; 400, 600 or 800 μmol/kg) or saline injections in rats previously treated systemically with capsaicin (B) or its injection vehicle (A). Tests were conducted in undeprived rats during light phase of circadian light cycle, using animals' maintenance diet (a fat-supplemented, high carbohydrate ration). Means ± are shown. (Used with permission by *Am. J Physiol.*, from Ritter, S. and Taylor, J.S.[60])

Systemic administration of antimetabolic drugs potentially impairs energy metabolism in all cells dependent on glucose or fatty acids as energy substrates. However, the effects of these drugs on food intake are clearly mediated by particular cells uniquely equipped by their neural connections for arousal of feeding behavior. These cells will be referred to as metabolic receptors for glucoprivic and lipoprivic feeding. In searching for metabolic receptor cells controlling food intake, it is encouraging that neurons which change their firing rate in response to metabolic stimuli have been identified in sites important for feeding behavior, such as the vagus nerve, the nucleus of the solitary tract (NTS) and the hypothalamus.[37,43,45] However, extensive anatomical and behavioral analysis will be required before metabolically responsive neurons in any of these sites can be considered to be mediators of the specific controls of food intake we are investigating.

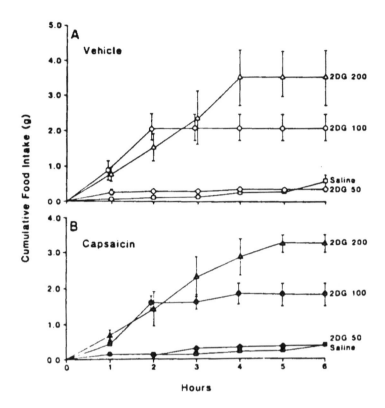

FIGURE 2. Cumulative food intake in a 6-hr test after 2-deoxy-D-glucose (2DG; 50, 100, and 200 mg/kg sc) or saline injections in rats previously treated systemically with capsaicin (B) or its injection vehicle (A). Tests were conducted in undeprived rats during light phase of circadian photoperiod, using animals' maintenance diet (a fat-supplemented, high-carbohydrate ration). Means ± SE are shown. (Used with permission by *Am. J Physiol.*, from Ritter, S. and Taylor, J.S.[60])

LIPOPRIVIC FEEDING: EVIDENCE FOR INVOLVEMENT OF VAGAL SENSORY NEURONS

Soon after their initial description of lipoprivic feeding, Langhans and Scharrer[29] found that feeding in response to MA was impaired by hepatic branch vagotomy. Their evidence prompted us to conduct a series of experiments using systemic capsaicin treatment and central and peripheral surgical vagotomies[60,61] to further assess the importance of the vagus nerve, of vagal sensory neurons in particular, and of specific vagal branches, in glucoprivic and lipoprivic feeding.

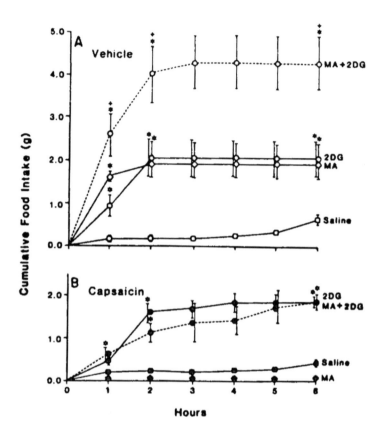

FIGURE 3. Cumulative food intake in 6-hr tests after mercaptoacetate (MA; 400 μmol/kg, ip), 2-deoxy-D-glucose (2DG; 100 mg/kg, sc), MA plus 2DG (400 μmol/kg and 100 mg/kg, respectively), or saline in rats previously treated systemically with capsaicin (B) or its injection vehicle (A). Tests were conducted in undeprived rats during light phase of circadian photoperiod, using animals' maintenance diet (a fat-supplemented, high carbohydrate ration). Means ± SE are shown. +Differs from intake after saline, 2DG, and MA (P < 0.01). *Differs from intake after saline for vehicle-treated rats and from both saline and MA for capsaicin-treated rats (P < 0.01). (Used with permission by *Am. J Physiol.*, from Ritter, S., and Taylor, J.S.[60])

Systemic Capsaicin Treatment Impairs Lipoprivic but not Glucoprivic Feeding

Capsaicin is a neurotoxin known to damage a subpopulation of primary sensory neurons possessing small diameter unmyelinated processes, including many vagal sensory neurons.[56,57] In addition, capsaicin treatment causes impairment or loss of certain behavioral and physiological responses mediated by vagal sensory neurons[51,81] (for reviews see Maggi and Meli[33] and Holzer[21]). Motor neurons do not appear to be damaged by capsaicin.[36] Because of these properties, capsaicin seemed the ideal tool with which to investigate the importance of visceral sensory neurons in the mediation of glucoprivic and lipoprivic feeding. Therefore, anesthetized rats were treated systemically with capsaicin and their food intake in response to MA and 2DG was subsequently examined.[60]

Figure 1 shows that MA stimulated feeding in vehicle-treated controls in a dose-related manner (panel A). Capsaicin-treated rats, however, did not increase their food intake to MA at any dose tested (panel B). In contrast, Figure 2 shows that capsaicin did not impair feeding induced by 2DG. The fact that capsaicin abolished MA feeding without impairing 2DG feeding indicates that feeding induced by glucoprivation and lipoprivation are mediated by separate neural substrates. Furthermore, in vehicle-treated rats, feeding responses to combined administration of low suprathreshold doses of 2DG (100 mg/kg) and MA (400 μmol/kg) were additive in their effects on feeding (Figure 3A). However, capsaicin-treated rats ate the same amount after 2DG plus MA as they did in response to 2DG alone (Figure 3B). This is exactly the result to be expected if capsaicin disables receptors involved exclusively in lipoprivic control. This result therefore reinforces the hypothesis that separate and independent receptor populations exist for monitoring the utilization of glucose and fatty acids.

Total Subdiaphragmatic Vagotomy Abolishes Lipoprivic but not Glucoprivic Feeding

Capsaicin damages small diameter unmyelinated primary sensory neurons of both vagal and nonvagal origin[21,26] as well as neurons within the brain and retina.[56,57,58] For this reason, we cannot conclude that lipoprivic feeding is mediated by vagal sensory neurons on the basis of the capsaicin results alone. Therefore, we also examined glucoprivic and lipoprivic feeding in rats with total surgical transections of both subdiaphragmatic vagal trunks.[61] We found that subdiaphragmatic vagotomy completely blocked feeding in response to MA (Figure 4). Vagotomy did not block the response to 2DG (Figure 4), although feeding in response to the higher dose was slightly attenuated compared to control. Like the selective impairment of lipoprivic feeding by capsaicin, the selective effects of subdiaphragmatic vagotomy illustrate that the neural substrates for glucoprivic and lipoprivic feeding are different: vagal sensory neurons are necessary for lipoprivic but not for glucoprivic feeding.

It is important to note that subdiaphragmatic vagotomized rats in our experiments were maintained on a medium-fat liquid diet or on a gelatinized, low-fiber diet beginning prior to surgery. Since both diets empty from the stomach as a liquid meal would do, they avoid the chronic gastric distention and impaction that complicate interpretation of feeding studies in vagotomized rats on solid diets. In addition, the ability of these vagotomized rats to increase their food intake in response to an acute challenge is evident from the sizable intakes of these same rats in the 2DG test. Therefore, we are fairly confident that the absence of MA-induced feeding in subdiaphragmatic vagotomized rats was not a spurious result of impaired gastric emptying, impaction or other pathology that accompanies vagal motor denervation of the gastrointestinal tract. Rather,

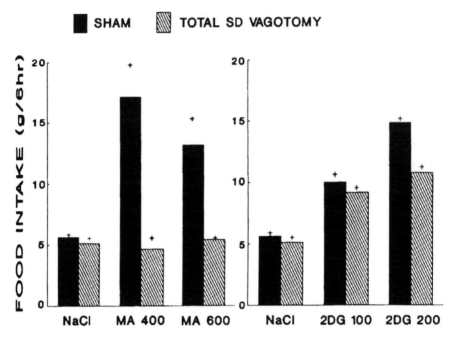

FIGURE 4. Food intake of subdiaphragmatic vagotomized rats and controls during 6-hr tests after injection of NaCl (0.9%, mean of 4 tests), MA (400 and 600 μmol/kg, ip) and 2DG (100 and 200 mg/kg, sc). Rats were maintained and tested on a medium-fat, gelatin-based diet. Means ± are shown.

the results support the hypothesis that neurons in the subdiaphragmatic vagus nerve are necessary for lipoprivic feeding.

Lipoprivic Feeding is Abolished by Lesion of the Vagal Sensory Terminal Field in the Area Postrema and Nucleus of the Solitary Tract (AP/NTS)

The dependence of lipoprivic feeding specifically on the sensory neurons of the vagus was further assessed in rats with selective lesions of the central terminals of vagal sensory neurons in the AP/NTS.[61] These lesions were made by gentle aspiration under direct visual guidance and were shown subsequently to have completely spared the dorsal motor nucleus of the vagus (DMV). Behavioral tests revealed that AP/NTS lesions abolished lipoprivic feeding (Figure 5). Loss of lipoprivic feeding after surgical destruction of central vagal sensory terminals, after selective capsaicin-induced destruction of visceral sensory neurons, and after total subdiaphragmatic vagotomy, together indicate that the lipoprivic control of feeding is dependent on vagal sensory neurons.

In contrast to capsaicin or subdiaphragmatic vagotomy, lesions of the AP/ NTS region abolished glucoprivic as well as lipoprivic feeding (Figure 5). Since glucoprivic feeding survives both capsaicin treatment and vagotomy, it is unlikely that damage to viscerosensory terminals of peripheral neurons is

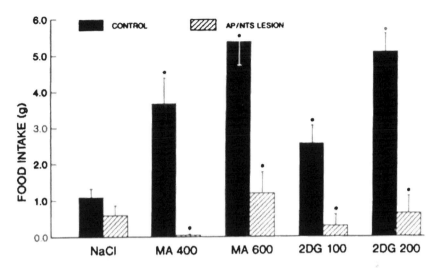

FIGURE 5. Food intake of AP/NTS-lesioned rats and controls during 6-hr tests after injection of NaCl (0.9%, mean of 4 tests), MA (400 and 600 μmol/kg, ip) and 2DG (100 and 200 mg/kg, sc). Rats were maintained and tested on a medium-fat powdered diet. Means ± are shown.

responsible for the deficits produced by the AP/NTS lesion. It seems more likely, as discussed below, that this region contains actual receptor cells important for glucoprivic feeding.

Sensory Neurons Important for Lipoprivic Feeding are Distributed in More than One Vagal Branch

In recent experiments Bruce Hutton, Thu Dinh and I have tested MA-induced feeding in rats with subtotal subdiaphragmatic vagotomies hoping to localize the participating vagal fibers to a specific branch.[59] The distribution of that vagal branch, we hoped, would then lead us to the specific visceral sites where fatty acid oxidation is monitored. This approach has been only partially successful and, as discussed below, considerable work remains to be done before the receptive sites for lipoprivic feeding can be precisely identified.

The subdiaphragmatic vagus distributes in two trunks, dorsal and ventral. The dorsal (posterior) trunk supplies the coeliac and dorsal gastric branches. The ventral (anterior) trunk supplies the hepatic, accessory coeliac and ventral gastric branches.[48] In our experiments, each trunk and each of the branches was transected individually or in combination with other branches. In addition, we examined the effect of total liver denervation on 2DG and MA feeding. At the experiment's conclusion, vagotomies were assessed anatomically by retrograde transport of fluorogold or cholera toxin conjugated to horseradish peroxidase, as described by Powley *et al.*[47] or by visual inspection where these techniques were not applicable. Retrograde transport of fluorogold from the gastric wall was also used to detect inadvertent damage to the right gastric branch during transection of the coeliac branch (with which it is closely associated).

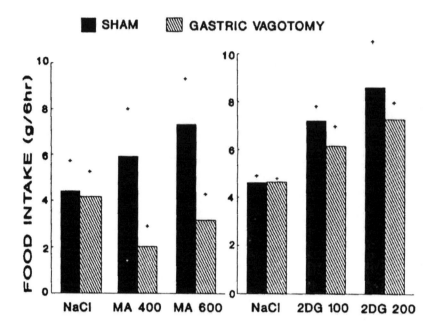

FIGURE 6. Food intake of rats with bilateral gastric branch transections or sham vagotomies in a 6-hr test following injection of saline (0.9%), MA (400 and 600 µmol/kg, ip) and 2DG (100 and 200 mg/kg, sc). Rats were maintained and tested on a moist, medium-fat, gelatin-based diet. Means ± SE are shown.

The only subtotal vagotomy which totally and permanently abolished lipoprivic feeding was bilateral gastric branch vagotomy (Figure 6, left panel).[59] Thus, the gastric branches appear to be essential for the feeding response. However, sensory fibers important for lipoprivic feeding are not located exclusively in the gastric branches. Some also appear to travel in the coeliac branch. Coeliac vagotomy alone or combined with transection of the accessory coeliac and hepatic branches caused a significant, though transient, impairment of MA-induced feeding (Figure 7). In addition, transection of one vagal trunk caused a greater impairment than transection of a single gastric branch (Figure 8).

The importance of the gastric branches was further demonstrated by the fact that bilateral gastric vagotomy caused a permanent (at least 6 months) loss of MA-induced feeding, whereas deficits caused by other partial vagotomies were temporary. Recovery of MA-induced feeding occurred within 2-3 months postsurgery in all lesioned animals with at least one intact gastric branch. Since our anatomical data show no evidence of regrowth from transected vagal branches in animals that recovered from initial deficits in lipoprivic feeding, we suspect that recovery of lipoprivic feeding in these cases was due to functional reorganization of or reinnervation from remaining vagal fibers.

Results from the partial vagotomies suggest that fibers important for lipoprivic feeding are distributed in multiple, possibly all, subdiaphragmatic vagal

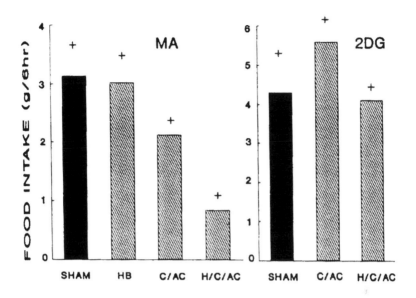

FIGURE 7. Intake of a medium-fat diet in a 6-hr test after MA (600 μmol/kg, ip) or 2DG (200 mg/kg, sc). Mean intake above saline baseline (± SE) is shown for each group. Rats had recovered for approximately 3 weeks at the start of testing from sham vagotomy (SHAM), hepatic branch (HB) transection, transection of the coeliac and accessory coeliac (C/AC) branches, or transection of all three of these branches (H/C/AC).

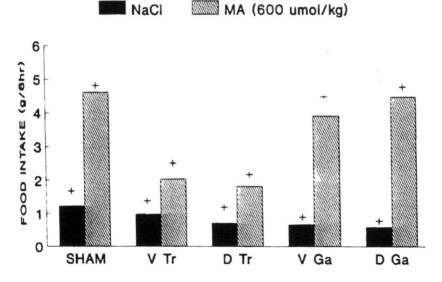

FIGURE 8. Intake of a medium-fat diet in a 6-hr test after MA (600 μmol/kg, ip) injection. Rats were sham-operated (SHAM) or partially vagotomized by transection of the ventral vagal trunk (V Tr), dorsal vagal trunk (D Tr), ventral gastric branch (V Ga) or dorsal gastric branch (D Ga). Means ± SE are shown.

branches. Based on the fiber counts in the individual vagal branches,[49] one way of interpreting our results is that the magnitude of the deficit produced by transection of a particular branch is related to the total numbers of fibers destroyed. Lipoprivic feeding was permanently abolished by bilateral transection of the gastric branches, which together contain approximately 75% of the total population of unmyelinated subdiaphragmatic vagal fibers in the rat.[49] Transection of either the dorsal or ventral vagal trunk separately, a procedure which destroys approximately 50% of the unmyelinated subdiaphragmatic vagal fibers, produced less impairment than gastric vagotomy and reduced the feeding response to approximately 50% of control. Dorsal coeliac plus accessory coeliac transection, destroying 32% of unmyelinated vagal fibers, respectively, produced even smaller deficits. And transection of the hepatic branch, destroying only 13% of the unmyelinated subdiaphragmatic vagal fibers, produced no detectable deficit in lipoprivic feeding.

The apparently diffuse distribution of vagal sensory neurons involved in lipoprivic feeding has made it difficult to determine the location of metabolic receptors for this control. One possibility is that receptors for lipoprivic feeding are in fact diffusely distributed in the abdominal viscera. Another possibility is that these receptors are located in one of the abdominal sites, such as the upper duodenum and pyloris, which is jointly innervated by several vagal branches.[5] (See also, Powley, chapter 3 of this volume.)

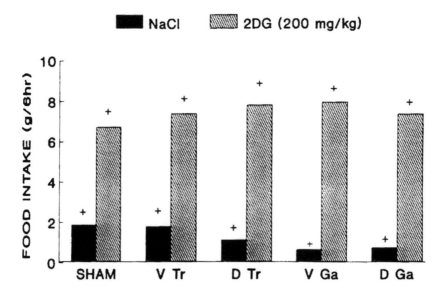

FIGURE 9. Intake of a medium-fat diet in a 6-hr test after 2DG (200 mg/kg, sc) injection. Rats were sham-operated (SHAM) or partially vagotomized by transection of the ventral vagal trunk (V Tr), dorsal vagal trunk (D Tr), ventral gastric branch (V Ga) or dorsal gastric branch (D Ga). Means ± SE are shown.

It was apparent from the partial vagotomies, as from previous work, that subdiaphragmatic vagal fibers are not required for glucoprivic feeding. Neither bilateral gastric vagotomy (Figure 6, right panel), transection of all the subdiaphragmatic branches except the gastrics (Figure 7, right panel), nor transection of the individual vagal trunks (Figure 9) impaired feeding in response to 2DG.

Does the Liver Contain Sensory Neurons Important for Lipoprivic Feeding?

The liver plays a key role in metabolism and is innervated by both afferent and efferent vagal fibers responsive to metabolic stimuli or infused nutrients.[40,42,43] For these reasons, several investigators have hypothesized that the liver is a receptive site for monitoring nutrient fluxes controlling food intake, including nutrient fluxes related specifically to lipoprivic feeding.[15,29] Indeed, one laboratory has reported deficits in lipoprivic feeding in hepatic vagotomized rats using vagotomy and testing procedures similar to ours.[29] However, the hypothesis that the hepatic branch of the vagus contains fibers essential for lipoprivic feeding is not supported by our data. In our experiments, transection of the hepatic branch, along with any other visible fascicles passing between the liver and the paraesophageal vagal trunk, did not cause deficits in lipoprivic feeding. In addition, transection of the ventral vagal trunk, which includes the hepatic branch, produced no greater deficit than transection of the dorsal trunk (Figure 8). Furthermore, in bilateral gastric vagotomized rats, lipoprivic feeding could not be elicited, as discussed above, even though the hepatic branch had not been damaged. These results clearly indicate that the hepatic vagal branch *per se* is neither necessary nor sufficient for lipoprivic feeding.

It is conceivable that both the failure of our hepatic vagotomy to significantly impair lipoprivic feeding and the impairment we observed after transection of other vagal branches is attributable to a diffuse distribution in our rats of hepatic sensory fibers in multiple vagal branches or fascicles. The hepatic branch has been described as having multiple small branches in some rats.[48,49] Furthermore, some sensory fibers en route to the brain from the liver may join branches other than the hepatic branch.[31,44] Indeed, there is some evidence for a functionally homologous hepatic branch emerging contralaterally from the dorsal vagal trunk.[34,41] If hepatic vagal fibers are not confined to the hepatic branch, selective transection of the hepatic branch obviously would not result in complete vagal denervation of the liver.

These anatomical caveats encouraged us to pursue a different strategy to assess the role of the liver as a receptive site for lipoprivic control of feeding. Using procedures adapted from Bellinger and Williams[3] and Lautt and Carroll,[30] we attempted to totally denervate the liver. Total liver denervation, like hepatic branch transection, did not attenuate the feeding response (Figure 10). Because the success of total liver denervation procedures are difficult to confirm, these findings can not exclude the participation of the hepatic innervation in lipoprivic

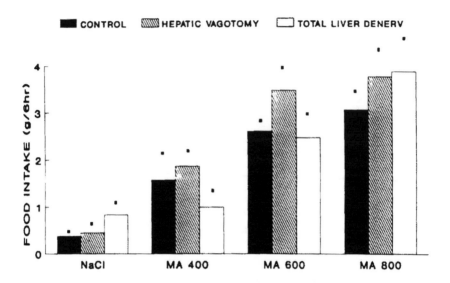

FIGURE 10. Intake of a medium-fat powdered diet by hepatic branch vagotomized, liver denervated and sham-operated control rats in a 6-hr test following injection of NaCl (0.9%) or MA (400, 600 and 800 µmol/kg, ip). Food intake of hepatic branch vagotomized and liver denervated rats did not differ significantly from intake of controls for any drug dose.

feeding. However, in light of these results, it seems highly unlikely that the liver is the exclusive recipient of sensory fibers involved in the arousal of lipoprivic feeding.

Summary

Lipoprivic feeding appears to be mediated by capsaicin-sensitive abdominal vagal sensory neurons that travel in more than one vagal branch. The precise location of receptors for lipoprivic feeding remains to be determined.

GLUCOPRIVIC FEEDING: EVIDENCE FOR MEDIATION BY CENTRAL METABOLIC RECEPTOR CELLS

Evidence for Central Glucoreceptors

In contrast to lipoprivic feeding, receptor cells important for glucoprivic feeding appear to be located in the brain. The strongest evidence for a central location of receptors for glucoprivic feeding is that injection of glucoprivic agents directly into the brain stimulates feeding at doses that do not produce systemic glucoprivation and that do not stimulate feeding when injected systemically.[6,38,52] Convergent results from a number of experiments suggest that these receptors may be located in the AP/NTS region. The glucoprivic agent, 5TG, is more effective in stimulating feeding when injected into the fourth ventricle than when injected into the lateral ventricle.[53] In addition, cerebral aqueduct obstruction by injection of a silicone grease plug blocks the feeding response to lateral ventricular injection of 5TG. The feeding response to fourth ventricular injection is not blocked by the aqueduct plug, suggesting that the cells responsive to both lateral and fourth ventricular 5TG are located in the hindbrain caudal to the plug.[53] Moreover, feeding in response to both central and systemic glucoprivation is severely impaired or abolished by AP/NTS lesions.[6,10,25,61] And finally, decerebrate rats with supracollicular brainstem transections increase their food intake in response to insulin-induced glucoprivation, indicating that the basic circuitry for detecting and responding to the glucoprivic challenge is present in the caudal hindbrain.[14]

Do Peripheral Receptors Contribute to Glucoprivic Feeding?

Although the data discussed above clearly demonstrate the existence of central glucoreceptors that are independently capable of stimulating feeding, they do not rule out the potential contribution of peripheral mechanisms. However, evidence for the existence of peripheral glucoreceptors controlling food intake has not been compelling. The potential contribution of spinal afferents to glucoprivic feeding has not been evaluated. However, if spinal afferents are involved, they are not capsaicin-sensitive, since our systemic capsaicin treatments did not impair glucoprivic feeding.[60] The possible contribution of vagal fibers has been more thoroughly investigated, but results are not conclusive.

In our own work, as shown above in Figure 4, rats with total subdiaphragmatic vagotomy did not differ from controls in their response to a low suprathreshold dose of 2DG (100 mg/kg), indicating that their sensitivity to this challenge had not been altered by the vagotomy. Only at the higher dose (200 mg/kg) was the magnitude of the response in vagotomized rats slightly attenuated compared to the controls. This pattern of deficits was also observed in our gastric vagotomized rats. The attenuation of intake at high, but not low, 2DG doses suggests that the attenuated intake at the higher drug dose was due to the physical limitation of intake imposed by impaired gastric emptying rather than to destruction of vagal fibers specifically involved in glucoprivic feeding.

The role of the hepatic branch of the vagus in glucoprivic feeding has also been specifically examined by several investigators. Most results indicate that the hepatic innervation is not required for glucoprivic feeding: hepatic denervation[3] (see above), hepatic branch vagotomy,[44,59,74] transection of the ventral vagal trunk (which includes the fibers giving rise to the hepatic branch) and total subdiaphragmatic vagotomy[61] do not abolish the response to 2DG.

Despite this negative evidence, a number of tantilizing experiments have suggested a role for peripheral (perhaps hepatic) mechanisms in glucoprivic feeding. Novin and his colleagues showed that in rabbits (although not in rats) 2DG stimulated feeding more effectively when injected into the hepatic portal vein than when injected into the jugular vein and the response was attenuated by subdiaphragmatic vagotomy.[44] In rats, however, the two routes of injection were equally effective in stimulating feeding.[62,70]

More recently, Delprete and Scharrer[11] reported that hepatic vagotomy attenuated the response to 2DG injected intraperitoneally 1 hr after the onset of the dark period and 0-0.5 hr after presentation of food. However, the amount of food consumed by each group in the period prior to the injection and the exact time of the injections after the meal were not specified in this report. Since dark onset is a period of very rapid rates of eating and characteristically high intakes, slight difference in procedure could produce very different results. These are crucial pieces of information since and amount eaten just prior to the test may have affected the development and potency of the glucoprivic challenge[70] or the amount consumed in the control condition. Nevertheless, the possibility that a role for the hepatic innervation in glucoprivic feeding might be expressed under highly specific behavioral, circadian or metabolic conditions, such as those described by Delprete and Scharrer, is a line of investigation that should be pursued.

Using a different approach, Tordoff and his colleagues[75,76] have shown that feeding can be stimulated with the antimetabolic fructose analogue, 2,5-anhydro-D-mannitol (2,5-AM). Like fructose itself, this analogue does not appear to pass the blood-brain barrier, and therefore, its direct antimetabolic actions would be restricted to peripheral tissues and circumventricular organs. Rats began eating sooner and ate more food during intraportal than during intrajugular infusions of 2,5-AM. The stimulation of feeding evoked by intragastric intubation of a low, but not a high, dose of 2,5-AM was blocked by hepatic vagotomy. The data were interpreted as indicating a role for the liver in feeding stimulated by low doses of the fructose analogue. The investigators speculated that perhaps a role for peripheral mechanisms in stimulation of feeding is more clearly demonstrated with low 2,5-AM doses than with 2DG because the contribution of the peripheral mechanisms is not masked by the activation of central receptors. These results are consistent with our early work indicating that insulin-induced glucoprivic feeding could be significantly attenuated, but not blocked, by intravenous infusion of fructose.[2] If these interpretations hold when more is known about the metabolic actions of 2,5-AM, this compound could prove to be an extremely valuable tool in defining the role of peripheral metabolic receptors in stimulation of feeding and in elucidating the interactions of central and peripheral mechanisms.

It is tantilizing to speculate that peripheral receptors for glucoprivic feeding, if they exist, might be low threshold receptors that mediate feeding in response to small local changes in fuel availability (in the liver or elsewhere) that are not necessarily detectable in the systemic circulation. Receptors with such a function could conceivably exert a glucoprivic control of meal initiation under the usual preprandial metabolic conditions in which glucose deficits are not in evidence.

Summary

Glucoprivic feeding is mediated by a population of metabolic receptors which appears to be different from those which mediate lipoprivic feeding.

Unlike lipoprivic feeding, glucoprivic feeding does not require vagal sensory neurons, is not capsaicin sensitive and can be stimulated by independent activation of metabolic receptors within the brain. The exact location of these receptors is not known, but several lines of evidence suggest that they are located in the caudal hindbrain, possibly in the AP/NTS region. Whether peripheral receptors contribute to to glucoprivic feeding has been difficult to demonstrate, possibly because their action is often masked by the simultaneous activation of the receptors in the brain.

CENTRAL NEURAL PATHWAYS FOR GLUCOPRIVIC AND LIPOPRIVIC FEEDING: EFFECT OF BRAIN LESIONS

As discussed below, a number of central lesions have been studied for their effect on glucoprivic feeding. In contrast, ours is the only work to date which has attempted to identify central neural pathways for lipoprivic feeding. In one line of investigation, we have used brain lesions to identify brain regions potentially involved in the glucoprivic and lipoprivic controls. Our lesion strategy was based on the fact that the AP/NTS region is important for both controls. The AP/NTS lesion impairs the metabolic control of feeding by destroying the central terminals of vagal sensory neurons important for lipoprivic feeding[60,61] and presumed receptor cells for glucoprivic feeding. Therefore, in order to trace the pathways for these controls rostrally in the brain, Noel Calingasan, Bruce Hutton and I placed electrolytic lesions in areas known to be innervated by projections from the AP/NTS.[19,20,50,65,78] Our studies so far[9] have included the lateral parabrachial nucleus (LPBN), the central nucleus of the amygdala (CNA) and the paraventricular nucleus of the hypothalamus (PVN). This approach has been a fruitful one, particularly with regard to central pathways important for lipoprivic feeding.

The Central Pathways for Glucoprivic and Lipoprivic Feeding Appear to Differ

The main findings of our central mapping studies to date are summarized in Figure 11. Despite the confluence of pathways for both controls in the AP/NTS, the figure shows that lesions in some brain sites affected feeding responses to 2DG and MA differentially. Relatively small bilateral lesions damaging portions of the external lateral, dorsal and central LPBN subnuclei abolished lipoprivic feeding but did not impair glucoprivic feeding. These specific subnuclei in which lesions impair lipoprivic feeding are known to be reciprocally connected with the AP/NTS region.[19,20]

Amygdaloid lesions also abolished lipoprivic feeding. Lipoprivic feeding was impaired only by lesions which destroyed the CNA bilaterally. This subnucleus of the amygdala is known to be interconnected with both the LPBN and the AP/NTS.[19,20] Lesions sparing the CNA on one or both sides did not produce feeding deficits in lipoprivic feeding, regardless of the extent of the damage to other areas of the amygdala.

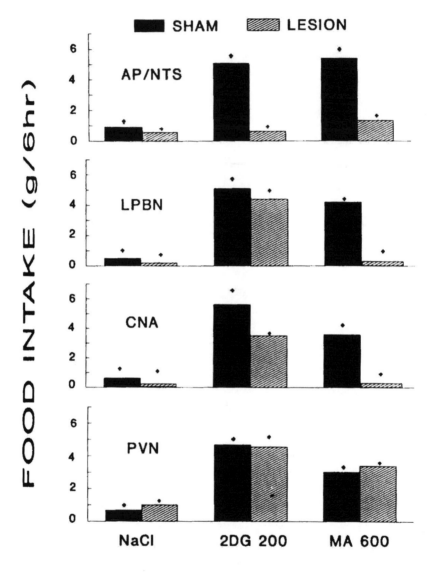

FIGURE 11. Intake of a medium-fat powdered diet by brain-lesioned rats and sham-operated controls in response to 2DG (200 mg/kg, sc) and MA (600 μmol/kg) and saline (NaCl, 0.9%). The four panels show responses of rats with lesions in the area postrema and portions of the underlying nucleus of the solitary tract (AP/NTS), the lateral parabrachial nucleus (LPBN), the central nucleus of the amygdala (CNA) and the paraventricular nucleus of the hypothalamus (PVN). Food intake in response to 2DG was significantly impaired by AP/NTS and CNA lesions, but not by LPBN or PVN lesions. Feeding induced by MA was significantly impaired by AP/NTS, LPBN and CNA lesions, but not by PVN lesions. Means ± SE are shown.

Glucoprivic feeding was not impaired by LPBN lesions that abolished lipoprivic feeding. However, CNA lesions did impair glucoprivic feeding. Lesioned rats did not eat in response to 100 mg/kg of 2DG and had an attenuated response to 200 mg/kg, compared to the controls. Although attenuated, the response to the higher dose was nevertheless significantly above the intake after saline injection. Impairment of 2DG-induced feeding by CNA lesions, very similar to that we observed, has been reported previously.[73] In our studies so far, we have not been able to determine whether precisely the same lesion site is important for both glucoprivic and lipoprivic feeding deficits. Analysis of lesions aimed at more precise targets within the amygdala is currently underway in our laboratory.

In contrast to the LPBN and CNA lesions, large lesions destroying the entire PVN, another major projection site for AP/NTS neurons, had no effect on either glucoprivic or lipoprivic feeding (Figure 11). The failure of PVN lesions to impair glucoprivic feeding is consistent with results reported previously.[66] Nevertheless, the failure of this lesion to impair either control is puzzling in view of the apparent importance of this structure in feeding behavior.[32]

Are Lesion Effects Specific?

It is important to realize that brain lesions may impair behaviors non-specifically or they may produce changes in the animal's responses to particular aspects of the behavioral testing environment that may lead to an erroneous conclusion regarding the true nature of the deficit produced. However, the ingestive responses elicited in control animals by the doses of 2DG and MA used in our experiments are similar in magnitude and time course, as shown previously in Figures 1A and 2A. Therefore, the fact that glucoprivic and lipoprivic feeding responses were differentially impaired by certain lesions suggests that the impairment was probably not due to non-specific behavioral incompetence. Also, it is important to mention that at the time of behavioral testing, all of the lesioned animals were healthy and able to maintain their body weights.

Summary

Lesion studies indicate that specific subnuclei within areas innervated by rostral projections of AP/NTS neurons are important for lipoprivic feeding. Thus, the neural pathway for lipoprivic feeding begins with vagal sensory neurons terminating in the AP/NTS. Higher order neurons appear to ascend with other visceral sensory neurons to the LPBN and CNA, but not to the PVN. Lesions had differential effects on lipoprivic and glucoprivic feeding, indicating that the central pathway for glucoprivic feeding is not identical to the pathway for lipoprivic feeding. However, the pathways for the two controls appear to overlap anatomically at in the AP/NTS region and perhaps to some extent in the amygdala.

C-FOS-LIKE IMMUNOREACTIVITY (FOS-LI) IS INCREASED IN SPECIFIC BRAIN AREAS BY SYSTEMIC 2DG AND MA: EFFECTS OF TOTAL SUBDIAPHRAGMATIC VAGOTOMY

Recently we have used Fos immunohistochemistry to identify specific brain structures with potential importance for glucoprivic and lipoprivic feeding. Fos is the protein product of a proto-oncogene (c-fos) that appears to be involved in the "immediate early" response of many neurons to stimulation. Fos protein increases in the nucleus of the activated neuron beginning within minutes, has a half life of about 2 hr,[39] and can be detected by standard immunohistochemical techniques.

MA and 2DG Induce Fos-li in Specific Brain Nuclei

We examined the distribution of Fos-li in rat brain after systemic adminis-tration of 2DG (200 and 600 mg/kg) and MA (600, 800 and 1200 µmol/kg) and vehicle solutions.[55] Rats were implanted with jugular catheters and allowed to recover for at least 1 week prior to the test. On the test day, drugs and vehicle solutions equated with drug solutions for tonicity and pH were infused remotely through jugular catheters in the absence of food. Animals were killed 2 hrs later, a time determined in pilot studies to be optimal for observing Fos-li with these stimuli.

Both MA and 2DG induced Fos-li in specific brain regions. Vehicle injec-tions did not induce Fos-li in any of these areas. The staining was remarkably specific and reproducible for both drugs. MA increased Fos-li immunoreactiv-ity markedly in the AP/NTS, dorsal motor nucleus of X (DMX), the LPBN (central, dorsal and external subnuclei), and central lateral subnucleus of the amygdala. It is noteworthy that MA did not appear to induce Fos-li in the PVN, a result which is consistent with the fact that PVN lesions do not impair lipoprivic feeding. Mercaptoacetate-induced immunoreactivity in the AP/NTS region is shown in Figure 12A.

After 2DG, Fos-li was present in the AP/NTS (Figure 12C), DMV, external LPBN, LC, CNA, the ventral lateral hypothalamus (vLH), arcuate nucleus, the supraoptic nucleus (SON) and the PVN. Occasionally very light staining was present in the dorsal raphe and in the olfactory portions of the amygdala. It is interesting that many of these same brain regions (DMV, LC, LPBN, PVN, SON and median eminence) were reported recently to be activated by electrical stimulation of the AP, as revealed by 2DG autoradiography.[17]

Subdiaphragmatic Vagotomy Blocks Induction of Fos-li in Brain by MA but not by 2DG

Since subdiaphragmatic vagotomy blocks MA- but not 2DG-induced feed-ing, we wanted to know whether induction of c-fos by these drugs would also be differentially affected by subdiaphragmatic vagotomy. Therefore, vagotomized

SHAM   VAGOTOMY

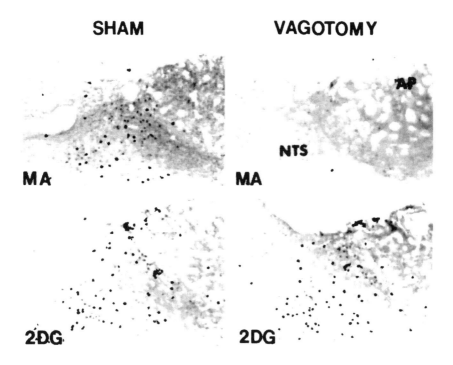

FIGURE 12. Photomicrographs at the level of the AP/NTS (coronal plane) showing Fos-li induced in control rats by remote intravenous infusion of MA (600 µmol/kg, *top left*) and 2DG (200 mg/ kg, *bottom left*). Subdiaphragmatic vagotomy blocked induction of Fos-li by MA (*top right*), but not by 2DG (*bottom right*). Fos-li was not induced in these areas by infusion of control solutions. Abbreviations: AP, area postrema; NTS, nucleus of the solitary tract.

and sham-operated control rats were surgically prepared and allowed to recover from surgery for 2 months. Both vagotomized rats and controls were maintained on our gelatinized medium-fat diet beginning prior to surgery. Staining induced by remote intrajugular infusion of MA was greatly attenuated or abolished by subdiaphragmatic vagotomy in all of the immunoreactive areas observed in controls. In contrast to MA, 2DG-induced activation of Fos-li was not abolished in any of the immunoreactive sites by subdiaphragmatic vagotomy. Our impression from the data is that the subnuclear distribution of 2DG-induced immunoreactivity within the AP/NTS may have been altered by vagotomy, but we have not yet carried our analysis far enough to confirm this. The blockade of MA-induced but not 2DG-induced Fos-li by vagotomy is shown for the AP/NTS region in Figure 12.

Fos Immunohistochemistry is Consistent with Lesion Effects

Fos-li was induced by MA specifically in those brain sites where lesions produce deficits in MA-induced feeding. In addition, subdiaphragmatic vagotomy blocks both the central induction of Fos-li and the stimulation of feeding by

MA. Thus, some of the brain neurons identified by the c-fos technique as being activated by MA may form an afferent pathway which originates with vagal sensory neurons and is responsible for arousal of appetite in response to lipoprivation.

We have made less progress in defining the central pathway(s) for glucoprivic feeding. However, results of the fos-immunohistochemistry are consistent with behavioral results showing that 2DG is capable of activating brain neurons in the absence of the subdiaphragmatic vagus. In addition, 2DG does induce Fos-li in the AP/NTS and CNA where lesions produce deficits in 2DG-induced feeding. However, the correspondence between areas where Fos-li is induced by 2DG and areas where lesions cause deficits in glucoprivic feeding is less precise than we have seen for MA. The PVN and LPBN, for example, are areas where 2DG induces Fos-li but where lesions do not cause deficits in glucoprivic feeding. Therefore, it appears from our present data that many neurons which express Fos-li in response to 2DG are not involved in or are not essential for the feeding response. Some activated neurons may be involved in other physiological responses to glucoprivation (e.g., sympathoadrenal and gastric secretory responses to glucoprivation). Alternatively, glucoprivation may activate multiple or redundant pathways, each of which is independently capable of stimulatiang food intake. It is also important to note that some areas such as the dorsomedial and lateral hypothalamus, where excitotoxin lesions have been reported to produce deficits in glucoprivic feeding,[4,18] did not contain 2DG-induced Fos-li. Such results remind us that some neurons essential for the the glucoprivic feeding response may not express Fos-li.

Summary

Systemic injection of MA induced Fos-li in the AP/NTS and in areas innervated by AP/NTS projections, including some sites where lesions cause deficits in lipoprivic feeding. Fos-li in the brain, like feeding, is not induced by MA in subdiaphragmatic vagotomized rats. These results demonstrate that MA causes activation of neurons in specific brain areas important for lipoprivic feeding and that this activation requires the subdiaphragmatic vagus nerve. Fos-li was induced in these same brain areas, as well as in several additional brain sites, by 2DG. However, like 2DG-induced feeding, 2DG-induced immuno-staining was not detectably altered by subdiaphragmatic vagotomy.

ROLE OF THE VAGUS IN MONITORING METABOLITES THAT INHIBIT FEEDING

Increased Levels of Some Blood-borne Metabolites Inhibit Feeding

This chapter has focused primarily on the stimulation of feeding by deficits in metabolic fuels. Recent work has suggested, however, that excesses in certain blood-borne metabolites may exert inhibitory effects on feeding that are also vagally-mediated. Langhans, *et al.*[28] have shown that subcutaneous injections of glycerol, D-3 hydroxybutyrate, L-malate, L-lactate and pyruvate reduced feeding. A role for vagal sensory neurons was suggested because the hypophagic effect of these substances was abolished by hepatic vagotomy, but not by intraperitoneal injection of atropine methylnitrate, which blocks cholinergically-mediated vagal motor actions. The investigators interpret their findings as indicating that the hypophagic effects of these nutrients is mediated by vagally-transmitted metabolic signals from the liver. However, the participation of a nonhepatic innervation site cannot be entirely ruled out since the hepatic branch of the vagus innervates both hepatic and nonhepatic sites.[5]

Additional work by these investigators suggested that the hypophagic effect of subcutaneous injections of the above metabolites was related to the generation of reducing equivalents by their mitochondrial oxidation. Glycerol, L-malate and L-lactate were compared to their immediate oxidation products (dihydroxyacetone, oxaloacetate and pyruvate, respectively) for their hypophagic potency. Glycerol and L-malate suppressed feeding, whereas their oxidation products did not. Both lactate and pyruvate suppressed feeding, suggesting that the oxidative decarboxylation of pyruvate, which requires the enzyme pyruvate dehydrogenase, may be crucial for the hypophagic effect of both lactate and pyruvate. This hypothesis is supported by their finding that neither lactate nor pyruvate suppresses feeding in rats maintained on high dietary fat. High dietary fat is known to decrease pyruvate dehydrogenase activity and thus inhibit pyruvate oxidation in favor of the gluconeogenic pathway.

Suppression of Feeding by Ketone Bodies is Mediated by a Capsaicin-insensitive Mechanism

Although vagal sensory neurons appear to be involved both in the stimulation of feeding by decreased fatty acid oxidation and in the suppression of feeding by oxidation of various metabolic fuels, it is not yet clear whether the same metabolic receptors or the same vagal sensory neurons are involved in all of these events (i.e., whether all the fuels are monitored by the same system and whether stimulatory and inhibitory effects on feeding are mediated by the same neural pathways). However, inhibition of feeding by beta-hydroxybutyrate is not mediated by the same vagal sensory neurons responsible for stimulation of feeding by MA, even though ketone bodies bypass the MA-induced metabolic blockade. We injected B-OHB at a dose (20 mmol/kg) sufficient to achieve plasma levels within the range of those seen in rats on medium- to high-fat diets.[71] This dose did not appear to make the animals sick, as indicated by the fact that it did not serve as a stimulus for conditioned taste aversion. Nevertheless, this dose did produce a potent suppression of both palatability- and deprivation-induced eating in both normal and capsaicin-treated rats but did not suppress feeding in AP/NTS-lesioned rats (Figure 13).

The fact that B-OHB suppressed feeding to a similar degree in both capsaicin-treated rats with confirmed deficits in lipoprivic feeding and controls suggests that its suppressive effect is not dependent on capsaicin-sensitive neurons; in particular, those involved in the lipoprivic control. Since B-OHB did not

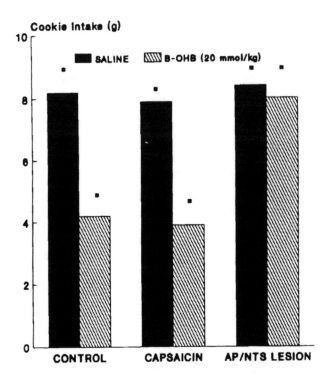

FIGURE 13. Intake of a palatable food (cookies, 'Nilla Wafers) in capsaicin-treated, AP/NTS-lesioned and control rats after administration of beta-hydroxybutyrate (B-OHB) and saline. Cookie intake was suppressed by B-OHB both in controls and in capsaicin-treated rats, but not in AP/NTS-lesioned rats. Means ± SE are shown.

suppress feeding in the AP/NTS-lesioned rats, it is possible that B-OHB may act at metabolic receptor cells in the AP region or on capsaicin insensitive visceral sensory neurons that innervate this region. Both possibilities are consistent with our finding that intravenous infusion of B-OHB induces Fos-li in the AP/NTS region. However, the latter possibility seems more likely in view of results of Langhans et al.[28] showing that hepatic branch vagotomy blocks the inhibition of feeding by B-OHB.

The liver may be a source of signals which suppress food intake in response to increased oxidation of metabolic fuels. In addition, certain nutrients appear to inhibit feeding by an action occurring in the intestine.[81,82] It is not yet known, however, whether the latter effect is mediated by the nutrients directly or by metabolites of these nutrients formed prior to or during intestinal absorption. These results are discussed by R.C. Ritter et al., in chapter 10 of this volume.

Summary

The vagus nerve contains neurons capable of evoking both inhibitory and stimulatory effects on food intake in response to signals potentially generated by metabolic events. The liver and the intestine are two sites where metabolic fuels or specific nutrients may act on vagal sensory neurons to exert these effects on food intake, although other abdominal sites and circumventricular organs are potential contributors.

CONCLUSION AND PERSPECTIVE

Since the adaptive value of hunger is to seek and ingest calories to supply energy to the organism and to maintain the special functions of specific organs, understanding how and where the principle sources of energy are monitored is essential for understanding how food intake is controlled and consequently how energy balance is maintained. Results presented in this chapter demonstrate that the two main macronutrients used for energy metabolism are monitored by distinct neural systems located in physiologically appropriate areas of the body. Sensory neurons of the abdominal vagus are essential for the arousal of appetite by decreased fatty acid oxidation, while receptors within the brain play a predominant role in stimulating glucoprivic feeding.

The location of receptors for glucoprivic and lipoprivic feeding in the brain and abdominal viscera, respectively, is intuitively pleasing. Brain cells use glucose, but not fatty acids, for energy metabolism and require uninterrupted delivery of glucose by the blood for survival. Similarly, it is reasonable that receptors monitoring fatty acid utilization would be located in peripheral tissues for which fatty acids are an important metabolic substrate.

The presence in the body of distinct neural systems for monitoring fatty acid and glucose utilization is compatible with the fact that carbohydrates and fatty acids are in effect in separate metabolic compartments.[13] Glucose cannot be made from fatty acids. Thus, availability of each fuel must be independently monitored in order to achieve energy balance and to meet the needs of metabolically nonfacultative tissues such as brain. In addition, the evidence that independent systems monitor fat and glucose utilization is consistent with new data revealing fundamental differences in the way in which carbohydrate and fat oxidation are controlled.[13] Finally, the fact that systems responsive to deficits in fatty acid and glucose are distinct provides the opportunity for animals to call upon each system separately to serve the needs of particular tissues or specific physiological states.

Future challenges include the precise localization and characterization of metabolic receptor cells or receptive nerve endings specifically and directly involved in control of glucoprivic and lipoprivic feeding. In addition, it will be important to elucidate the sites at which metabolic signals generated in separate sensory systems are integrated to produce appropriate feeding behavior and other homeostatic responses. Furthermore, the relative importance of the metabolic controls of feeding in the overall regulation of food intake, and their possibly concurrent roles in subserving the metabolic requirements of specific organs or tissues, will need to be addressed.

REFERENCES

1. Bauche, F., Sabourault, D., Giudicelli, Y., Nordmann, J., and Nordmann, R., Inhibition *in vitro* of acyl-CoA-dehydrogenases by 2-mercaptoacetate in rat liver mitochondria, *Biochem. J.*, 215, 457-464, 1983.

2. Bellin, S.I., and Ritter, S., Disparate effects of infused nutrients on delayed glucoprivic feeding and hypothalamic norepinephrine turnover, *J. Neurosci.*, 1, 1347-1353, 1981.

3. Bellinger, L.L., and Williams, F.E., Liver denervation does not modify feeding responses to metabolic challenges or hypertonic NaCl induced water consumption, *Physiol. Behav.*, 30, 463-470, 1983.

4. Bellinger, L.L., Williams, F.E., Aphagia and adipsia after kainic acid lesioning of the dorsomedial hypothalamic area, *Am. J. Physiol.*, 244, R389-R399, 1983.

5. Berthoud, H.-R., Carlson, N.R., and Powley, T.L., Topography of efferent vagal innervation of the rat gastrointestinal tract, *Am. J. Physiol.*, 260, R200-R207, 1991.

6. Bird, E., Cardone, C.C., and Contreras, C.C., Area postrema lesions disrupt food intake induced by cerebroventricular infusions of 5-thioglucose in the rat, *Brain Res.*, 270, 193-196. 1983.

7. Booth, D.A., Modulation of the feeding response to peripheral insulin, 2-deoxyglucose or 3-O-methyl glucose injection, *Physiol. Behav.*, 8, 1069-1076, 1972.

8. Brown, J., Effects of 2-deoxy-D-glucose on carbohydrate metabolism: review of the literature and studies in the rat, *Metabolism*, 11, 1098-1112, 1962.

9. Calingasan, N., Hutton, B.W., and Ritter, S., Effects of lesioning the amygdala, parabrachial nucleus and hypothalamic paraventricular nucleus on lipoprivic and glucoprivic feeding, *Neurosci. Abstr.*, 16, 1251 (513.6), 1990.

10. Contreras, R.J., Fox, E., and Drugovich, M.L., Area postrema lesions produce feeding deficits in in the rat: effects of preoperative dieting and 2-deoxy-D-glucose, *Physiol. Behav.*, 29, 875-884, 1982.

11. Delprete, E., and Scharrer E., Hepatic branch vagotomy attenuates the feeding response to 2-deoxy-d-glucose in rats, *Exper. Physiol.*, 75, 259-261, 1990.

12. Epstein, A.N., Nicolaidis, S., and Miselis, R., The glucoprivic control of food intake and the glucostatic theory of feeding behavior, in *Neural Integration of Physiological Mechanisms and Behavior*, Mogenson, G.J., and Calarescu, F.R., Eds., University Press, Toronto, 1975, 148-168.

13. Flatt, J.P., Opposite effects of variations in food intake on carbohydrate and fat oxidation in ad libitum fed mice, *J. Nutr. Biochem.*, 2, 186-192, 1991.

14. Flynn, F.W., and Grill, H., Insulin elicits ingestion in decerebrate rats, *Science*, 221, 188-190, 1982.

15. Friedman, M.I., Tordoff, M.G., and Ramirez, I., Integrated metabolic control of food intake, *Brain Res. Bull.*, 17, 855-859, 1986.

16. Geary, N., and Smith, G.P., Selective hepatic vagotomy blocks pancreatic glucagon's satiety effect, *Physiol. Behav.*, 31, 391-394, 1983.

17. Gross, P.M., Wainman, D.S., Shaver, S.W., Wall, K.M., and Ferguson, A.V., Metabolic activation of efferent pathways from the rat area postrema, *Am. J. Physiol.*, 258, R788-R797, 1990.

18. Grossman, S.P., and Grossman, L., Iontophoretic injections of kainic acid into the rat lateral hypothalamus: effects on ingestive behavior, *Physiol. Behav.*, 29, 553-559, 1982.

19. Herbert, H., Moga, M.M., and Saper, C.B., Connections of the parabrachial nucleus with the nucleus of the solitary tract and the medullary reticular formation in the rat, *J. Comp. Neurol.*, 293, 540-580, 1990.

20. Herbert, H., and Saper, C.B., Cholecystokinin-, galanin-, and corticotropin-releasing factor-like immunoreactive projections from the nucleus of the solitary tract to the parabrachial nucleus in the rat, *J. Comp. Neurol.*, 293, 581-598, 1990.

21. **Holzer, P.,** Capsaicin: cellular targets, mechanisms of action, and selectivity for thin sensory neurons, *Pharmacol. Rev.*, 43, 143-210, 1991.
22. **Houpt, T.R.,** Stimulation of food intake in ruminants by 2-deoxy-D-glucose and insulin, *Am. J. Physiol.*, 227, 161-167, 1974.
23. **Houpt, T.R., and Hance, H.E.,** Threshold levels of 2-deoxy-D-glucose for the hyperglycemic response: Dog and goat compared, *Life Sci.*, 21, 513-518, 1977.
24. **Houpt, K.A., Houpt, T.R., and Pond, W.G.,** Food intake control in the suckling pig: Glucoprivation and gastrointestinal factors, *Am. J. Physiol.*, 232, E510-E514, 1977.
25. **Hyde, T.A., and Miselis, R.R.,** Effects of area postrema/caudal medial nucleus of solitary tract lesions on food intake and body weight, *Am. J. Physiol.*, 244, R577-R587, 1983.
26. **Jancso, G., and Kiraly, E.,** Distribution of chemosensitive primary sensory afferents in the central nervous system of the rat, *J. Comp. Neurol.*, 90, 781-792, 1980.
27. **Kiorpes, T.C., Hoerr, D., Ho, W., Weaner, L.E., Inman, M.G., and Tutwiler, G.F.,** Identification of 2-tetradecylglycidyl coenzyme A as the active form of methyl 2-tetradecylglycidate (methyl palmoxirate) and its characterization as an irreversible, active site-directed inhibitor of carnitine palmitoyltransferase A in isolated rat liver mitochondria, *J. Biol. Chem.*, 259, 9750-9755, 1984.
28. **Langhans, W., Egli, G., and Scharrer, E.,** Selective hepatic vagotomy eliminates the hypophagic effect of different metabolites, *J. Autonom. Nerv. Syst.*, 13, 255-262, 1985.
29. **Langhans, W., and Scharrer, E.,** Evidence for a vagally mediated satiety signal derived from hepatic fatty acid oxidation, *J. Autonom. Nerv. Syst.*, 18, 13-18, 1987.
30. **Lautt, W.W., and Carroll, A.M.,** Evaluation of topical phenol as a means of producing autonomic denervation of the liver, *Can. J. Physiol. Pharmacol.*, 62, 849-853, 1984.
31. **Legros, G., and Griffith, C.A.,** The abdominal vagal system in rats, *J. Surg. Res.*, 9, 183-186, 1969.
32. **Leibowitz, S.F., and Stanley, G.B.,** Neurochemical controls of appetite, in *Feeding Behavior: Neural and Humoral Controls*, Ritter, R.C., Ritter, S., and Barnes, C.D., Eds., Academic Press, NY, 1986, 191-234.
33. **Maggi, C.A., and Meli, A.,** The sensory-efferent function of capsaicin-sensitive sensory neurons, *Gen. Pharmacol.*, 19, 1-43, 1988.
34. **Magni, F., and Carobi, C.,** The afferent and preganglionic parasympathetic innervation of the rat liver, demonstrated by the retrograde transport of horseradish peroxidase, *J. Auton. Nerv. Syst.*, 8, 237-260, 1983.
35. **Makay, E.M., Calloway, J.W., and Barnes, R.H.,** Hyperalimentation in normal animals produced by protamine insulin, *J. Nutr.*, 20, 59-66, 1940.
36. **McDougal, D.B. Jr., Yuan, M.J.C., Dargar, R.V., and Johnson, E.M. Jr.,** Neonatal capsaicin and guanethidine and axonally transported organelle-specific enzymes in sciatic nerve and in sympathetic and dorsal root ganglia, *J. Neurosci.*, 3, 124-132, 1983.
37. **Melone, J.,** Vagal receptors sensitive to lipids in the small intestine of the cat, *J. Autonom. Nerv. Syst.*, 17, 231-241, 1986.
38. **Miselis, R.R., and Epstein, A.N.,** Feeding induced by intracerebroventricular 2-deoxy-D-glucose in the rat, *Am. J. Physiol.*, 229, 1438-1447, 1975.
39. **Morgan, J.I., and Curran, D.R.,** Calcium and proto-oncogene involvement in the immediate early response in the nervous system, *Ann. N.Y. Acad. Sci.*, 568, 283-290, 1989.
40. **Niijima, A.,** Glucose sensitive afferent nerve fibers in the liver and regulation of blood glucose, *Brain Res. Bull.*, 5 (Suppl. 4), 175-179, 1980.
41. **Niijima, A.,** Electrophysiological study on nervous pathway from splanchnic nerve to vagus nerve in rat, *Am J. Physiol.*, 244, R888-R890, 1983.
42. **Niijima, A.,** Suppression of afferent activity of the hepatic vagus nerve by anomers of D-glucose, *Am. J. Physiol.*, 244, R611-R614, 1983.
43. **Niijima, A.,** Nervous regulation of metabolism. *Prog. Neurobiol.*, 33, 135-147, 1989.
44. **Novin, D., Vander Weele, D.A., and Rezek, M.,** Infusion of 2-deoxy-D-glucose into the hepatic portal system causes eating: evidence for peripheral glucoreceptors, *Science*, 181, 859-860, 1973.

45. **Oomura, Y.**, Glucose as a regulator of neuronal activity, in *CNS Regulation of Carbohydrate Metabolism*, Szabo, A.J., Ed., Academic Press, New York, 1983, 31-65.

46. **Powley, T.L., and Berthoud, H.-R.**, Participation of the vagus and other autonomic nerves in the control of food intake, in *Feeding Behavior: Neural and Humoral Controls*, Ritter, R.C., Ritter, S., and Barnes, C.D., Eds., Academic Press, Orlando, FL, 1986, 67-101.

47. **Powley, T.L., Fox, E.A., and Berthoud, H.-R.**, Retrograde tracer technique for assessment of selective and total subdiaphragmatic vagotomies, *Am. J. Physiol.*, 253, R361-R370, 1987

48. **Powley, T.L., Prechtl, J.C., Fox, E.A., and Berthoud, H.-R.**, Anatomical considerations for surgery of the rat abdominal vagus: distribution, paraganglia and regeneration, *J. Autonom. Nerv. Syst.*, 9, 79-97, 1983.

49. **Prechtl, J.C., and Powley, T.L.**, The fiber composition of the abdominal vagus of the rat, *Anat. Embryol.*, 181, 101-1155, 1990.

50. **Ricardo, J.A., and Koh, E.T.**, Anatomical evidence of direct projections from the nucleus of the solitary tract to the hypothalamus, amygdala, and other forebrain structures, *Brain Res.*, 153, 1-26, 1978.

51. **Ritter, R.C., and Ladenheim, E.E.**, Capsaicin pretreatment attenuates suppression of food intake by cholecystokinin octapeptide, *Am. J. Physiol.*, 248, R501-R504, 1985.

52. **Ritter, R.C., and Slusser, P.G.**, 5-thio-D-glucose causes increased feeding and hyperglycemia in the rat, *Am. J. Physiol.*, 238, E141-E144, 1980.

53. **Ritter, R.C., Slusser, P.G., and Stone, S.**, Glucoreceptors controlling feeding and blood glucose: location in hindbrain, *Science*, 213, 451-453, 1981.

54. **Ritter, S.**, Glucoprivation and the glucoprivic control of food intake, in *Food Intake: Neural and Humoral Controls*, Ritter, R.C., Ritter, S., and Barnes, C.D., Eds, Academic Press, Orlando, 1986, 268-299.

55. **Ritter, S., Calingasan, N.Y., Dinh, T.T., and Taylor, J.S.**, Expression of c-fos protein is induced in specific brain neurons by metabolic inhibitors that increase food intake, *Neurosci. Abstr.*, 17, 192, 1991.

56. **Ritter, S., and Dinh, T.T.**, Capsaicin-induced neuronal degeneration: silver impregnation of cell bodies, axons and terminals in the central nervous system of the adult rat, *J. Comp. Neurol.*, 271, 79-90, 1988.

57. **Ritter, S., and Dinh, T.T.**, Capsaicin-induced neuronal degeneration in the brain and retina of preweanling rats, *J. Comp. Neurol.*, 296, 447- 461, 1990.

58. **Ritter, S., and Dinh, T.T.**, Prior optic nerve transection reduces capsaicin-induced degeneration in rat subcortical visual structures, *J. Comp. Neurol.*, 308, 79-90, 1991.

59. **Ritter, S., Hutton, B.W., and Dinh, T.T.**, Neurons required for lipoprivic feeding are not limited to a single vagal branch, *Neurosci. Abstr.*, 16, 295, 1990.

60. **Ritter, S., and Taylor, J.S.**, Capsaicin abolishes lipoprivic but not glucoprivic feeding in rats, *Am. J. Physiol.*, 256, R1232-R1239, 1989.

61. **Ritter, S., and Taylor, J.S.**, Vagal sensory neurons are required for lipoprivic but not glucoprivic feeding in rats, *Am. J. Physiol.*, 258, R1395-R1401, 1990.

62. **Russell, P.J.D., and Mogenson, G.J.**, Drinking and feeding induced by jugular and portal infusions of 2-deoxy-D-glucose, *Am. J. Physiol.*, 229, 1014-1018, 1975.

63. **Sakata, T., Tsutsui, K., Fukushima, M., Arase, K., Kita, H., Oomura, Y., Ohki, K., and Nicolaidis, S.**, Feeding and hyperglycemia induced by 1,5-anhydroglucitol in the rat, *Physiol. Behav.*, 27, 401-405, 1981.

64. **Scharrer, E., and Langhans, W.**, Control of food intake by fatty acid oxidation, *Am. J. Physiol.*, 250, R1003-R1006, 1986.

65. **Shapiro, R.E., and Miselis, R.R.**, The central neural connections of the area postrema of the rat, *J. Comp. Neurol.*, 234, 344-364, 1985.

66. **Shor-Posner, G., Azar, A., Insinga, S., and Leibowitz, S.**, Deficits in the control of food intake after hypothalamic paraventricular nucleus lesions, *Physiol. Behav.*, 35, 883-890, 1985.

67. **Smith G.P., and Epstein, A.N.**, Increased feeding in response to decreased glucose utilization in the rat and monkey, *Am. J. Physiol.*, 217, 1083-1087, 1969.

68. **Smith, G.P., Jerome, C., Cushin, B.J., Eterno, R., and Simansky, K.J.,** Abdominal vagotomy blocks the satiety effect of cholecystokinin in the rat, *Science*, 213, 1036-1037, 1981.

69. **Smith, G.P., and Root, A.,** Effect of feeding on hormonal responses to 2-deoxy-D-glucose in conscious monkeys, *Endocrinol.*, 85, 963-966, 1969.

70. **Stricker, E.M., and Rowland, N.,** Hepatic versus cerebral origin of stimulus for feeding induced by 2-deoxy-D-glucose in rats, *J. Comp. Physiol. Psychol.*, 92, 126-132, 1978.

71. **Taylor, J.S., and Ritter, S.,** Suppression of food intake by ketone bodies is not mediated by visceral sensory neurons controlling lipoprivic feeding, *Proc. Soc. Exp. Biol. Med.*, 190, 306, 1989.

72. **Thompson, D.A., and Campbell, R.G.,** Hunger in humans induced by 2-deoxy-D-glucose: Glucoprivic control of taste preference and food intake, *Science*, 198, 1065-1068, 1977.

73. **Tordoff, M.G., Geiselman, P.J., Grijalva, C.V., Keifer, S.W., and Novin, D.,** Amygdaloid lesions impair ingestive responses to 2-deoxy-D-glucose but not insulin, *Am. J. Physiol.*, 242, R129-R135, 1982.

74. **Tordoff, M.G., Hopfenbeck, J., and Novin, D.,** Hepatic vagotomy (partial hepatic denervation) does not alter ingestive responses to metabolic challenges, *Physiol. Behav.*, 28, 417-424, 1982.

75. **Tordoff, M.G., Rafka, R., DiNovi, M.J., and Friedman, M.I.,** 2,5-Anhydro-D-mannitol: a fructose analogue that increases food intake in rats, *Am. J. Physiol.*, 254, R150-R153, 1988.

76. **Tordoff, M.G., Rawson, N., and Friedman, M.I.,** 2,5-Anhydro-D-mannitol acts in the liver to initiate feeding, *Am. J. Physiol.*, 261, R283-R288, 1991.

77. **Tutwiler, G.F., Brentzel, H.J., and Kiorpes, T.C.,** Inhibition of mitochondrial carnitine palmitoyl transferase A *in vivo* with methyl 2-tetradecylglycidate (methyl palmoxirate) and its relationship to ketonemia and glycemia, *Proc. Soc. Exper. Biol. Med.*, 178, 288-296, 1985.

78. **Van der Kooy, D., and Koda, L.Y.,** Organization of the projections of a circumventricular organ: the area postrema in the rat, *J. Comp. Neurol.*, 219, 328-338, 1983.

79. **Weatherford, S.C., and Ritter, S.,** Lesion of vagal afferent terminals impairs glucagon-induced suppression of food intake, *Physiol. Behav.*, 43, 645-650, 1988.

80. **Wick, A.N., Dury, D.R., Nakada, H.I., and Wolfe, J.B.,** Localization of the primary metabolic block produced by 2-deoxyglucose, *J. Biol. Chem.*, 224, 963-969, 1957.

81. **Yox, D.P., and Ritter, R.C.,** Capsaicin attenuates suppression of sham feeding induced by intestinal nutrients, *Am. J. Physiol.*, 255, R569-R574, 1988.

82. **Yox, D.P., Stokesberry, H., and Ritter, R.C.,** Vagotomy attenuates suppression of sham feeding induced by intestinal nutrients, *Am. J. Physiol.*, 260, R503-R508, 1991.

Chapter 12

A PROTECTIVE ROLE FOR
VAGAL AFFERENTS: AN HYPOTHESIS

P.L.R. Andrews and I.N.C. Lawes

TABLE OF CONTENTS

INTRODUCTION

The extensive distribution of the vagus nerve was recognized from the earliest systematic dissections undertaken by Galen (129-199). From his studies of the Barbary apes and humans he attended in his post as physician to the gladiators at Pergamon and Rome, he described "the sixth pair of nerves" which can be recognized from his descriptions as comprising what are now known as the glossopharyngeal, spinal accessory and vagus nerves (see Sheehan[108]). Galen's description of this "sixth pair of nerves" concludes that "the viscera thereby receive from the brain an exquisite sensitivity and from the spinal cord their motor power."

Galen's descriptions really formed the basis for the future studies of the vagal distribution carried out by Vesalius (1555), Eustachio (1552) and Willis (1664) (see Pick[97] for references) who provided the most extensive and accurate description of the vagus, describing it as the "wandering" nerve. This anatomical work laid the foundations for the histological, physiological and pharmacological studies of Gaskell,[43] Langley,[78] Dale (review)[32] and Cannon[21] which led to our current view of the "autonomic nervous system" and its division into sympathetic and parasympathetic components.

Classically, the autonomic nervous system is considered to be an efferent or motor system, but this was based on the fact that no single histological marker could be found for the afferent fibers traveling in the autonomic nerve trunks rather than on denying their existence (see Prechtl and Powley[99] for recent review). The problem of the afferents in the autonomic nerves is primarily one of semantics although the "no afferents" dogma is reinforced by diagrams of the autonomic nervous system in virtually all textbooks with some going further (e.g., "the results of vagotomy prove that the vagi do not carry afferent fibers from the alimentary canal"[118]). In this review we will call sensory afferents which have their cell bodies in the nodose (and other) ganglia and travel in the vagus nerve, "vagal afferents." Histological studies have quantified the magnitude of the afferent contribution to the vagus, particularly in its abdominal course. Electrophysiological studies extending back over 50 years (e.g., Partridge and Wilson[95]) have revealed the richness of information conveyed to the medulla.[53]

The function of vagal afferents has usually been considered in terms of visceral autonomic reflexes that regulate processes such as blood pressure, respiratory tract secretion and diameter, and gastrointestinal secretion and motility. More recently attention has focused on the involvement of vagal afferents, particularly those from the gut, in the generation of visceral sensation in both health and disease.[6,86] Studies have also shown an involvement of these afferents in the control of aspects of behavior such as food ingestion, particularly in hunger and satiety signals (see R. Ritter *et al.* and S. Ritter *et al.*, chapters 10 and 11 of this volume). It is apparent from the literature stretching back over a number of years, however, that vagal afferents are capable of modulating activity in a large number of systems that regulate a wide variety of visceral and somatic functions.

In this review we present an hypothesis which brings all these diverse functions of vagal afferents, particularly those from the gut, together into one coherent scheme. We will argue that the unifying concept underlying these diverse functions is that vagal afferents constitute the major intero-protective system for the body.

The Functional Correlates of Vagal Afferents

The abdominal vagus supplies the following abdominal structures with afferents: the abdominal esophagus and lower esophageal sphincter, abdominal paraganglia (pO_2 sensitive glomus tissue), the stomach, pyloric sphincter, duodenum, jejunum, ileum, proximal colon (some species), liver, biliary tree, gall bladder and adrenal gland (for references see Christensen,[28] Andrews,[5] Andrews et al.,[9] Mei,[88,89] Howe et al.,[67] and Coupland et al.[30]). The extent of this distribution is particularly impressive when it is remembered that in most cases the vagus supplies both the muscular and mucosal layers of the gut. In addition, when one considers the extra-abdominal structures supplied by vagal afferents (upper esophageal sphincter, esophageal body, aortic arch and carotid artery chemo- and baro-receptors, atria and ventricles, airways and lungs), it is apparent that the vagus monitors most of the crucial bodily functions.

Before outlining the functional roles of vagal afferents, we should address what might seem to be a rather trivial question but one which is fundamental to a proper understanding of the functions of vagal afferents: why do we have afferents from the gut to the brain?

Why Do We Have Afferents from the Gut to the Brain?

In this section we attempt to rationalize the extensively ramified projections of the vagal afferents in general terms before discussing numerous specific examples. The functions may be classified hierarchically, as follows.

Interactions Between Components within a System

The question of why the gastrointestinal tract should project a wealth of afferent information to the central nervous system is complicated by the fact that the gut possesses an extensive enteric nervous system (ENS) containing as many neurons as the spinal cord. The ENS has all the components required for the generation of reflexes such as peristalsis, secretion of hormones and gastric acid, and modulation of absorption and secretion in the small intestine. Why, then, are extrinsic reflexes mediated by the central nervous system required?

The answer is probably that they enable rapid communication between separate regions of the gut for feed back and feed forward control mechanisms. For example, the presence of food in the stomach stimulates the secretion of pancreatic juice, partly by a vagal mechanism. The gastro-colic reflex and the slowing of gastric emptying by duodenal distension are other examples.

Interactions Between Systems

Different organ systems may communicate with each other by hormones but neural pathways are also exploited where they exist. There are several examples where interaction between the gastrointestinal tract and other systems is required. For example, following a meal the gastrointestinal tract may receive 20% of the cardiac output and adjustments to the systemic circulation must be made to accommodate this. The vomiting reflex also provides a good example of such interactions since emetic activation of the abdominal vagal afferents produces reflex changes in the cardiovascular, respiratory and gastrointestinal systems and in addition may alter secretion of pituitary hormones (e.g. vasopressin).

Interactions of Visceral Events with the External Environment

It could be argued that the main evolutionary pressure for the projection of visceral information to the central nervous system is to facilitate the coordination of visceral events with behaviors which impact upon them. The best example relating to the gut is the regulation of ingestive behavior.

The presence or absence of food in the gastrointestinal tract has effects that permeate several aspects of behavior. Lack of food enhances exploratory behavior which is likely to lead to discovery of a food source; ingestion of food reduces levels of arousal and activity that would compete with the demands of the gastrointestinal tract on cardiovascular capacity; food has effects on memory and learning, presumably related to a capacity to find nutrition and avoid poison. In fact, the effects of food on general central neural processes is so extensive that it has been argued that the brain may have evolved primarily to direct feeding behavior.[121] The considerable differences between the cerebral cortices of carnivores and herbivores is a striking example of the effects of feeding patterns on the nature of the brains even from within the same order of animals.

How are Vagal Afferent Functions Organized?

Having seen from the above discussion that there are numerous fundamental reasons for conveying visceral information to the brain, we will now review the components involved. In particular, attention will focus on the generation of conscious sensations. (An anatomical description of these connections by Leslie *et al.* is available in chapter 4 of this volume).

FUNCTIONS SUBSERVED BY GASTROINTESTINAL VAGAL AFFERENTS

This section examines the range of bodily functions which can be influenced by abdominal vagal afferents so that the enormous extent of their influence can be appreciated.

Gastrointestinal Reflexes

Gastrointestinal reflexes are reviewed extensively by H.E. Raybould in chapter 9 of this volume, hence this section will be confined to more general aspects. Since the original demonstration by Harper *et al.*[56] that electrical stimulation of the central end of the abdominal vagus evoked reflex changes in gastric and intestinal motility mediated by vagal efferents, numerous vago-vagal reflexes regulating motility and secretion have been identified. Some examples include: adaptive relaxation of the gastric body,[69] antral mechano- or chemoreceptor induced relaxation of the gastric body,[1,15] distension- and food-induced secretion of gastrin and gastric acid, entero-pancreatic endocrine (insulin) and exocrine secretory reflexes. Esophageal vagal afferents are also capable of modulating gastrointestinal motility; for example, esophageal distension induces relaxation of the proximal stomach by activation of vagally driven non-adrenergic, non-cholinergic intramural neurons.[2] In addition to vago-vagal reflexes the vagal afferents have also been shown to be involved in reflexes in which the splanchnic sympathetic efferents form the motor pathway.[12]

Although vagal efferents clearly have an extensive influence on gastrointestinal function, there are only a few thousand efferent motor fibers in the abdominal vagus. Vagal afferents outnumber the efferents by about ten to one, hence there is a considerable degree of convergence of information between afferents and efferents. This convergence is highlighted by the neurophysiological studies of Grundy *et al.*[52] which demonstrate that individual vagal efferent fibers could be modulated by inputs from the stomach, small intestine and colon. More recent studies demonstrated convergence between abdominal vagal and splanchnic afferents in the nucleus tractus solitarius (NTS).[16]

In addition to vago-vagal reflexes, vagal afferents are also involved in the regulation of motility, secretion and blood flow via local axon reflexes.[34,35] Such reflexes appear to be mainly involved in protection of the gastric mucosa against damage; for example capsaicin treatment of the vagus nerve facilitates the damage induced by ethanol.[65]

Abdominal Visceral Sensation

A wide variety of sensations arise from, or are associated with, the abdominal viscera. These include sensations associated with normal gut function such as emptiness, comfortable fullness and temperature, as well as contrasting sensations associated with disordered function or disease such as pain, bloating and cramping. The mechanisms underlying some of these sensations are outlined below, but it must be emphasized that our knowledge of the signalling and central processing of non-painful visceral sensations is poor and requires considerable experimental investigation.

Pain

The origin of painful sensations has been most extensively investigated and numerous clinical and animal studies have concluded that such sensations are the result of splanchnic or pelvic afferent activation.[24,82] Abdominal vagal afferents have no direct role in visceral pain. However, in the thorax, investigation of patients with high spinal cord lesions or sympathetic chain removal has revealed some indirect evidence for an involvement of vagal afferents in the genesis of esophageal pain and heartburn.

Temperature

In the studies on his fistulous patient Tom, Wolf[117] reported that thermal sensations could be elicited from the gastric mucosa by stimuli above 40°C and below 18°C. The lower esophagus appears more temperature sensitive than the stomach.[62] While formal studies have not been undertaken to show that vagal afferents are responsible for these sensations, the characteristics of vagal afferent thermoreceptors[38] are consistent with such a role. The purpose of such visceral thermoreception is unclear as oropharyngeal thermoreceptors should presumably prevent ingestion of food in these temperature ranges if they were considered undesirable.

Emptiness and Fullness

These sensations associated with the upper abdomen may be regarded as the extremes of a range of normal sensations which are used by the animal to regulate its feeding behavior. The sensations are not generated solely by vagal afferents as studies in humans have shown that sensation is reduced but not abolished by truncal vagotomy.[74] Similar conclusions have been reached from animal studies where the behavioral correlates of the sensations were studied. It appears likely that vagal afferents are responsible for the more acute phase and that other endocrine or central mechanisms are responsible for the more chronic phase.

If vagal afferents are involved, what is the nature of the afferent signal? To answer this question we need to consider first the state of the stomach under the two conditions of fullness and emptiness. The sensation of hunger arises some time after the stomach is emptied and it has long been known that the stomach in food deprived animals is not flaccid but may be quite contracted. In animals deprived of food overnight, gastric vagal afferent receptors with receptive fields in the gastric body or antrum spontaneously discharge.[10] Mucosal receptors may also be involved, since in the empty stomach the prominent rugal folds can rub against each other during gastric contractions. The sensation of emptiness giving rise to hunger can be reduced immediately or even abolished by eating a very small amount of food or even non-food material such as clay.[22] The most likely explanation for these effects is that swallowing evokes a vago-vagal reflex relaxation of the stomach[2] via activation of vagal non-adrenergic, noncholinergic inhibitory neurons which supply the gastric body and which induce a relaxation lasting several minutes, even after a brief period of activation.[13] Such relaxation will lead to decrease in activation of tension receptors. As the stomach fills with food the sensation of emptiness decreases. In humans gastric distension with food induces sensations of fullness and the presence of a gastric balloon decreases meal size both in humans[45] and the dog.[94] Such studies strongly implicate activation of vagal afferent muscle mechanoceptors in the genesis of sensations of normal post-prandial fullness. Mucosal vagal afferents may be involved, not only via their ability to signal the chemical nature of the luminal contents, but also because they signal the stretching of the gastric mucosa which occurs as the stomach fills.

From the preceding discussion it can be seen that the discharge in gastric muscle mechanoceptors (and possibly mucosal receptors) is involved in the genesis of sensations of both emptiness and fullness. At first sight this may seem strange, but it is likely that the precise nature of the afferent signal under the two conditions is subtly different. In addition, there is some evidence to suggest that other factors may modify the interpretation of the visceral afferent signal. In esophagostomized dogs, gastric distension 5-40 minutes prior to, and during, sham feeding has no satiety effect, but if the distension occurs once sham feeding has begun, feeding is curtailed.[68]

Convergence of orosensory and visceral afferent information occurs in the hypothalamus, an area where neurons are activated by circulating nutrients. Thus, there are likely to be complex interactions between inputs, which in turn will determine the nature of the signal reaching the visceral cortex and hence the sensation generated.

Although attention has focused on the role of gastric vagal mechanoceptors in the genesis of sensations, various animal studies have implicated vagal intestinal mucosal chemoceptors and hepatic portal vein osmoceptors in various types of satiety. It is possible that such afferents are also involved in the genesis of visceral sensations. The role of vagal afferent cues in hunger and satiety is extensively discussed in chapters 10 and 11 of this volume.

Nausea and Early Satiety

The involvement of vagal afferents in non-painful, but nevertheless unpleasant, sensations arising from the abdomen is currently under investigation because of its major clinical relevance to gastrointestinal disorders such as nonulcer dyspepsia. This section considers only the possibility of vagal afferents initiating these sensations and does not discuss the central generation of such sensations nor their "referral" to the gut.

Lewis[82] reported that electrical stimulation of the central end of the vagus in humans elicited nausea. In animals and humans high, but not painful, levels of gastric distension evoke nausea or its behavioral correlates, with vomiting ensuing if still higher levels of distension are used. While distension, particularly of the gastric antrum, is a nauseogenic stimulus, studies in humans suggest that nausea induced by a variety of stimuli is associated with antral hypomotility[73] and antral tachygastria (e.g. Geldof *et al.*[44]). It is unclear at present whether this association is causally linked. Although this section has focused on visceral afferents as the origin of the sensation, the focus is not meant to exclude an involvement of central sites such as the area postrema (see section on taste aversion below).

Early satiety, a feeling of fullness following a small meal, is a particularly interesting symptom as it may represent a heightened state of abnormal sensation. In the section on emptiness and hunger it was argued that these sensations are at least partly generated by abdominal vagal afferents and hence early satiety may result from a modification of such signals. This may occur in two main ways: muscle properties or afferent sensitization.

Muscle Properties

The mechanoceptors located in the gastric smooth muscle signal the wall tension. Factors which alter the wall tension will modify the discharge in these afferents as the stomach is distended. For example, "resting" tension could be increased by elevated activity in intrinsic or extrinsic cholinergic (vagal) neurons or by reduced activity in intrinsic or vagally driven non-adrenergic, noncholinergic pathways involved in adaptive gastric relaxation to a meal. Under these conditions a meal of normal size will cause a larger increase in wall tension and hence a higher vagal afferent discharge. If vagal afferent activity generates the sensation of fullness, then under these conditions it will be elicited with smaller meals than usual. It is possible that the aversion to food seen in anorexia nervosa may be the consequence of a learned aversion resulting initially from the generation of unpleasant sensations of early satiety and nausea by eating.

Afferent Sensitization

The properties of afferents may be directly affected by locally released chemicals such as 5-hydroxytryptamine and bradykinin acting on the afferent terminal to sensitize the transduction mechanism so that the afferent has an enhanced response to natural stimulation (see Andrews[6] for references). In addition, the perception of visceral events may also be modified by changes in the central processing of afferent signals. Some evidence for involvement of such mechanisms comes from clinical studies of patients with esophageal chest pain[105] and irritable bowel syndrome.[86]

Nausea and Vomiting

Although nausea and vomiting are most frequently encountered in a clinical context as a symptom of disease (particularly gastrointestinal) or as a result of therapies such as anti-cancer radio- and chemotherapy, they are also key components of the body's defense against ingested toxins. Accidental ingestion of toxins is avoided by using the senses of vision, taste and smell to avoid, for example, brightly colored bitter-tasting foods. If the animal has eaten the food before and illness (e.g., nausea, vomiting or pain) resulted, the animal remembers this and will subsequently reject the food. If, however, the presence of the toxin is somehow masked or the feeding habit precludes adequate tasting (such as when carnivores bolt their food), then the toxin must be identified in the upper gut.

There is a considerable body of evidence demonstrating a role for putative antral and duodenal mucosal vagal afferents in the activation of the emetic pathways:

1) Electrical stimulation of the central end of the abdominal vagus, but not of the greater splanchnic nerve, induces emesis.[7]

2) There is an emetic response to intra-gastric administration of hypertonic solutions or copper sulphate.[8]

3) Vomiting induced by the common food poisoning bacterium *Staphylococcus* is reduced or abolished by abdominal denervation.[37]

4) Vomiting induced by total body irradiation and systemically administered cytotoxic drugs can be reduced or abolished by abdominal vagotomy but not by greater splanchnic nerve section,[8] indicating that these stimuli act by vagal afferent activation.[8] These and other studies led to the proposal that 5-hydroxytryptamine -3 receptor antagonists, used as selective anti-emetic agents against radio- and chemotherapy induced emesis, have a vagal afferent site of action.[14]

The emetic reflex can also be activated by distension of the upper gut, particularly of regions such as the gastric antrum and duodenum which have little storage capacity (see Andrews and Hawthorn[11] for discussion)

The actual vomiting induced by abdominal vagal afferent activation is due to a compression of the stomach by the diaphragm and the anterior abdominal muscles leading to the expulsion of the contents of the upper gut. Before this happens, a number of other events occur, particularly in the gastrointestinal tract. These include relaxation of the proximal stomach under the influence of vagal efferents activating non-adrenergic, non-cholinergic inhibitory neurons.[77] The function of this relaxation is probably to delay the emptying of ingested contaminated food and to place the stomach in the most mechanically advantageous position for compression. In addition, a giant retrograde contraction originating in the small intestine sweeps toward the stomach.[77] This wave is initiated by vagal efferents and may serve to return contaminated contents to the stomach, the only place from which food can be expelled by vomiting. It has been argued that the bile and pancreatic juice which will also be returned may buffer the gastric contents prior to ejection.[77]

Thus, it can be seen that all the major components of the emetic reflex have a function contributing to its overall protective nature. In addition, the nausea which usually precedes vomiting will discourage the animal from continuing to ingest the food and will also lead to the formation of an aversive response to the food if encountered again.[42]

If toxins are not detected in the gut, they may be absorbed. Emesis may be triggered from the area postrema, or "chemoceptor trigger zone for emesis," a circumventricular organ located at the caudal part of the fourth ventricle (see Borison[19] for review). While there is little doubt that emesis can be induced from this structure, in a real biological context it is probably best regarded as the final line of detection in a hierarchially organized defensive system.[33]

Cardiovascular Influences

Increases in blood pressure due to noxious stimulation of the abdominal viscera by bradykinin or capsaicin are mediated predominantly via splanchnic afferents, the vagus having only a minor involvement.[83,84] Nevertheless, electrical stimulation of the central end of the abdominal vagus induces an increase in blood pressure in the ferret[7] and application of irritant chemicals (e.g., sodium hydroxide) to the antral mucosa increases blood pressure in animals treated with guanethidine and with the greater splanchnic nerve cut.[15] In the rat, Grundy and Davison[51] reported modulation of heart rate by large gastric contractions.

These cardiovascular influences of abdominal vagal afferents may be involved in the circulatory adjustments needed to cope with the increase in the proportion of the cardiac output taken by the gastrointestinal circulation following a meal.

Respiratory Effects

Stimulation of the abdominal visceral afferents produces a characteristic apnoeic response followed by depression of diaphragmatic activity. These changes are accompanied by an increase in intercostal and upper airway muscular activity (*alae nasi*, posterior cricoarytenoid). The apnoeic and diaphragmatic responses are mediated by splanchnic afferents whereas the intercostal and airway responses are vagally dependent.[49] In this study the levels of distension used were without effect on blood pressure and hence were unlikely to be in the noxious range. Thus, abdominal afferents may have a normal role in respiratory modulation in addition to the well-known apnoeic responses accompanying painful stimulation.

Besides intestinal afferents, esophageal vagal afferents also appear to have the capacity to modulate respiration, since esophageal distension induces a vagally dependent inhibition of the diaphragm and enhancement of inspiratory intercostal and upper airway muscle activity.[27]

As well as motor effects, abdominal vagal afferents can also reflexly induce secretion in the airways. In the cat, gastric distension induced an increase in fluid secretion from the submucosal mucous glands of the trachea. This response was abolished by abdominal vagotomy.[46] The function of this reflex is unknown, but German *et al.*[46] suggested that because gastric irritation is a potent stimulus for emesis, tracheal secretion may protect the airways and lungs from any aspirated vomitus. Interestingly, some agents used as expectorants, such as ipecacuanha syrup, are also used as orally administered emetic agents.

Endocrine Effects

Apart from the reflex release of gastrointestinal hormones, vagal afferents have also been implicated in the release of vasopressin. In the anesthetized ferret, electrical stimulation of the central end of the abdominal vagus leads to a large increase of plasma vasopressin but not of oxytocin.[58] The natural stimulus evoking this response is unknown, but in view of the link between vasopressin and nausea observed in primates, stimuli that induce emesis (e.g. over-distension) would appear likely candidates, although this is not supported by studies of gastric distension in humans.[90] In contrast, in the rat, oxytocin but not vasopressin is released in response to stimuli that induce emesis in other species (e.g., intragastric $CuSO_4$).[114] Gastric distension caused by isotonic saline or large volumes of food induce release of oxytocin but not of vasopressin.[104]

Taken together, these studies show that abdominal vagal afferent information reaches the paraventricular nucleus to evoke vasopressin or oxytocin secretion, depending on the species. The functional significance of the release remains unclear. Cholecystokinin octapeptide (CCK-OP) is thought to exert its satiety effect mainly by activation of abdominal vagal afferents. In humans and the monkey, CCK-OP induces a substantial release of vasopressin when given at doses producing aversive symptoms. Moreover, similar studies in the rat demonstrated release of oxytocin but not vasopressin. In the rat the response is attenuated by capsaicin. Gastric distension has been shown to activate oxytocinergic cells in the rat hypothalamus.[104]

Somatic Motor Reflexes

Although cardio-pulmonary vagal afferents have long been known to exert profound influences on somatic motor reflexes (see below), the influence of abdominal vagal afferents is less well studied.

One of the earliest studies indicating that abdominal visceral afferents could modulate somatic reflexes was the observation in humans by Cannon and Carlson[23] that during large gastric contractions there was an enhancement in the magnitude of the patellar reflex.

In the rabbit, Petorossi[96] demonstrated that the masseteric jaw reflex was reduced both by electrical stimulation of the central end of the abdominal vagus and by gastric distension, the latter effect depending upon an intact vagal innervation. It was proposed that this reflex may facilitate opening of the mouth prior to vomiting induced by emetic stimuli acting on gastric afferents.

Abdominal vagal afferents appear to have a more general modulatory effect on somatic reflexes, because peripherally administered caerulein induced a vagally dependent suppression of the crossed extensor reflex in the rat.[72] The response was mimicked by electrical stimulation of vagal afferents.

Exploratory Behavior and Locomotion

A hungry animal explores the environment, maximizing its chances of discovering food, whereas a sated animal rests, redirecting its physiological processes toward digestion while decreasing its exposure to predators and conserving energy. As the principal nerve monitoring the state of the gastrointestinal tract, the vagus is strategically situated to mediate the influence of recent ingestion, or its lack, on exploratory behavior.

The abdominal vagus is the route by which cholecystokinin, released in response to ingestion, engenders satiety and reduces exploration. Peripherally administered CCK-8 increases locomotor pauses, decreases movement and decreases investigative approaches, all by an action requiring the abdominal vagus.[31] The complex effects of cholecystokinin on central dopaminergic neurons, critically involved in locomotion, are heavily dependent on the vagus or the solitary nucleus for both mediation and modulation.[66] To add to this complexity, the degree of obesity alters the modulating or mediating influence of the vagus.[93]

Cerulatide, related to cholecystokinin, reduces central dopaminergic activity via an action on the abdominal vagus.[55] Interestingly, cerulatide also increases dopaminergic activity, presumably via an effect on area postrema or a related circumventricular organ, in the absence of the abdominal vagus.

It is apparent that the abdominal vagus not only affects the central nervous system at a level as low as simple reflexes, as indicated in the previous section, but also influences much higher levels of behavior, such as the action of at least two ingestion-related hormones on cortico-striato-cortical circuits.

Arousal

The effects of a heavy meal on drowsiness and of hunger on insomnia are well known. Tonically active tension receptors innervated by the abdominal vagus are alleged to contribute to the electroencephalographic sleep induced by rhythmic intestinal distension, although splanchnically innervated phasic receptors account for most of this influence.[75] Whereas the humoral effects of ingestion are mainly on paradoxical sleep, the viscerosensory contribution of the vagus is to increase the duration and decrease the latency of slow wave sleep.[76]

Serotonin (5-HT) has a central role in sleep mechanisms, and cholecystokinin, released in response to ingestion, alters central 5-HT metabolism by an action dependent on the vagus.[93]

Taste Perception

Olfaction and gustation give an early indication of the nature of ingested and inhaled substances before ingestion is complete. Coupled to past experience and reinforcement mechanisms, this provides a powerful protective system to which the vagus contributes in several ways.

There is a direct contribution to gustation provided by the vagal gustatory innervation of the epiglottis. A more subtle contribution is that the relevance of food is altered by recent ingestion and this effect is mediated by the vagus, together with the hypothalamus. Thus gastric distension, the nature of gastric luminal contents and the nutrients absorbed into the hepatic portal vein all modify central gustatory transmission. For example, gastric vagal mechanoceptors reduce the response to sapid stimuli in the rodent solitary nucleus,[48] depending on the length of food deprivation. Although this effect is not seen in monkeys,[119] intragastric loads reduce the hedonic value of food in humans.[20] Furthermore, interoceptors signaling visceral illness or deficiency can convert an initially innocuous taste into an aversive signal.[106]

Such modification of gustatory afference by vagal activity may reflect the frequent corepresentation of gustatory and vagal afference in central pathways, all the way from the solitary nucleus through parabrachial, thalamic and hypothalamic nuclei and the limbic system to the final destination in the cerebral cortex.[61] Thus, gustatory units in the orbitofrontal cortex,[119] but not in the anterior insula,[120] alter their response rates with varying degrees of satiation. Olfaction also converges on central vagal representation, an interaction being possible as far caudally as the parabrachial nuclei.[92]

Taste is a principal determinant of whether intraoral contents will be ingested or rejected. Ingestion and rejection share several of the same neuromuscular components, differing mainly in the sequence in which the components appear.[112] The particular sequence generated by an oral stimulus can be altered by visceral vagal afferents. The vagus, therefore, provides the context which gives an oral stimulus meaning, altering its signal from "ingest" to "reject."

Taste Aversion

Conditioned taste aversion is perhaps one of the best examples of the protective role of the vagus. Lesions of the vagus attenuate or abolish those conditioned taste aversions that depend on unconditioned gastrointestinal stimuli, such as low doses of intragastric copper sulphate.[29] Abdominal vagotomy also abolishes conditioned taste aversions where the unconditioned stimulus is rotation.[40] Since this topic is reviewed elsewhere, only a few comments pertinent to the current hypothesis will be made.

There is a specific affinity between visceral illness signaled by the vagus and taste, on the one hand, and a corresponding affinity between somatic nociception and exteroceptive modalities, on the other.[41] The effect of visceral illness signalled by the vagus is to produce a context free, primary change in the hedonic value of a gustatory stimulus. This is in contrast to the aversive properties of exteroceptive visual, somatic and auditory modalities, which depend for their effect on the context and are aversive only because of what they imply in that context. These differences may be related to the different anatomical routes to the amygdala taken by the two sets of information, one directly from first order solitary synapses, the others reaching the amygdala only after traversing the relevant sensory cortex. The anatomical differences may, in turn, reflect a different phylogenetic history for these two classes of aversive learning.

Conditioned taste aversion modifies the response at the first central synapse in the solitary nucleus[25] which, together with the parabrachial nuclei,[36] is a target for descending cerebral influences.[85] Perhaps these descending influences are part of the reason why decerebration abolishes conditioned taste aversions.[92] It is not yet clear which component of the cerebrum is essential.

Learning and Memory

Conditioned taste aversion is not the only link between food and learning. A meal increases the memory of all aversive learning.[39] Cholecystokinin, released in response to ingestion, has memory-enhancing effects mediated by the vagus. Vagal activity evokes the secretion of neurohypophyseal hormones and these have direct effects on aversive learning. For example, an intracerebroventricular injection of oxytocin attenuates, whereas arginine vasopressin enhances, passive avoidance; hypophysectomy impairs shuttle box avoidance; rats deficient in neurohypophyseal hormones have difficulty acquiring and maintaining avoidance responses. There are, therefore, several mechanisms whereby interoceptive states signaled by the vagus can influence the learning of avoidance behavior. This is clearly much more than would be expected of a purely autonomic or visceral nerve.

FUNCTIONS SUBSERVED BY EXTRA-GASTROINTESTINAL VAGAL AFFERENTS

Respiratory Reflexes

The lung inflation and deflation reflexes demonstrated by Hering and Breuer[60] were probably the first reflexes involving vagal afferents to be described. Since then many other reflexes activated by vagal afferents have been identified, such as the aortic arch chemoceptor reflexes described by Heymans and Heymans[63] in 1927. For a comparative review of respiratory reflexes see Widdicombe.[115]

Because this review is primarily concerned with the defensive roles of vagal afferents, this section will be confined to the involvement of the vagus in triggering involuntary coughing. Coughing is an important defensive reflex for the airways, analogous to vomiting for the gut. It is triggered primarily by mechanical or chemical stimulation of the larynx and upper tracheobronchial tree.[71,116]

Vagal afferents also participate in bronchoconstriction, another protective airway reflex, but the receptor type appears different from that involved in coughing.[71,116] The role of vagal afferents in the generation of sensations such as breathlessness is unclear.

In addition to an involvement in visceral and somatic reflexes, vagal airway afferents with unmyelinated axons have recently been shown to be involved in axon reflexes. These are involved in secretory, motor and vascular changes in the airways induced by inflammatory stimuli.[17]

Cardiovascular Reflexes

The involvement of vagal and glossopharyngeal afferents supplying the aortic arch and carotid sinus arterial baroreceptors in the reflex control of the circulation was first described by Hering and Heymans in the late 1920s (see Heymans and Neil[64]). Since then vagal afferents supplying the atria and ventricles have been identified and their influence on the cardiovascular system described (see Hainsworth *et al.*[54] for review). Although at first sight the cardiovascular receptors may not appear to have a defensive function, this is an incorrect impression. For example, they are critically involved in the short (e.g., maintenance of cardiac output) and longer term (fluid intake) responses to hemorrhage which may occur as a result of aggression or accident.

In addition, they are necessary for the cardiovascular adjustments required for the intense muscular activity needed to escape from a predator.

Stimulation of vagal cardiovascular receptors can evoke the classical defense reaction.[18] If the function of these vagal afferents were only to regulate blood pressure, heart rate and respiration, this would be a perplexing effect. An account of the connection between vagal activity and defense will be offered in the final section.

Nausea and Vomiting

One of the most intriguing phylogenetic mysteries is the link between the vagus, the transducer for orientation and for detection of oscillations in the surrounding medium, and nausea and vomiting. In fish, both orientation within the environment and the detection of objects by the vibrations they generate, are transduced by the lateral line system, which is innervated by facial, glossopharyngeal and vagal nerves. In terrestrial vertebrates, both functions are the province of the membranous labyrinth, which is innervated by the vestibulocochlear nerve, but the three lateral line nerves (facial, glossopharyngeal and vagal) retain an innervation of the structures surrounding the labyrinth, namely the outer and middle ears. That emesis and an increase in gastric capacity can be evoked by stimulation of the ears of feasting Romans and over-indulging aldermen has passed into legend, indicating that vagal aural receptors induce vomiting. At the same time, abnormal stimulation of the labyrinth is a strong stimulus for nausea and vomiting, as any nautical tyro will testify. It has been suggested that the brain uses mismatch between vestibular and visual input to detect poisoning,[113] and removal of the labyrinths impairs the effectiveness of some emetic agents.[91] Furthermore, it has been shown that vestibular stimulation evokes a vagal response.[4] Apart from aural vagal receptors, cardiac vagal receptors are also able to induce gastric relaxation and vomiting.[3]

Arousal

The cervical vagus contains rapidly conducting fibers that can induce electroencephalographic sleep, and more slowly conducting fibers that can induce desynchronization.[26] Aortic baroreceptors innervated by the vagus are capable of inducing the complete sleep cycle in encephale isole cats.[98] In REM-deprived animals, this is accompanied by cataplexy. Hypnogenic stimulation of the cervical vagus is accompanied by increased discharge rates in the reticular nucleus of the thalamus and decreased rates in the ventroposterior nucleus.[70]

Analgesia

Over the past ten years, neurophysiological and behavioral studies have demonstrated that vagal afferents, particularly those supplying cardio-pulmonary structures, modulate the nociceptive responses to a variety of painful stimuli. The most thoroughly studied nociceptive reflex is the tail-flick reflex induced by noxious levels of thermal stimulation. The latency of this reflex is increased by electrical stimulation of the cervical or abdominal vagus[100,111] or by chemical activation of cardiopulmonary afferents with veratridine, or with the opioid receptor agonist [D-Ala]-methionine enkephalinamide.[102] These behavioral studies are supported by neurophysiological studies which indicate that the pathway for this effect is vagal afferent activation of the nucleus tractus solitarius, which in turn activates a potent descending system modulating spinal nociceptive transmission in the dorsal horn of the spinal cord.[103] In addition to studies examining cutaneous noxious stimuli, Thies and Foreman[110] have demonstrated that vagal afferents can modulate transmission in the spinoreticular neurons noxiously activated by coronary artery occlusion or intracardiac bradykinin.

The function of vagal afferent modulation of nociceptive pathways is unclear but Randich and Maixner[102] propose that such pathways are involved in analgesia induced by stress and acupuncture. They propose that endogenous agents capable of activating these afferents are released. This is certainly a possibility as, for example, sympathetic stimulation of the adrenal gland releases enkephalin-like peptides.[50] They suggest that one group of vagal afferents involved are the baroreceptors, because volume expansion produces a long-lasting inhibition of the tail flick response, and many stressful events are accompanied by an elevation of blood pressure or central venous pressure.[101] This is supported by a recent study showing that, in patients with chronic pain syndromes, the pain rating was lower during carotid sinus baroreceptor activation by neck suction.[59]

A study in the rat demonstrated a naloxone-sensitive reduction in the tail flick response induced by mild food deprivation.[87] This may be the natural correlate of the abdominal vagal afferent modulation of the tail flick response reported by Thurston and Randich.[111]

Somatic Muscle Reflexes

Numerous studies dating back over fifty years have demonstrated that cervical vagal afferent stimulation can modulate somatic muscle reflex activity driven by a variety of stimuli. One of the earliest and most dramatic demonstrations of this effect was by Schweitzer and Wright,[107] who reported that electrical central vagal stimulation could abolish feline convulsions induced by strychnine. More recent studies have shown that both electrical and chemical (e.g. phenylbiguanide nicotine, lobeline) stimulation of vagal afferents supplying cardiopulmonary structures depress both alpha and gamma motoneuron activity.[47] The function proposed for such visceral modulation of somatic motor activity is to protect the organism against physical over exertion. Ginzel and

Eldridge[47] comment that this visceral afferent suppression of somatic muscular activity will encourage the animal to assume a recumbent position, which in itself may promote sleep. As described above, cardiopulmonary vagal afferents are able to induce alterations in the synchronization of the EEG.

In addition to modulating these postural somatic reflexes, cardiopulmonary afferents can also influence the somatic components of the coughing and vomiting reflexes involving the diaphragm and abdominal muscles. In the cat pulmonary C-fiber activation by capsaicin or phenylbiguanide inhibited the coughing and sneezing reflexes and reduced the aspiration reflex.[109] The retching induced by electrical stimulation of canine abdominal vagal afferents can be blocked by cervical vagal afferent stimulation[122] and in the conscious ferret, retching and vomiting induced by both central (opiate) and peripheral (radiation) emetic stimuli can be transiently reduced by activation of cardiopulmonary afferents by phenylbiguanide or 5-hydroxytryptamine (Andrews and Bhandari, unpublished observations).

The above section shows the powerful modulatory influences that vagal afferents have on somatic motor activity, but we have little idea of the natural circumstances under which such influences are exerted.

Endocrine Functions

Baroreceptors from the carotid sinus (glossopharyngeal afferents), aortic arch (vagal afferents) and the low pressure "volume" receptors in the atria (vagal afferents) all can suppress the release of vasopressin from the posterior pituitary, leading to a diuresis (see Harris and Loewy[57] for review). These afferents play a major role in postural cardiovascular adjustment, control of plasma volume and the adaptive responses to sudden hemorrhage.

The inhibition of vasopressin secretion contrasts with the effect of abdominal vagal afferent activation which induces an increase in plasma vasopressin.[58]

THE VAGUS AS THE INTERO-PROTECTIVE NERVE: AN HYPOTHESIS

Categorization of efferents as autonomic versus somatic, and then as parasympathetic versus sympathetic, has provided a useful framework for subsequent investigation. Unfortunately, the consequence of this particular categorization is that afferent nerves traveling with the vagus have no particular niche. Langley,[78] realizing that differences in function can rarely be isolated from differences in structure, avoided categorizing afferents because he could detect no histological marker identifying autonomic fibers. Dissatisfaction with this has recently led to alternative proposals contrasting A and B fibers, but excluding vagal afferents.[99] We feel that there is now sufficient evidence to supersede attempts to link afferents, on the basis of their peripheral distribution, to the efferents with which they travel. The dichotomy is not between somatic afferents projecting to somatic efferents, on the one hand, versus visceral afferents projecting to autonomic efferents, on the other, nor any variation of this. A major consequence of having a central nervous system, as opposed to a series of isolated ganglia, is that afferents from either source can evoke responses in both sets of efferents; there is no "fracture line" in the brain separating autonomic from somatic functions.

We suggest that a more profitable approach is to view structure and function from the perspective of possible phylogenetic history. One of us has suggested that the vagal afferents are a major portal of entry to a collection of subependymal and subpial nuclei that once served the function of generating escape from, and subsequent avoidance of, suboptimal conditions.[79,80,81] These nuclei may be called the paraventricular system. Efferent connections from the central nervous system to viscera were limited (vagal efferents not extending as far caudally as the stomach, for example), so central neural contributions to maintenance of homeostasis were restricted to escape and avoidance of perturbing stimuli. As autonomic efferents extended their peripheral influence, however, the paraventricular system acquired the capacity to substitute regulation via visceral efferents for regulation by somatic escape but retained its former functions.

Vagal afferents had a more extensive distribution than vagal efferents, and indeed still outnumber efferents even in mammals. Thus, originally vagal afferents could project only to the paraventricular system involved in protective and defensive somatic reflexes. We suggest that this was their primordial function, exemplified by vagal innervation of the lateral line system. Now that the paraventricular system can achieve the same protective ends by autonomic means, vagal afferents have also acquired the capacity to drive sympathetic and parasympathetic efferents. Protective and defensive responses have been supplemented by homeostatic reflexes, and vagal afferents have an obvious role to play in these. Less obvious (in the literature) is the contribution of the vagus to protective and defensive responses. The evidence presented above is intended to demonstrate that the vagus makes significant contributions to protective reflexes and responses, regardless of whether the responses are somatic or visceral. The contribution of the vagus to protection and defense is made at levels from simple axon reflexes confined to the periphery, through classical oligosynaptic reflexes limited to the brain stem, finally to complex behavioral responses involving the corpus striatum, thalamus and cerebral cortex. The common factor in all cases is that some noxious stimulus is detected by vagal afferents and a protective response made by any appropriate efferent system, be it somatic, autonomic or endocrine. The vagus nerve could be called "the wandering protector." In view of the remarkable extent of its distribution to respiratory, cardiovascular, gastrointestinal and other systems, covering a surface area many times larger than any other nerve, perhaps "great wandering protector" would be a more appropriate epithet.

REFERENCES

1. **Abrahamsson, H.,** Vagal relaxation of the stomach induced from the gastric antrum, *Acta Physiol. Scand.*, 89, 406-414, 1973.
2. **Abrahamsson, H., and Jansson, G.,** Reflex vagal relaxation of the stomach from the pharynx and oesophagus in the cat, *Acta Physiol. Scand.*, 77, 172-178, 1969.
3. **Abrahamsson, H., and Thoren, P.,** Vomiting and reflex vagal relaxation of the stomach elicited from heart receptors in the cat, *Acta Physiol. Scand.*, 88, 433-439, 1973.
4. **Akert, K., and Gernandt, B.E.,** Neurophysiological study of vestibular and limbic influences upon vagal outflow, *Electroencephalogr. Clin. Neurophysiol.*, 14, 904-914, 1962.
5. **Andrews, P.L.R.,** Vagal afferent innervation of the gastrointestinal tract, *Prog. Brain Res.*, 67, 65-86, 1986.
6. **Andrews, P.L.R.,** Modulation of visceral afferent activity as a therapeutic possibility for gastrointestinal disorders, in *Irritable Bowel Syndrome*, Read, N.W., Ed., Blackwell Scientific, London, 1991, 91-121.
7. **Andrews, P.L.R., Bingham, S., and Davis, C.J.,** Retching evoked by stimulation of abdominal vagal afferents in anesthetized ferrets, *J. Physiol.*, 358, 103P, 1985.
8. **Andrews, P.L.R., Davis, C.J., Bingham, S. Davidson, H.I.M., Hawthorn, J., and Maskell, L.,** The abdominal visceral innervation and the emetic reflex: Pathways, pharmacology and plasticity, *Can. J. Physiol. Pharmacol.*, 68, 325-345, 1990.
9. **Andrews, P.L.R., Grundy, D., and Scratcherd, T.,** The reflex activation of antral motility by gastric distension in the ferret, *J. Physiol.*, 298, 79-84, 1980.
10. **Andrews, P.L.R., Grundy, D., and Scratcherd, T.,** Vagal afferent discharge from mechanoreceptors in different regions of the ferret stomach, *J. Physiol.*, 298, 513-524, 1980.
11. **Andrews, P.L.R., and Hawthorn, J.,** The neurophysiology of nausea and vomiting, in *Neurophysiology of the Gut*, Read, N.J., and Grundy, D., Eds., Bailliere's Clinical Gastroenterology 2, Bailliere and Tindall, London, 1988, 141-168.
12. **Andrews, P.L.R., and Lawes, I.N.C.,** Interactions between the vagus and splanchnic nerves in the control of mean intragastric pressure in the ferret, *J. Physiol.*, 351, 473-490, 1984.
13. **Andrews, P.L.R., and Lawes, I.N.C.,** Characteristics of the vagally driven non-adrenergic, non-cholinergic inhibitory innervation of the ferret corpus, *J. Physiol.*, 1-20, 1985.
14. **Andrews, P.L.R., Rapeport, W.G., and Sanger, G.J.,** Neuropharmacology of emesis induced by anti-cancer therapy, *Trends in Pharmacological Sciences*, 9, 334-341, 1988.
15. **Andrews, P.L.R., and Wood, K.L.,** Vagally mediated gastric motor and emetic reflexes evoked by stimulation of the antral mucosa in anesthetized ferrets, *J. Physiol.*, 395, 1-16, 1988.
16. **Barber, W.D., and Yuan, C.,** Gastric vagal-splanchnic interactions in the brain stem of the cat, *Brain Res.*, 487, 1-8, 1989.
17. **Barnes, P.J.,** Neurogenic inflammation in the airways and its modulation, *Arch. Int. Pharmacodyn Ther.*, 303, 67-82, 1990.
18. **Bizzi, E., Libretti, A., Malliani, A., and Zanchetti, A.,** Reflex chemoceptive excitation of diencephalic sham rage behavior, *Am. J. Physiol.*, 200, 923, 1961.
19. **Borison, H.L.,** Area postrema: Chemoreceptor circumventricular organ of the medulla oblongata, *Prog. Neurobiol.*, 32, 351-390, 1989.
20. **Cabanac, M., and Duclax, R.,** Specificity of internal signals in producing satiety for taste stimuli, *Nature*, 227, 966-967, 1970.
21. **Cannon, W.B.,** *Bodily Changes in Pain, Hunger, Fear and Rage; an Account of Recent Researches into the Function of Emotional Excitement*, 2nd Ed., D. Appleton and Co., New York, 1929.
22. **Cannon, W.B., and Washburn, A.L.,** An explanation of hunger, *Am. J. Physiol.*, 24, 441-454, 1912.
23. **Cannon, W.B., Carlson, A.J.,** *The Control of Hunger in Health and Disease*, University of Chicago Press, 1916.

24. **Cervero, F.,** Neurophysiology of gastrointestinal pain, in *Neurophysiology of the Gut*, Read, N.J., and Grundy, D., Eds., Baillier's Clinical Gastroenterology 2, Bailliere and Tindal, London, 1988, 183-199.

25. **Chang, F-C.T., and Scott, T.R.,** Conditioned taste aversions modify neural responses in the rat nucleus tractus solitarius, *J. Neurosci*, 4, 1850-1862, 1984.

26. **Chase, M.H., Nakamura, Y., Clemente, C.D., and Sterman, B.,** Afferent vagal stimulation: Neurographic correlates of induced EEG synchronization, *Exp. Neurol.*, 5, 236-249, 1967.

27. **Cherniak, N.S., Haxhiu, M.A., Mitra, J., Strohl, K., and van Lunteren, E.,** Responses of upper airway, intercostal and diaphragm muscle activity to stimulation of oesophageal afferents in dogs. *J. Physiol.*, 349, 15-25, 1984.

28. **Christensen, J.,** Origin of sensation in the esophagus, *Am. J. Physiol.*, 246, 221-225, 1984.

29. **Coil, J.D., Rogers, R.C., Garcia, J., and Novin, D.,** Conditioned taste aversions: Vagal and circulatory mediation of the toxic unconditioned stimulus, *Behav. Biol.*, 24, 509-519, 1978.

30. **Coupland, R.E., Parker, T.L., Kesse, W.K., and Mohamed, A.A.,** The innervation of the adrenal gland. III. Vagal innervation, *J. Anat.*, 163, 173-181, 1989.

31. **Crawley, J.N., Hays, S.E., and Paul, S.M.,** Vagotomy abolishes the inhibitory effects of cholecystokinin on rat exploratory behaviours, *Eur. J. Pharmacol.*, 73, 379-380, 1981.

32. **Dale, H.H.,** *Adventures in Physiology*, The Wellcome Trust, London, 1965.

33. **Davis, C.J., Harding, C.J., Leslie, R.A., and Andrews, P.L.R.,** The organization of the vomiting reflex, in *Nausea and vomiting: Mechanisms and treatment*, Davis, C.J., Lake-Bakaar, G.V., and Grahame-Smith, D.G., Eds., Springer-Verlag, Berlin, 1986.

34. **Delbro, D., Fandriks, L., Rosell, S., and Folkers, K.,** Inhibition of antidromically induced stimulation of gastric motility by substance P receptor blockade, *Acta Physiol. Scand.*, 118, 309-316, 1983.

35. **Delbro, D., Lissander, B., and Andersson, S.A.,** Atropine sensitive smooth muscle excitation by mucosal nociceptive stimulation—the involvement of an axon reflex? *Acta Physiol. Scand.*, 122, 621-627, 1984.

36. **Di Lorenzo, P.M.,** Taste responses in the parabrachial pons of decerebrate rats, *J. Neurophysiol.*, 59, 1871-1887, 1988.

37. **Elwell, M.R., Liu, C.T., Spertzel, R.O., and Beisel, W.R.,** Mechanism of oral enterotoxin-B induced emesis in the monkey, *Proc. Soc. Exp. Biol. Med.*, 148, 424-427, 1975.

38. **El Ouazzani, T., and Mei, N.,** Electrophysiological properties and role of the vagal thermoreceptors of lower oesophagus and stomach, *Gastroenterology*, 83, 995-1001, 1982.

39. **Flood, J.F., Smith, G.E., and Morley, J.E.,** Modulation of memory processing by cholecystokinin: Dependence on the vagus nerve, *Science*, 236, 832-834, 1987.

40. **Fox, R.A., and McKenna, S.,** Conditioned taste aversion induced by motion is prevented by selective vagotomy in the rat, *Behav. Neural Biol.*, 50, 275-284, 1988.

41. **Garcia, J., and Ervin, F.R.,** Gustatory-visceral and telereceptor-cutaneous conditioning: Adaptation in internal and external milieus, *Commun. Behav. Biol.*, A1, 389-415, 1968.

42. **Garcia, J., Lasiter, P.S., Bermudez-Rattoni, F., and Deems, D.A.,** A general theory of aversion learning, *Ann. N.Y. Acad.*, *Sci.*, 443, 8-21, 1985.

43. **Gaskell, W.H.,** *The Involuntary Nervous System*, Longmans, Green, 1916.

44. **Geldof, H., van der Schee, E.J., van Blankenstein, M., and Grashuis, J.L.,** Electrogastrographic study of gastric myoelectrical activity in patients with unexplained nausea and vomiting, *Gut*, 27, 799-808, 1986.

45. **Geliebter, A.,** Gastric distension and gastric capacity in relation to food intake in humans, *Physiol. Behav.*, 44, 665-668, 1988.

46. **German, V.F., Corrales, R., Ueki, I.F., and Nadel, J.A.,** Reflex stimulation of tracheal mucus gland secretion by gastric irritation in cats, *J. Appl. Physiol.*, 52, 1153-1155, 1982.

47. **Ginzel, K.H., and Eldridge, E.,** Reflex depression of somatic motor activity from heart, lungs and carotid sinus, in *Respiratory Adaptations, Capillary Exchange and Reflex Mechanisms*, Paintal, A.S., and Gill-Kumar, P., Eds., Delhi, 1975, 358-395.

48. **Glenn, J.F., and Erickson, R.P.,** Gastric modulation of afferent activity, *Physiol. Behav.*, 16, 561-568, 1976.

49. **Gottfried, S.B., and Di Marco, A.,** Effect of intestinal afferent stimulation on pattern of respiratory muscle activation, *J. Appl. Physiol.*, 66, 1455-1461, 1989.

50. **Govoni, S., Hanbauer, I., Hexum, T.D., Yang, T., Kelly, G.D., and Costa, E.,** *In vivo* characterization of the mechanisms that secrete enkephalin-like peptide stored in dog adrenal medulla, *Neuropharmacology*, 20, 639-645, 1981.

51. **Grundy, D., and Davison, J.S.,** Cardiovascular changes elicited by vagal gastric afferents in the rat, *Q.J. Exp. Physiol.*, 66, 307-310, 1981.

52. **Grundy, D., Salih, A.A., and Scratcherd, T.,** Modulation of vagal efferent discharge by mechanoreceptors in the stomach, duodenum and colon in the ferret, *J. Physiol.*, 319, 43-52, 1981.

53. **Grundy, D., and Scratcherd, T.,** Sensory afferents from the gastrointestinal tract, in *Motility and Circulation of the Gastrointestinal Tract*, Wood, J.D., Ed., American Physiological Society, Bethesda, MD, 1989, 593-620.

54. **Hainsworth, R., Kidd, C., and Linden, R.J.,** Cardiac receptors, *C.U.P.*, 1979, 517.

55. **Hamamura, T., Kazahaya, Y., and Otsuki, S.,** Ceruletide suppresses endogenous dopamine release via vagal afferent system, studied by *in vivo* intracerebral dialysis, *Brain Res.*, 483, 78-83, 1989.

56. **Harper, A.A., Kidd, C., and Scratcherd, T.,** Vago-vagal reflex effects on gastric and pancreatic secretion and gastro-intestinal motility, *J. Physiol.*, 148, 417-436, 1959.

57. **Harris, M.C., and Loewy, A.D.,** Neural regulation of vasopressin containing hypothalamic neurons and the role of vasopressin in cardiovascular function, in *Central Regulation of Autonomic Functions*, Loewy, A.D., and Spyer, K.M, Eds., O.U.P. New York, 1990, 224-246.

58. **Hawthorn, J., Andrews, P.L.R., Ang, V.T.Y., and Jenkins, J.S.,** Differential release of vasopressin and oxytocin in response to abdominal vagal afferent stimulation and apomorphine in the ferret, *Brain Res.*, 438, 193-198, 1988.

59. **Herbert, M.K., Kniffki, K., Mengel, M.K.C., and Sprotte, G.,** Pain perception in chronic pain patients can be reduced by activation of carotid sinus baroreceptors, *Pain*, Suppl. 5, S310, 1990.

60. **Hering, E., and Breuer, J.,** *Die Selbststeuerung der Atmung Durch den Nerven Vagus*, Sitzungsb. Akad. Wissensch. Wein., 57, 1868.

61. **Hermann, G.E., Kohlerman, N.J., and Rogers, R.C.,** Hepatic-vagal and gustatory afferent interactions in the brainstem of the rat, *J. Auton. Nerv. Syst.*, 9, 477-495, 1983.

62. **Hertz, A.F.,** *The Sensibility of the Alimentary Canal*, Hodder and Stoughton, London, 1911.

63. **Heymans, J.F., and Heymans, C.,** Sur les modifications directes et sur la regulation reflexe de l'activite du centre respiratoire de la tete isolee du chein, *Arch. Int. Pharmacodyn.*, 33, 273-372, 1927.

64. **Heymans, C., and Neil, E.,** *Reflexogenic areas of the cardiovascular system*, J.A. Churchill Ltd., London, 1958, 271.

65. **Holzer, P., and Sametz, W.,** Gastric and mucosal protection against ulcerogenic factors in the rat mediated by capsaicin sensitive afferent neurons, *Gastroenterology*, 91, 975-981, 1986.

66. **Hommer, D.W., Palkovits, M., Crawley, J.N., Paul, S.M., and Skirboll, R.L.,** Cholecystokinin-induced excitation in the substantia nigra: Evidence for peripheral and central components, *J. Neurosci.*, 5, 1387-1392, 1985.

67. **Howe, A., Pack, R.J., and Wise, J.C.M.,** Arterial chemoreceptorlike activity in the abdominal vagus of the rat, *J. Physiol.*, 320, 309-318, 1981.

68. **Janowitz, H.D., and Grossman, M.I.,** Some factors affecting food intake of normal dogs and dogs with esophagostomy and gastric fistula, *Am. J. Physiol.*, 159, 143-148, 1949.

69. **Jansson, G.,** Vago-vagal relaxation of the stomach, *Acta Physiol. Scand.*, 75, 245-252, 1969.

70. **Juhasz, G., Detari, L., and Kukorelli, T.,** Effects of hypnogenic vagal stimulation on thalamic neuronal activity in cats, *Brain Res. Bull.*, 15, 437-441, 1985.

71. **Karlsson, J., Sant'Ambrogio, G., and Widdicombe, J.,** Afferent neural pathways in cough and reflex bronchoconstriction, *J. Appl. Physiol.*, 65, 1007-1023, 1988.

72. **Kawasaki, K., Kodama, M., and Matsushita, A.,** Caerulein a cholecystokinin-related peptide, depresses somatic function via the vagal afferent system, *Life Sci.*, 33, 1045-1050, 1983.
73. **Kerlin, P.,** Postprandial antral hypomotility in patients with idiopathic nausea and vomiting, *Gut*, 30, 54-59, 1989.
74. **Kral, J.G.,** Behavioural effects of vagotomy in humans, in *Vagal Nerve Functions: Behavioural and Methodological Considerations*, Kral, J.G., Powley, T.L., and Brooks, C.McC., Eds., Elsevier, Amsterdam, 1983, 273-281.
75. **Kukorelli, T., and Juhasz, G.,** Electroencephalographic synchronization induced by stimulation of small intestine and splanchnic nerve in cats, *Electroencephalogr. Clin. Neurophysiol.*, 44, 491-500, 1976.
76. **Kukorelli, T., and Juhasz, G.,** Sleep induced by intestinal stimulation in cats, *Physiol. Behav.*, 19, 355-358, 1977.
77. **Lang, I.M.,** Digestive tract motor correlates of vomiting and nausea, *Can. J. Physiol. Pharmacol.*, 68, 242-253, 1990.
78. **Langley, J.N.,** The autonomic nervous system, *Brain*, 26, 1-26, 1903.
79. **Lawes, I.N.C.,** Nucleus tractus solitarius - a point of entry to the paraventricular system, *Neurosci. Lett.*, 26S, 438, 1986.
80. **Lawes, I.N.C.,** The origin of the vomiting response: A neuroanatomical hypothesis, *Can. J. Physiol. Pharmacol.*, 68, 254-259, 1990.
81. **Lawes, I.N.C.,** The central connections of area postrema define the paraventricular system involved in anti-noxious behaviours, in *Nausea and Vomiting*, Kucharcyzck, J., and Stewart, D., Eds., CRC Press, Florida, 1991.
82. **Lewis, T.,** *Pain*, MacMillan, London, 1942.
83. **Longhurst, J.C., Ashton, J.H., and Iwamoto, G.A.,** Cardiovascular reflexes resulting from capsaicin stimulated gastric receptors in anesthetized dogs, *Circ. Res.*, 46, 780-788, 1980.
84. **Longhurst, J.C., Stebbins, C.L., and Ordway, G.A.,** Chemically induced cardiovascular reflexes arising from the stomach in the cat, *Am. J. Physiol.*, 247, 459-466, 1984.
85. **Mark, G.P., Scott, T.R., Chang, F-C.T., and Grill, H.J.,** Taste responses in the nucleus tractus solitarius of the chronic decerebrate rat, *Brain Res.*, 443, 137-148, 1988.
86. **Mayer, E.A., and Raybould, H.E.,** Role of visceral afferent mechanisms in functional bowel disorders, *Gastroenterology*, 99, 1688-1704, 1990.
87. **McGivern, R.F., and Bernston, G.G.,** Mediation of diurnal fluctuations in pain sensitivity in the rat by food intake patterns: Reversal by naloxone, *Science*, 210, 210-211, 1980.
88. **Mei, N.,** Sensory structures in the viscera, in *Progress in Sensory Physiology* 4, Springer-Verlag, Berlin, 1983, 1-44.
89. **Mei, N.,** Intestinal chemosensitivity, *Physiol. Rev.*, 65, 211-237, 1985.
90. **Miaskiewicz, S.L., Striker, E.M., and Verbalis, J.G.,** Neurohypophyseal secretion in response to cholecystokinin but not meal induced gastric distension in humans, *J. Clin. Endocrinol. Metab.*, 68, 837-843, 1989.
91. **Money, K.E., and Cheung, B.S.,** Another function of the inner ear: Facilitation of the emetic response to poisons. *Aviat. Space Environ. Med.*, 208-211, 1983.
92. **Norgren, R., and Leonard, C.M.,** Taste pathways in rat brainstem, *Science*, 173, 1136-1139, 1971.
93. **Orosco, M., Rybarczyk, M.C., Rouch, C., Cohen, Y., and Jacquot, C.,** Cholecystokinin and bombesin in vagotomized or intact lean and obese rats: Effects of neurotransmitters in brain, *Neuropharmacology*, 26, 575-579, 1987.
94. **Pappas, T.N., Melendez, R.L., and Debas, H.T.,** Gastric distension is a physiologic satiety signal in the dog, *Dig. Dis. Sci.*, 34, 1489-1493, 1989.
95. **Partridge, R.C., and Wilson, M.J.,** Gastric impulses in the vagus, *J. Cell Comp. Physiol.*, 123-126, 1933.
96. **Petorossi, V.E.,** Modulation of the masseteric reflex by gastric vagal afferents, *Arch. Ital. Biol.*, 121, 67-79, 1983.

97. **Pick, J.,** *The Autonomic Nervous system, Morphological, Comparative, Clinical and Surgical Considerations,* J.B. Lippincott, Philadelphia, 1970.

98. **Puizillout, J.J., and Foutz, A.S.,** Characteristics of the experimental reflex sleep induced by vago-aortic nerve stimulation, *Electroencephalogr. Clin. Neurophysiol.,* 42, 552-563, 1977.

99. **Prechtl, J.C., and Powley, T.L.,** B-afferents: A fundamental division of the nervous system mediating homeostasis, *Behavioural and Brain Sciences,* 13, 289-331, 1990.

100. **Randich, A., and Aicher, S.,** Medullary substrata mediating anti-nociception produced by electrical stimulation of the vagus, *Brain Res.,* 445, 68-76, 1988.

101. **Randich, A., and Hartunian, C.,** Activation of sinoaortic baroreceptor reflex arc induces analgesia: Interaction between cardiovascular and endogenous pain inhibition systems, *Physiol. Psychol.,* 11, 214-220, 1983.

102. **Randich, A., and Maixner, W.,** [D-Ala]-methionineenkephalinamide reflexively induces anti-nociception by activating vagal afferents, *Pharmacol. Biochem. Behav.,* 21, 441-448, 1984.

103. **Ren, K., Randich, A., and Gebhart, G.F.,** Modulation of spinal nociceptive transmission from nuclei tractus solitarii: A relay for effect of vagal afferent stimulation, *J. Neurophysiol.,* 63, 971-986, 1990.

104. **Renaud, L.P., Tang, M., McCann, M.J., Striker, E.M., and Verbalis, J.G.,** Cholecystokinin in and gastric distension activate oxytocinergic cells in rat hypothalamus, *Am. J. Physiol.,* 253, 661-665, 1987.

105. **Richter, J.E., Barish, C.F., and Castell, D.O.,** Abnormal sensory perception in patients with esophageal chest pain, *Gastroenterology,* 91, 845-852, 1986.

106. **Rozin, P., and Kalat, J.W.,** Specific hungers and poison avoidance as adaptive specializations of learning, *Phychol. Rev.,* 78, 459-486, 1971.

107. **Schweitzer, A., and Wright, S.,** The anti-strychnine action of acetylcholine, prostigmine and related substances and of central vagus stimulation, *J. Physiol.,* 90, 310-329, 1937.

108. **Sheehan, D.,** Discovery of the autonomic nervous system, *Arch. Neurol. Psych.,* 35, 1081-1115, 1936.

109. **Tatar, M., Webber, S.E., and Widdicombe, J.G.,** Lung C-fibre receptor activation and defensive reflexes in anesthetized cats, *J. Physiol.,* 402, 411-420, 1988.

110. **Thies, R., and Foreman, R.D.,** Inhibition and excitation of thoracic spinoreticular neurons by electrical stimulation of vagal afferent fibres, *Exp. Neurol.,* 82, 1-16, 1983.

111. **Thurston, C.L., and Randich, A.,** Intrathecal methysergide antagonises anti-nociception produced by subdiaphragmatic vagal stimulation, *Pain,* Suppl. 5, S450, 1990.

112. **Travers, J.B., and Norgren, R.,** An electromyographic analysis of the ingestion and rejection of sapid stimuli in the rat, *Behav. Neurosci.,* 100, 544-555, 1986.

113. **Triesman, M.,** Motion sickness: An evolutionary hypothesis, *Science,* 197, 493-495, 1977.

114. **Verbalis, J.G., McCann, M.J., McHale, C.M., and Striker, E.M.,** Oxytocin secretion in response to cholecystokinin in food: Differentiation of nausea from satiety, *Science,* 232, 1417-1419, 1986.

115. **Widdicombe, J.G.,** Respiratory reflexes in man and other mammalian species, *Clin. Sci.,* 21, 163-170, 1961.

116. **Widdicombe, J.G.,** Physiology of cough, in *Cough,* Braga, P.C., and Allegra, L., Eds., Raven Press, New York, 1989, 3-25.

117. **Wolf, S.,** *The Stomach,* Oxford University Press, New York, 1965.

118. **Wright, S.,** *Applied Physiology,* Oxford University Press, Humphry Milford, 1971.

119. **Yaxley, S., Rolls, E.T., Sienkiewicz, Z.J., and Scott, T.R.,** Satiety does not affect gustatory activity in the nucleus of the solitary tract of the alert monkey, *Brain Res.,* 347, 85-93, 1985.

120. **Yaxley, S., Rolls, E.T., Sienkiewicz, Z.J.,** The responsiveness of neurons in the insular gustatory cortex of the macaque monkey is independent of hunger, *Physiol. Behav.,* 42, 223-229, 1988.

121. **Young, J.Z.,** Influence of the mouth on the evolution of the brain, in *Biology of the Mouth,* American Association for the Advancement of Science, 1968, 21-35.

122. **Zabara, J., Chaffee, R.B., and Tansy, M.F.,** Neuroinhibition in the regulation of emesis, *Space Life Sci.,* 3, 282-292, 1972.

INDEX

Printed and bound by CPI Group (UK) Ltd, Croydon, CR0 4YY

17/10/2024

01775690-0013